....
Bacterial Flora in Digestive Disease

Bacterial Flora in Digestive Disease

Focus on Rifaximin

Editors

C. Scarpignato   *Parma, Italy*
Á. Lanas   *Zaragoza, Spain*

60 figures, 13 in color, and 48 tables, 2006

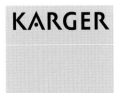

Basel · Freiburg · Paris · London · New York ·
Bangalore · Bangkok · Singapore · Tokyo · Sydney

....
Carmelo Scarpignato, MD, DSc (Hons),
PharmD (h.c.), FRCP (London), FCP, FACG
Laboratory of Clinical Pharmacology
School of Medicine and Dentistry
University of Parma
Via Volturno, 39
43100 Parma (Italy)

Ángel Lanas, MD, PhD
Servicio de Aparato Digestivo
Hospital Clínico 'Lozano Blesa'
50009 Zaragoza (Spain)

Reprint of 'Digestion' (ISSN 0012-2823)
    Vol. 73, Suppl. 1, 2006

Library of Congress Cataloging-in-Publication Data

Bacterial flora in digestive disease : focus on rifaximin / editors, C.
Scarpignato, A. Lanas.
    p. ; cm.
    Published also as v. 73, suppl. 1, 2006, of Digestion.
    Includes bibliographical references and indexes.
    ISBN 3-8055-8083-5 (hard cover : alk. paper)
    1. Digestive organs–Diseases. 2. Digestive organs–Microbiology. 3.
Rifamycins. 4. Bacteria.
    [DNLM: 1. Digestive System Diseases–microbiology. 2. Anti-Bacterial
Agents–therapeutic use. 3. Digestive System Diseases–drug therapy. 4.
Rifamycins–therapeutic use. WI 140 B131 2006] I. Scarpignato, C. II.
Lanas, A. (Ángel) III. Digestion.
    RA645.D54B332 2006
    616.3–dc22

                                                2006004546

Bibliographic Indices. This publication is listed in bibliographic services, including Current Contents® and Index Medicus.

Disclaimer. The statements, options and data contained in this publication are solely those of the individual authors and contributors and not of the publisher and the editor(s). The appearance of advertisements in the book is not a warranty, endorsement, or approval of the products or services advertised or of their effectiveness, quality or safety. The publisher and the editor(s) disclaim responsibility for any injury to persons or property resulting from any ideas, methods, instructions or products referred to in the content or advertisements.

Drug Dosage. The authors and the publisher have exerted every effort to ensure that drug selection and dosage set forth in this text are in accord with current recommendations and practice at the time of publication. However, in view of ongoing research, changes in government regulations, and the constant flow of information relating to drug therapy and drug reactions, the reader is urged to check the package insert for each drug for any change in indications and dosage and for added warnings and precautions. This is particularly important when the recommended agent is a new and/or infrequently employed drug.

© Copyright 2006 by S. Karger AG, P.O. Box, CH–4009 Basel (Switzerland)
www.karger.com
Printed in Switzerland on acid-free paper by Reinhardt Druck, Basel
ISBN 3–8055–8083–5

Contents

Foreword

As a medical student, I still remember being lectured about 'intestinal dysbacteriosis' and the bygone theories of 'autointoxication' that prevailed in the early 20th century and which were expounded so convincingly by Elie Metchnikoff who thought that the ample reservoir of microbial flora present in the gut would generate toxins that would disseminate in the organism and inevitably cause its degeneration and senescence. A positive indican urine test which was in vogue at that time purportedly established an excessive metabolic activity of the intestinal flora. While some clinicians prescribed massive colonic irrigations to 'clean the 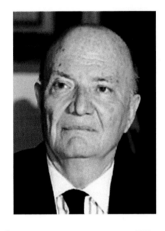 intestine' of microbes, Metchnikoff advocated yoghurt as a means to modify some adverse effects of the gut flora. He thus started the current probiotic mode. The role of the gastrointestinal bacterial flora in health and disease has attracted researchers for more than a century.

The gut is a rather unique example of an organ harbouring an abundant commensal bacterial colony which is often bound to interact with foreign pathogenic germs ingested via contaminated food or water. As the oxygen tension in the large bowel is very low, anaerobic bacteria grow at the expense of other organisms such as streptococci and enterobacteria. The growth of some species may be inhibited or promoted by the products of others. Changes in intestinal pH may also induce growth of some acid-tolerant species over other organisms.

The workshop showed that 60–80% of the identified intestinal flora cannot be cultivated and that the molecular structure of intestinal bacteria has been identified in only 24% of them. I was really impressed by the fact that in Crohn's disease, 30% of intestinal bacteria belong to species that are yet to be identified. We were also reminded that there are differences between the flora present in the colon and that excreted in the faeces: for instance, lactobacilli are not found in faeces. Thus the microbiological study of a faecal sample does not entirely reflect the composition of the intestinal flora.

The study of gastrointestinal flora has clarified the pathogenesis of intestinal bacterial overgrowth and other intestinal infections, the role of *Clostridium difficile* in antibiotic-related colitis, or the usefulness of antimicrobial therapy in such varied disorders as traveler's diarrhea, inflammatory bowel disease, diverticular disease of the colon, the irritable bowel syndrome or seemingly unrelated problems such as hepatic encephalopathy. Some of these conditions are causing heavy economic burdens on the delivery of health services in most countries. In the year 2000 in the USA, the cost of colonic diverticulitis reached the impressive figure of 2,667 million dollars while the global cost of intestinal infections gave a figure of 2,238 million dollars. On the other hand, the large decrease in the costs of peptic ulcer disease can be rightly attributed to the identification of *Helicobacter pylori* as a major component of gastric pathology. This has been a true landmark in the history of medical science in the 20th century.

The current management of these frequent gastroenterological conditions and the role of the poorly absorbed antibiotic, rifaximin, has been at the centre of this worthwhile workshop on *Bacterial Flora in Digestive Disease – Focus on Rifaximin*, in which these topics and their therapeutic options have been discussed in depth by a distinguished group of Italian and Spanish clinicians and investigators. The workshop provided extremely useful information not easily available in this format on the pathogenesis and the therapy of a variety of conditions related to the microbiota of the gut. All presentations were followed by lively discussions, skilfully moderated by Professor Scarpignato. I am especially grateful to him and to Professor Angel Lanas for preparing such an interesting programme and selecting so appropriately a group of outstanding speakers from Italy and Spain. Moreover, the final texts of the proceedings which Carmelo Scarpignato has been so talented in editing, certainly represent much more than the usual congress proceedings. This is a true 'the state of the art' that includes comprehensive reviews for a large variety of topics. It will be useful for many years to come.

It was a great honour to preside this first encounter between Italian and Spanish gastroenterologists which, it is hoped, will have an adequate follow-up.

Francisco Vilardell
MD, DSc, FRCP, FRCP (E), FACP, FACG
Director Emeritus
Postgraduate School of Gastroenterology Hospital de Sant Pau
Universitat Autonoma, Barcelona, Spain
Past President, World Organization of Gastroenterology (OMGE)

Preface

Hundreds of bacterial species make up human gut flora. The intestine has at least 400 different species of bacteria totalling over 10^{12} organisms. Of these, 99% are anaerobic bacteria. The gastrointestinal tract is then exposed to countless numbers of bacterial species and foreign antigens and has embedded a unique and complex network of immunological and non-immunological mechanisms to protect the host from potentially harmful pathogens.

Altered gut microecology, reported in many gut-related inflammatory diseases, is clearly a common phenomenon. Inflammation is accompanied by imbalances in the intestinal microbiota. When the host-microbe interaction is disturbed, resident bacteria can induce an immune response. Healthy individuals are generally tolerant to their own microbiota, but such tolerance is impaired in patients with both organic and functional GI diseases. Altered gut microbiota is also found in patients with extra GI disturbances (like, for instance, rheumatoid arthritis and allergic disease), indicating that the normal gut microbiota constitutes an ecosystem responding to and regulating inflammation both in the gut and elsewhere in the body.

The advancement of the knowledge on microbial-gut interactions in health and disease has allowed a more pathophysiologically-oriented approach to several challenging clinical conditions. There are currently two ways to manipulate enteric flora. Antibiotics can selectively decrease tissue invasion and eliminate aggressive bacterial species or globally decrease luminal and mucosal bacterial concentrations, depending on their spectrum of activity. Alternatively, administration of beneficial bacterial species (probiotics), poorly absorbed dietary oligosaccharides (prebiotics), or combined probiotics and prebiotics (symbiotics) can restore a predominance of beneficial commensal flora. These two therapeutic approaches are not, of course, mutually exclusive.

Rifaximin, a poorly absorbed antibiotic targeted at the GI tract, has been long used in Italy for the treatment of infectious diarrhea in both adults and children. During the past few years the appreciation of the pathogenic role of gut bacteria in several organic and functional GI diseases has increasingly broadened its clinical use, which now covers hepatic encephalopathy, small intestine bacterial overgrowth, inflammatory bowel disease and colonic diverticular disease. Other potential clinical indications are being explored and look promising. The drug has been recently made available for clinical practice in Spain and we took this opportunity to review its clinical use together with the role of bacterial flora in digestive disease. We therefore decided to get together leading scientists (both Spanish and Italian) in order to exchange ideas and experience during one full day of face-to-face confrontation. The meeting was held in Barcelona (Spain), in January 2005, under the Presidency of Professor Francisco Vilardell and aroused strong interest both on account of the issues addressed and on the outstanding quality of the presentations.

In light of the consent obtained, we felt it worthwhile to compile a series of reviews to further consolidate the mass of general and scientific information existing in the field. Our original idea was to collect manuscripts of the speeches presented at the symposium to merely publish the proceedings. Later, we realized that a more complete work could be of help for all the colleagues involved in everyday care of patients with disturbed gut microecology. All the faculty members enthusiastically accepted the challenge to provide us with state-of-the-art reviews covering both pathophysiology and therapeutics. We thank all of them for their excellent contribution, made despite numerous other calls on their time.

The Spanish-Italian cooperation is certainly not new and dates back to the 12th century, when people from Barcelona and Genoa drew up mutually fruitful commercial and travel agreements. At the beginning of the third millennium we are proud to present the reader the result of this Spanish-Italian scientific cooperation. This volume, which includes much of the information collected from scattered sources, will be useful to both scientists and clinicians interested in this rapidly evolving field.

Some of the concepts presented in this issue are still in an evolutionary state. The precise mechanisms on how gut bacteria interact with host to cause digestive symptoms and diseases are not completely understood. The reader, therefore, will have to be tolerant of some lack of clear-cut explanations for many of the clinical observations. It cannot be expected that this publication will quiet all controversies. However, data are presented that should aid any practitioner in making therapeutic decisions.

We would like to thank Mr. Patrick Näf and the whole team of S. Karger AG for their excellent cooperation during the publication of this supplement. We would also acknowledge the help of Mrs Monse Tort, Edicciones Mayo (Barcelona, Spain) in the logistic organization of the meeting which gave rise to this publication. Moreover, we are grateful to Bama-Geve (Barcelona, Spain) for supporting the conference and backing the publication costs. Last but not least, our sincere gratitude goes to Dr. Giampiero Piccinini at the Alfa Wassermann, International Division (Milan, Italy), who rendered this publication possible. He greatly and enthusiastically helped us in every step of our *puzzling* editorial work.

Carmelo Scarpignato
MD, DSc (Hons), PharmD (h.c.), FRCP (London), FCP, FACG
Professor of Pharmacology & Therapeutics
Associate Professor of Gastroenterology
School of Medicine & Dentistry University of Parma, Italy

Ángel Lanas
MD, PhD
Associate Professor of Gastroenterology
Chief of the Gastrointestinal Oncology Unit
School of Medicine & Surgery
University of Zaragoza, Spain

Scarpignato C, Lanas Á (eds): Bacterial Flora in Digestive Disease.
Focus on Rifaximin.

....

Enteric Flora in Health and Disease

Francisco Guarner

Digestive System Research Unit, University Hospital Vall d'Hebron,
Barcelona, Spain

Abstract

The human gut is the natural habitat for a large and dynamic bacterial community.
Recently developed molecular biology tools suggest that a substantial part of these bacterial
populations are still to be described. However, the relevance and impact of resident bacteria
on host's physiology and pathology is well documented. Major functions of the gut
microflora include metabolic activities that result in salvage of energy and absorbable nutrients, protection of the colonized host against invasion by alien microbes, and important
trophic effects on intestinal epithelia and on immune structure and function. Gut bacteria
play an essential role in the development and homeostasis of the immune system. It is important to underscore that the specialized lymphoid follicles of the gut mucosa are the major
sites for induction and regulation of the immune system. On the other hand, there is evidence
implicating the gut flora in certain pathological conditions, including multisystem organ
failure, colon cancer and inflammatory bowel diseases.

The Gut Flora

The term 'microflora' or 'microbiota' refers to the community of living
microorganisms assembled in a particular ecological niche of a host individual
[1]. The human gut is the natural habitat for a large, diverse and dynamic population of microorganisms, mainly bacteria, that have adapted to live on the
mucosal surfaces or in the lumen [2]. Gut bacteria include native species that
permanently colonize the tract, and a variable set of living microorganisms that
transit temporarily through the tract. Native bacteria are mainly acquired at
birth and during the first year of life, whereas transient bacteria are continuously being ingested from the environment (food, drinks, etc.).

The stomach and duodenum harbour very low numbers of microorganisms
adhering to the mucosal surface or in transit, typically less than 10^3 bacteria

cells per gram of contents. Acid, bile, and pancreatic secretions kill most ingested microbes, and the phasic propulsive motor activity impedes stable colonisation of the lumen. There is a progressive increase in numbers of bacteria along the jejunum and ileum, from approximately 10^4 in the jejunum to 10^7 colony-forming units per gram of contents at the ileal end, with predominance of Gram-negative aerobes and some obligate anaerobes. In contrast, the large intestine is heavily populated by anaerobes and bacteria counts reach densities around 10^{12} colony-forming units per gram of luminal contents (100,000-fold higher concentrations than in the ileal lumen). In the upper gut, transit is rapid and bacterial density is low, but the impact on immune function is thought to be important by interactions of bacteria with organized lymphoid structures of the small intestinal mucosa. In the colon, however, transit time is slow and microorganisms have the opportunity to proliferate by fermenting available substrates derived from either the diet or endogenous secretions.

The intestinal habitat of an adult individual contains 300–500 different species of bacteria, with 30–40 species comprising up to 99% of the total population. Conventional bacteriological analysis of the faecal flora by isolation of bacteria on selective growth media shows that strict anaerobic bacteria outnumber aerobes by a factor of 100 to 1,000. The dominant genera are *Bacteroides, Bifidobacterium, Eubacterium, Clostridium, Lactobacillus, Fusobacterium* and various anaerobic Gram-positive cocci. Bacteria present in lower numbers include *Enterococcus*, and *Enterobacteriaceae*. Every individual has a particular combination of predominant and subdominant species that is distinct from that found in other individuals. However, over 50% of bacteria cells that are observed by microscopic examination of faecal specimens cannot be grown in culture media. Molecular biology techniques have been developed to characterize nonculturable bacteria, and previously unknown strains are now being identified [3, 4]. These techniques show differences in predominant species between proximal and distal colon, and between mucosal and faecal communities [5]. Some data even suggest that each individual harbours unique strains [6].

Some of the bacteria in the gut are pathogens or potential pathogens when the integrity of the mucosal barrier is functionally breached (fig. 1). However, the normal interaction between gut bacteria and their host is a symbiotic relationship, defined as mutually beneficial for both partners [7]. The host provides a nutrient-rich habitat and the bacteria can infer important benefits on host's health.

Primary Functions of the Microflora

Comparison of animals bred under germ-free conditions with their conventionally raised counterparts (harbouring microflora) has revealed a series

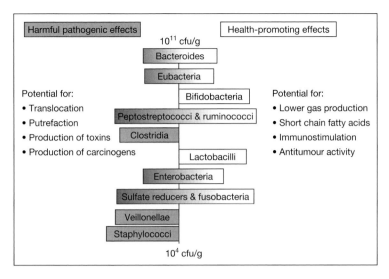

Fig. 1. Generalized scheme of predominant groups of colonic bacteria, indicating how the genera may exhibit potentially harmful and beneficial functions (from Salminen et al. [56]).

of anatomic characteristics and physiological functions that are associated with the presence of the microflora [1, 4]. Organ weights (heart, lung, and liver), cardiac output, intestinal wall thickness, intestinal motor activity, serum γ-globulin levels, lymph nodes, among other characteristics, are all reduced or atrophic in germ-free animals, suggesting that gut bacteria have important and specific functions on the host (fig. 2). These functions are ascribed into three categories, i.e. metabolic, protective and trophic functions [2].

The *metabolic functions* of the enteric flora consist in the fermentation of non-digestible dietary substrates and endogenous mucus. Gene diversity among the microbial community provides a variety of enzymes and biochemical pathways that are distinct from the host's own constitutive resources. Fermentation of carbohydrates is a major source of energy in the colon for bacterial growth and produces short chain fatty acids (SCFA) that can be absorbed by the host. This results in salvage of dietary energy, and favours the absorption of ions (Ca, Mg, Fe) in the caecum. Metabolic functions also include the production of some vitamins (K, B_{12}, biotin, folic acid, pantothenate) and synthesis of amino acids from ammonia or urea [7]. Anaerobic metabolism of peptides and proteins (putrefaction) by the microflora also produces SCFA but, at the same time, it generates a series of potentially toxic substances including ammonia, amines, phenols, thiols and

- **Metabolic functions**
  Fermentation of non-digestible dietary residue and endogenous mucus: salvage of energy as SCFA, production of vitamin K, absorption of calcium, iron, etc.

- **Protective functions**
  Protection against pathogens (the barrier effect)

- **Trophic functions**
  Control of epithelial cell proliferation and differentiation; development and homeostasis of the immune system

Fig. 2. Primary functions of the enteric microflora.

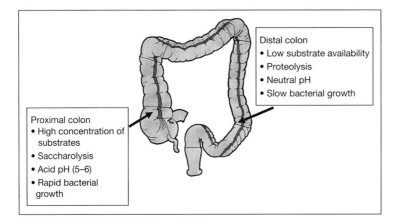

Fig. 3. Fermentation in the colon (from Guarner and Malagelada [2]).

indols [8, 9]. Available proteins include elastin and collagen from dietary sources, pancreatic enzymes, sloughed epithelial cells and lysed bacteria. Interestingly, in the caecum and right colon, fermentation is very intense with high SCFA production, acidic pH (around 5–6), and rapid bacterial growth. In contrast, in the left or distal colon there is lower concentration of available substrate, the pH is close to neutral, putrefactive processes become quantitatively more important, and bacterial populations are close to static (fig. 3).

The *protective functions* of the microflora include the barrier effect that prevents invasion by pathogens. The resident bacteria represent a crucial line of resistance to colonization by exogenous microbes or opportunistic bacteria that are present in the gut, but their growth is restricted. The equilibrium between species of resident bacteria provides stability in the microbial population. The barrier effect is based on the ability of certain bacteria to secrete antimicrobial substances, like bacteriocins, that inhibit the growth of other bacteria, and also on the competition for nutrients and attachment to ecological niches [10–12].

Finally, the *trophic functions* of the gut microflora are a major field of scientific research in recent years. Gut bacteria can control the proliferation and differentiation of epithelial cells. Epithelial cell turnover is reduced in colonic crypts of germ-free animals as compared with colonized controls [1]. Cell differentiation is highly influenced by the interaction with resident microorganisms as shown by the expression of a variety of genes in germ-free animals mono-associated with specific bacteria strains [13]. Bacteria also play an essential role in the development of the immune system. Animals bred in a germ-free environment show low densities of lymphoid cells in the gut mucosa, specialized follicle structures are small, and circulating immunoglobulin levels are low. Immediately after exposure to microbes, the number of mucosal lymphocytes expands, germinal centres and immunoglobulin producing cells appear rapidly in follicles and in the lamina propria, and there is a significant increase in serum immunoglobulin levels [1, 14, 15]. Multiple and diverse interactions between microbes, epithelium and gut lymphoid tissues are constantly reshaping local and systemic mechanisms of immunity.

Host-Bacteria Relationships in the Gut

The possibility of controlling or modulating the immune system by acting at gut mucosal interfaces is attracting particular attention from the scientific community. The gastrointestinal tract constitutes a sensitive interface for fine and sophisticated contact and communication between the individual and the external environment. The large mucosal surface (300–400 m^2) is adapted to the main functions of the gut that include not only the well-known processes leading to the digestion of food and absorption of nutrients, but also a series of activities aimed at establishing a strong line of defence against aggressions from the external environment. Three essential constituents interacting in the gut accomplish this important defensive task of the gut: the microflora, the mucosal barrier and the immune system [16]. Homeostasis of the individual with the external environment critically depends on the dynamic balance between the three constituents.

Intestinal epithelial cells are in close contact with luminal contents and play a crucial role in signalling and mediating host innate and adaptive mucosal immune responses. Activation of innate host defence mechanisms is based on the rapid recognition of conserved molecular patterns in microbes by preformed receptors recently recognized (toll-like and NOD-family receptors) [17]. In response to invading bacteria, the signals converge to transcription factors (NF-κB and others), which start the transcription of genes responsible for the synthesis of proinflammatory proteins [18]. Hence, epithelial cells secrete mediators including chemoattractants for neutrophils and proinflammatory cytokines and express inducible enzymes for the production of nitric oxide, prostaglandins and leukotrienes at a large scale. Intestinal epithelial cells also express MHC class II and non-classical MHC class I molecules, suggesting that they can function as antigen-presenting cells [19]. However, non-pathogenic bacteria may also elicit cytokine responses that are transmitted to underlying immunocompetent cells [20]. Interestingly, responses to non-pathogenic bacteria involve regulatory cytokines such as TGF-β or IL-10, and appear to be related with the induction regulatory pathways of the immune system [20, 21]. Some commensal *Lactobacillus* strains can downregulate the spontaneous release of TNF-α by inflamed tissue, and also the inflammatory response induced by *Escherichia coli* [22]. These effects on cytokine release are associated with changes in the expression of activation markers by lamina propria T lymphocytes [22], and with induction of apoptosis of activated lymphocytes, which is a major homeostatic mechanism in the gut mucosa [23]. Thus, signals generated at the mucosal surface can promote changes in the phenotype of lamina propria lymphocytes. Taken together, epithelial cells produce the essential signals for the onset of mucosal innate responses and recruitment of appropriate cell populations for induction of memory pathways of acquired immunity (fig. 4).

Acquired immune responses develop in specialized lymphoid tissues. Gut-associated lymphoid tissues (GALT) are located in three compartments: organized structures (Peyer's patches and lymphoid follicles), the lamina propria, and the surface epithelium [24]. The organized structures are believed to represent the inductive sites and the lamina propria and epithelial compartment principally constitute effector sites. The organized structures are covered by follicle-associated epithelium, which contains M cells. They are specialized epithelial cells that transport microorganisms as well as dead antigens from the gut lumen into the organized lymphoid tissue. Stimuli from the gut lumen via the M cells (dendritic cells at the epithelial layer also contribute) induce mucosal immune responses. Antigens are presented to naïve T cells by antigen-presenting cells after intracellular processing. In addition, luminal antigens may be taken up and presented by epithelial cells directly to various subsets of intra- and subepithelial T lymphocytes. Expansion of T cell clones occur after antigen priming in the GALT, but interestingly, they may differentiate into Th1, Th2 or T-regulatory cells, with different effector capabilities [25]. The mechanisms which determine the differentiation of T-helper cells are not well understood, but certainly depend on the cytokine

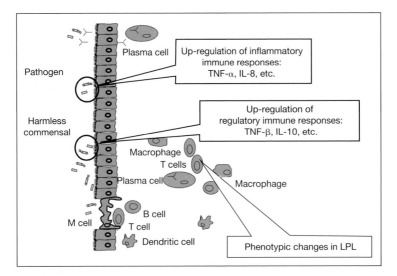

Fig. 4. Intestinal epithelial cells play a crucial role in signalling and mediating host innate and adaptive mucosal immune responses. Activation of innate host defence mechanisms is based on the rapid recognition of conserved molecular patterns in microbes by preformed toll-like and NOD-family receptors expressed by intestinal epithelial cells. The signals converge to transcription factors which start the transcription of genes for the synthesis of proteins or peptides that mediate inflammatory (pathogens) or regulatory (harmless commensals) responses. Signals generated at the epithelial surface can promote changes in the phenotype of lamina propria lymphocytes (LPL).

environment during antigen presentation and clonal induction. Mucosal antigen-specific B cells differentiate to predominantly IgA-secreting plasma cells. Primed B cells migrate via draining lymphatics to mesenteric lymph nodes where they are further stimulated; they may then reach peripheral blood and become seeded by preferential homing mechanisms into distant mucosal effector sites, particularly the intestinal lamina propria where they finally develop to plasma cells. An essential message to remember is that *induction of effector and regulatory pathways of the immune system takes place primarily in the specialized follicles of the gut mucosa.*

The indigenous microbial flora of the gut is essential for the development and homeostasis of the immune system. Abnormalities in the development of the immune system may be due to defects in the interaction of the flora with the mucosal immune compartments. According to the hygiene hypothesis, the increasing incidence of allergy in westernized societies may to some extent be explained by a reduced microbial load early in infancy [26]. In this context, an appropriate composition of the commensal flora is needed. Exposure to food-borne and orofaecal non-pathogenic microbes probably exerts a homeostatic impact. The feeding to which the newborn is subjected, as well as its nutritional state, exerts a significant influence on the composition of its indigenous microbiota and eventually on the development of a healthy immune system.

Disease States Associated with Dysfunction of the Enteric Flora

Several disorders are associated with changes in the composition or metabolic function of the enteric flora [2]. For instance, several acute diarrheal diseases are due to pathogens that proliferate and invade or produce toxins. Antibiotic-associated diarrhea is due to imbalance in the gut flora composition with overgrowth of pathogenic species, as some *Clostridium difficile* strains that produce toxins and cause pseudomembranous colitis. It is believed that gut bacteria play a role in the pathogenesis of the irritable bowel syndrome [27]. Symptoms of abdominal pain, bloating, and flatulence are commonly seen in patients with irritable bowel syndrome. Fermentations taking place in the colon generate a variable volume of gas. Likewise, putrefaction of proteins by bacteria within the gut lumen is associated with the pathogenesis of hepatic encephalopathy in patients with chronic or acute liver failure.

Mucosal barrier dysfunction can cause bacterial translocation. Translocation of viable or dead bacteria in minute amounts constitutes a physiologically important boost to the immune system. However, dysfunction of the gut mucosal barrier may result in translocation of a conspicuous quantity of viable microorganisms, usually belonging to Gram-negative aerobic genera. After crossing the epithelial barrier, bacteria may travel via the lymph to extraintestinal sites, such as the mesenteric lymph nodes, liver and spleen. Subsequently, enteric bacteria may disseminate throughout the body producing sepsis, shock, multisystem organ failure, or death of the host. Bacterial translocation may occur in haemorrhagic shock, burn injury, trauma, intestinal ischaemia, intestinal obstruction, severe pancreatitis, acute liver failure, and cirrhosis [28]. The three primary mechanisms promoting bacterial translocation are: (a) small bowel bacterial overgrowth, (b) increased permeability of the intestinal mucosal barrier, and (c) deficiencies in host immune defences.

It has been shown in experimental models that intestinal bacteria may play a role in the initiation of colon cancer through production of carcinogens, cocarcinogens, or pro-carcinogens. The molecular genetic mechanisms of human colorectal cancer are well established, but epidemiological evidence suggests that environmental factors such as diet play a major role in the development of sporadic colon cancer. Dietary fat and high consumption of red meat, particularly processed meat, are associated with high risk in case-control studies. In contrast, a high intake of fruits and vegetables, whole grain cereals, fish and calcium has been associated with reduced risk. Dietary factors and genetic factors interact in part via events taking place in the lumen of the large bowel [29]. The influence of diet on the carcinogenic process may be mediated by changes in metabolic activity and composition of the colonic microflora.

There is evidence implicating the resident bacterial flora as an essential factor in driving the inflammatory process in human inflammatory bowel diseases. In Crohn's disease and ulcerative colitis, clinical evidence suggests that abnormal activation of the mucosal immune system against the enteric flora is the key event triggering inflammatory mechanisms that lead to intestinal injury [30]. Patients show an increased mucosal secretion of IgG antibodies against commensal bacteria [31], and mucosal T lymphocytes are hyperreactive against antigens of the common flora, suggesting that local tolerance mechanisms are abrogated [32]. In fact, faecal stream diversion has been shown to prevent recurrence of Crohn's disease, whereas infusion of intestinal contents to the excluded ileal segments reactivated mucosal lesions [33]. In ulcerative colitis, short-term treatment with an enteric-coated preparation of broad-spectrum antibiotics rapidly reduced metabolic activity of the flora and mucosal inflammation [34]. Several factors may contribute to the pathogenesis of the aberrant immune response towards the autologous flora, including genetic susceptibility [35], a defect in mucosal barrier function, and a microbial imbalance. Recent data suggest that gut bacteria populations in patients with Crohn's disease differ from that in healthy subjects [36].

Therapeutic Manipulation of the Intestinal Flora

Symbiosis between microbiota and host can be improved and optimized by pharmacological or nutritional intervention. Wise use of antibiotic drugs can control bacterial overgrowth and prevent translocation of gut bacteria in specific conditions of increased risk, as mentioned above. Other contributions to this issue review in depth the use of antibiotics to prevent or treat diseases due to gut bacteria. On the other hand, some bacteria may provide specific health benefits when consumed as a food component or in the form of specific preparations of viable microorganisms. A consensus definition of the term 'probiotic' was issued a few years ago and states that oral probiotics are living microorganisms that upon ingestion in certain numbers, exert health benefits beyond those of inherent basic nutrition [37]. The term 'prebiotic' refers to a non-digestible food ingredient that beneficially affects the host by selectively stimulating growth and/or activity of one or a limited number of bacteria in the colon [38]. The prebiotic effect is linked to three essential conditions. A prebiotic should not be hydrolyzed by human intestinal enzymes, it should be selectively fermented by beneficial bacteria, and this selective fermentation should result in a beneficial effect on health or well-being of the host.

A number of clinical trials have tested the efficacy of probiotics in the prevention of acute diarrheal conditions. Two meta-analyses concluded that probiotics can be used to prevent antibiotic-associated diarrhea in children and adults [39, 40]. Prophylactic use of probiotics has proven useful for the prevention of acute diarrhea in infants admitted into hospital wards for a chronic disease condition [41–43]. Probiotics may also be useful in the prevention of community-acquired diarrhea [44, 45]. Several studies have investigated the efficacy of probiotics in the prevention of travelers' diarrhea in adults, but methodological drawbacks, such as low compliance with the treatment and problems in the follow-up, limit the validity of these conclusions [46].

The benefit of probiotics as a treatment for acute diarrhea in children has also been demonstrated. Three meta-analyses of controlled clinical trials have been published [47–49]. It is evident that probiotic therapy shortens the duration of acute diarrheal illness in children by approximately 1 day.

Prebiotics have been proven useful for the prevention of gastrointestinal infections. Inulin and oligofructoses are well-defined prebiotics that increase counts of lactobacilli and bifidobacteria in the human colonic lumen [50]. A number of controlled clinical trials have shown that prebiotics are safe and may be effective in the prevention of acute gastrointestinal conditions, such as community-acquired diarrhea and traveler's diarrhea [51, 52].

Prebiotics and probiotics have also been shown to improve the gut mucosal barrier function. In critical disease states, translocation of gut bacteria is associated with septic complications, and synbiotic preparations, including probiotics and prebiotics, have been used to preserve barrier function. Randomized controlled trials suggest that these preparations can reduce the rate of postoperative infections in liver transplant patients and the occurrence of septic complications in severe acute pancreatitis [53, 54].

Probiotics and prebiotics have been tested for therapeutic efficacy in clinical trials with patients with ulcerative colitis, Crohn's disease or chronic relapsing pouchitis. However, with the exception of the studies on pouchitis, results of controlled clinical trials published so far are poor and below the expectations raised [55]. Further research is needed to optimize the use of probiotics or prebiotics for these indications.

Conclusions

A large and diverse community of commensal bacteria is harboured in the human gut, in a symbiotic arrangement that influences both physiology and pathology in the host. Furthermore, knowledge about the relevance of the microbial flora for host well-being is advancing rapidly as exemplified by two recent developments. First, molecular biology techniques have dramatically improved our means to investigate actual bacterial colonization of the gut, and myriads of strains that were elusive to conventional microbiological culture can now be described. Second, convincing evidence suggests that immune mechanisms taking place within the gut play a major role in the constitution and reshaping of host's immunity. As a consequence, a better understanding of our relations with the microbial world may be achieved. This certainly could help in the prevention of disease states (atopy, cancer, and inflammatory bowel diseases) afflicting modern societies that neglected an ecological role for bacteria in human life.

References

1   Falk PG, Hooper LV, Midtvedt T, Gordon JI: Creating and maintaining the gastrointestinal ecosystem: what we know and need to know from gnotobiology. Microbiol Mol Biol Rev 1998;62: 1157–1170.
2   Guarner F, Malagelada JR: Gut flora in health and disease. Lancet 2003;361:512–519.
3   Suau A, Bonnet R, Sutren M, Godon JJ, Gibson G, Collins MD, Dore J: Direct rDNA community analysis reveals a myriad of novel bacterial lineages within the human gut. Appl Environ Microbiol 1999;65:4799–4807.
4   Tannock GW: Molecular assessment of intestinal microflora. Am J Clin Nutr 2001;73(suppl): 410S–414S.
5   Zoetendal EG, von Wright A, Vilpponen-Salmela T, Ben-Amor K, Akkermans ADL, de Vos WM: Mucosa-associated bacteria in the human gastrointestinal tract are uniformly distributed along the colon and differ from the community recovered from feces. Appl Environ Microbiol 2002;68: 3401–3407.
6   Kimura K, McCartney AI, McConnell MA, Tannock GW: Analysis of fecal populations of bifidobacteria and lactobacilli and investigation of the immunological responses of their human hosts to the predominant strains. Appl Environ Microbiol 1997;63:3394–3398.
7   Hooper LV, Midtvedt T, Gordon JI: How host-microbial interactions shape the nutrient environment of the mammalian intestine. Annu Rev Nutr 2002;22:283–307.
8   Macfarlane GT, Cummings JH, Allison C: Protein degradation by human intestinal bacteria. J Gen Microbiol 1986;132:1647–1656.
9   Smith EA, Macfarlane GT: Enumeration of human colonic bacteria producing phenolic and indolic compounds: effects of pH, carbohydrate availability and retention time on dissimilatory aromatic amino acid metabolism. J Appl Bacteriol 1996;81:288–302.
10 Hooper LV, Xu J, Falk PG, Midtvedt T, Gordon JI: A molecular sensor that allows a gut commensal to control its nutrient foundation in a competitive ecosystem. Proc Natl Acad Sci USA 1999;96:9833–9838.
11 Brook I: Bacterial interference. Crit Rev Microbiol 1999;25:155–172.

12 Lievin V, Peiffer I, Hudault S, Rochat F, Brassart D, Neeser JR, Servin AL: *Bifidobacterium* strains from resident infant human gastrointestinal microflora exert antimicrobial activity. Gut 2000;47: 646–652.

13 Hooper LV, Wong MH, Thelin A, Hansson L, Falk PG, Gordon JI: Molecular analysis of commensal host-microbial relationships in the intestine. Science 2001;291:881–884.

14 Butler JE, Sun J, Weber P, Navarro P, Francis D: Antibody repertoire development in fetal and newborn piglets. III. Colonization of the gastrointestinal tract selectively diversifies the preimmune repertoire in mucosal lymphoid tissues. Immunology 2000;100:119–130.

15 Fagarasan S, Muramatsu M, Suzuki K, Nagaoka H, Hiai H, Honjo T: Critical roles of activation-induced cytidine deaminase in the homeostasis of gut flora. Science 2002;298:1414–1427.

16 Bourlioux P, Braesco V, Koletzko B, Guarner F: The intestine and its microflora are partners for the protection of the host. Am J Clin Nutr 2003;78:675–683.

17 Aderem A, Ulevitch RJ: Toll-like receptors in the induction of the innate immune response. Nature 2000;406:782–787.

18 Elewaut D, DiDonato JA, Kim JM, et al: NF-kappa B is a central regulator of the intestinal epithelial cell innate immune response induced by infection with enteroinvasive bacteria. J Immunol 1999;163:1457–1466.

19 Maaser C, Kagnoff MF: Role of the intestinal epithelium in orchestrating innate and adaptive mucosal immunity. Z Gastroenterol 2002;40:525–529.

20 Haller D, Bode C, Hammes WP, Pfeifer AM, Schiffrin EJ, Blum S: Non-pathogenic bacteria elicit a differential cytokine response by intestinal epithelial cell/leucocyte co-cultures. Gut 2000;47: 79–87.

21 Borruel N, Casellas F, Antolín M, Carol M, Llopis M, Espín E, Naval J, Guarner F, Malagelada JR: Effects of nonpathogenic bacteria on cytokine secretion by human intestinal mucosa. Am J Gastroenterol 2003;98:865–870.

22 Borruel N, Carol M, Casellas F, Antolín M, de Lara F, Espín E, Naval J, Guarner F, Malagelada JR: Increased mucosal TNF-α production in Crohn's disease can be downregulated ex vivo by probiotic bacteria. Gut 2002;51:659–664.

23 Carol M, Borruel N, Antolín M, Casellas F, Guarner F, Malagelada JR: *Lactobacillus casei* can overcome resistance to apoptosis in lymphocytes from patients with Crohn's disease. Gastroenterology 2003;124:A321.

24 Brandtzaeg PE: Current understanding of gastrointestinal immunoregulation and its relation to food allergy. Ann NY Acad Sci 2002;964:13–45.

25 Cummings JH, Antoine JM, Azpiroz F, Bourdet-Sicard R, Brandtzaeg P, Calder PC, Gibson GR, Guarner F, Isolauri E, Pannemans D, Shortt C, Tuijtelaars S, Watzl B: PASSCLAIM – gut health and immunity. Eur J Nutr 2004;43(suppl 2):118–173.

26 Rook GA, Brunet LR: Give us this day our daily germs. Biologist (London) 2002;49:145–149.

27 Lin HC: Small intestinal bacterial overgrowth: a framework for understanding irritable bowel syndrome. JAMA 2004;292:852–858.

28 Lichtman SM: Bacterial translocation in humans. J Pediatr Gastroenterol Nutr 2001;33:1–10.

29 Rafter J, Glinghammar B: Interactions between the environment and genes in the colon. Eur J Cancer Prev 1998;7(suppl 2):S69–S74.

30 Shanahan F: Inflammatory bowel disease: immunodiagnostics, immunotherapeutics, and ecotherapeutics. Gastroenterology 2001;120:622–635.

31 Macpherson A, Khoo UY, Forgacs I, Philpott-Howard J, Bjarnason I: Mucosal antibodies in inflammatory bowel disease are directed against intestinal bacteria. Gut 1996;38: 365–375.

32 Pirzer U, Schönhaar A, Fleischer B, Hermann E, Meyer zum Büschenfelde KH: Reactivity of infiltrating T lymphocytes with microbial antigens in Crohn's disease. Lancet 1991;338: 1238–1239.

33 D'Haens GR, Geboes K, Peeters M, Baert F, Penninckx F, Rutgeerts P: Early lesions of recurrent Crohn's disease caused by infusion of intestinal contents in excluded ileum. Gastroenterology 1998;114:262–267.

34 Casellas F, Borruel N, Papo M, Guarner F, Antolín M, Videla S, Malagelada JR: Anti-inflammatory effects of enterically coated amoxicillin-clavulanic acid in active ulcerative colitis. Inflammatory Bowel Dis 1998;4:1–5.

35 Hampe J, Cuthbert A, Croucher PJ, Mirza MM, Mascheretti S, Fisher S, Frenzel H, King K, Hasselmeyer A, MacPherson AJ, Bridger S, van Deventer S, Forbes A, Nikolaus S, Lennard-Jones JE, Foelsch UR, Krawczak M, Lewis C, Schreiber S, Mathew CG: Association between insertion mutation in NOD2 gene and Crohn's disease in German and British populations. Lancet 2001;357:1902–1904.

36 Seksik P, Rigottier-Gois L, Gramet G, Sutren M, Pochart P, Marteau P, Jian R, Doré J: Alterations of the dominant faecal bacterial groups in patients with Crohn's disease of the colon. Gut 2003;52:237–242.

37 Guarner F, Schaafsma G: Probiotics. Int J Food Microbiol 1998;39:237–238.

38 Gibson GR, Roberfroid MB: Dietary modulation of the human colonic microbiota: introducing the concept of prebiotics. J Nutr 1995;125:1401–1412.

39 D'Souza AL, Rajkumar C, Cooke J, Bulpitt CJ: Probiotics in prevention of antibiotic associated diarrhoea: meta analysis. Br Med J 2002;324:1361–1366.

40 Cremonini F, Di Caro S, Nista EC, Bartolozzi F, Capelli G, Gasbarrini G, Gasbarrini A: Meta-analysis: the effect of probiotic administration on antibiotic-associated diarrhoea. Aliment Pharmacol Ther 2002;16:1461–1467.

41 Saavedra JM, Bauman NA, Oung I, Perman JA, Yolken RH: Feeding of *Bifidibacterium bifidum* and *Streptococcus termophilus* to infants in hospital for prevention of diarrhoea and shedding of rotavirus. Lancet 1994;334:1046–1049.

42 Szajewska H, Kotowska M, Mrukowicz JZ, Armanska M, Mikolajczyk W: Efficacy of *Lactobacillus* GG in prevention of nosocomial diarrhea in infants. J Pediatr 2001;138:361–365.

43 Mastretta E, Longo P, Laccisaglia A, Balbo L, Russo R, Mazzaccara A, Gianino P: Effect of *Lactobacillus* GG and breast-feeding in the prevention of rotavirus nosocomial infection. J Pediatr Gastroenterol Nutr 2002;35:527–531.

44 Oberhelman RA, Gilman RH, Sheen P, Taylor DN, Black RE, Cabrera L, Lescano AG, Meza R, Madico G: A placebo-controlled trial of *Lactobacillus* GG to prevent diarrhea in undernourished Peruvian children. J Pediatr 1999;134:15–20.

45 Pedone CA, Arnaud CC, Postaire ER, Bouley CF, Reinert P: Multicentric study of the effect of milk fermented by *Lactobacillus casei* on the incidence of diarrhoea. Int J Clin Pract 2000; 54:568–571.

46 Marteau P, Seksik P, Jian R: Probiotics and intestinal health effects: a clinical perspective. Br J Nutr 2002;88(suppl 1):S51–S57.

47 Szajewska H, Mrukowicz JZ: Probiotics in the treatment and prevention of acute infectious diar-rhea in infants and children: a systematic review of published randomized, double-blind, placebo-controlled trials. J Pediatr Gastroenterol Nutr 2001;33:S17–S25.

48 Van Niel CW, Feudtner C, Garrison MM, Christakis DA: *Lactobacillus* therapy for acute infec-tious diarrhea in children: a meta-analysis. Pediatrics 2002;109:678–684.

49 Huang JS, Bousvaros A, Lee JW, Diaz A, Davidson EJ: Efficacy of probiotic use in acute diarrhea in children: a meta-analysis. Dig Dis Sci 2002;47:2625–2634.

50 Gibson GR, Beatty ER, Wang X, Cummings JH: Selective stimulation of bifidobacteria in the human colon by oligofructose and inulin. Gastroenterology 1995;108:975–982.

51 Saavedra JM, Tschernia A: Human studies with probiotics and prebiotics: clinical implications. Br J Nutr 2002;87(suppl 2):S241–S246.

52 Cummings JH, Christie S, Cole TJ: A study of fructo-oligosaccharides in the prevention of trav-ellers' diarrhoea. Aliment Pharmacol Ther 2001;15:1139–1145.

53 Olah A, Belagyi T, Issekutz A, Gamal ME, Bengmark S: Randomized clinical trial of specific lac-tobacillus and fibre supplement to early enteral nutrition in patients with acute pancreatitis. Br J Surg 2002;89:1103–1107.

54 Rayes N, Seehofer D, Theruvath T, Schiller RA, Langrehr JM, Jonas S, Bengmark S, Neuhaus P: Supply of pre- and probiotics reduces bacterial infection rates after liver transplantation – a ran-domized, double-blind trial. Am J Transplant 2005;5:125–130.

55   Sartor RB: Therapeutic manipulation of the enteric microflora in inflammatory bowel diseases: antibiotics, probiotics, and prebiotics. Gastroenterology 2004;126:1620–1633.
56   Salminen S, Bouley C, Boutron-Ruault MC, Cummings JH, Franck A, Gibson GR, Isolauri E, Moreau MC, Roberfroid M, Rowland I: Functional food science and gastrointestinal physiology and function. Br J Nutr 1998;80(suppl 1):S147–S171.

Francisco Guarner, MD, PhD
Digestive System Research Unit
University Hospital Vall d'Hebron
Passeig Vall d'Hebron, 119–129
ES–08035 Barcelona (Spain)
Tel. +34 93274 6282, Fax +34 93489 4456
E-Mail fguarnera@medynet.com

This chapter should be cited as follows:

Guarner F: Enteric Flora in Health and Disease. Digestion 2006;73(suppl 1):5–12.

Scarpignato C, Lanas Á (eds): Bacterial Flora in Digestive Disease.
Focus on Rifaximin.

....

Experimental and Clinical Pharmacology of Rifaximin, a Gastrointestinal Selective Antibiotic

Carmelo Scarpignato, Iva Pelosini

Laboratory of Clinical Pharmacology, Department of Human Anatomy,
Pharmacology and Forensic Sciences, School of Medicine and Dentistry,
University of Parma, Parma, Italy

Abstract

Rifaximin (4-deoxy-4'-methylpyrido[1',2'-1,2]imidazo[5,4-c]rifamycin SV) is a product of synthesis experiments designed to modify the parent compound, rifamycin, in order to achieve low gastrointestinal (GI) absorption while retaining good antibacterial activity. Both experimental and clinical pharmacology clearly show that this compound is a non-systemic antibiotic with a broad spectrum of antibacterial action covering Gram-positive and Gram-negative organisms, both aerobes and anaerobes. Being virtually non-absorbed, its bioavailability within the GI tract is rather high with intraluminal and fecal drug concentrations that largely exceed the minimum inhibitory concentration values observed in vitro against a wide range of pathogenic organisms. The GI tract represents therefore the primary therapeutic target and GI infections the main indication. This antibiotic has therefore little value outside the enteric area and this will minimize both antimicrobial resistance and systemic adverse events. Indeed, the drug proved to be safe in all patient populations, including young children. The appreciation of the pathogenic role of gut bacteria in several organic and functional GI diseases has increasingly broadened its clinical use, which is now extended to hepatic encephalopathy, small intestine bacterial overgrowth, inflammatory bowel disease and colonic diverticular disease.

Introduction

Infectious diseases still represent a leading cause of morbidity and mortality worldwide. It is not possible to adequately protect the health of a nation without addressing infectious disease problems that are occurring elsewhere in the

Table 1. Primary reasons for prescribing antimicrobial agents for enteric infections (from Pickering [9])

To reduce symptoms and duration of disease
To prevent serious sequelae
To prevent mortality
To eradicate fecal shedding
To prevent pathogen transmission

world. In an age of expanding air travel and international trade, infectious agents are transported across borders every day, carried by infected people, animals, and insects, and contained within commercial shipments of contaminated food [1, 2]. Since their discovery, antibiotics have completely transformed humanity's approach to infectious disease. Today, the use of antibiotics combined with improvements in sanitation, housing, and nutrition, alongside the advent of widespread vaccination programs, have led to a dramatic drop in once common infectious diseases that formerly laid low entire populations. However, emerging infectious pathogens, increasing antimicrobial resistance (mediated primarily through horizontal transfer of a plethora of mobile DNA transfer factors) and the appearance of diseases that decrease the host defense have increased the need for more effective and safe antimicrobial treatments [3]. Like elsewhere, these drugs have an important place in the management of GI disease [4–6]. Antibiotic use in gastroenterology falls into three general settings [5]:

- GI infections (e.g. bacterial diarrhea, cholangitis, diverticulitis)
- GI diseases that may involve infectious agents but are not 'classic' infectious diseases (e.g. *Helicobacter pylori*-positive peptic ulcer, Whipple's disease, inflammatory bowel disease)
- Antibiotic prophylaxis for GI procedures.

Enteric infections generally are self-limited conditions that require only fluid and electrolyte therapy [7]. However, patients with diarrhea associated with certain bacterial and protozoal agents may benefit from therapy with an antimicrobial agent [8]. In some instances, specific antimicrobial therapy may reduce morbidity and mortality associated with enteric illnesses or prevent future complications, but antimicrobial agents should be prescribed with an appreciation for their limitations [9]. The primary reasons for prescribing antimicrobial agents for enteric infections are listed in table 1.

The proliferation of new antibacterial agents has made the choice of antibiotics increasingly complex. General consideration in selecting antibiotic therapy include (1) the identity and susceptibility pattern of the infecting organisms, (2) the anatomic localization of the infection, (3) the antimicrobial spectrum of the drug, and (4) its pharmacokinetic properties. Other important considerations include the possible selection of resistant organisms, interactions with other drugs, toxicity and cost [5].

The anatomic location of the GI infection influences the selection of the antimicrobial agent and the route of administration. For instance, oral administration of a poorly absorbable antibiotic may be used for eradication of non-invasive enteric pathogens [10]. Although the importance of attaining high biliary concentrations of antimicrobial agents in treating patients with cholangitis is still debated, it has been suggested that agents undergoing biliary secretion have higher efficacy in the treatment of these infections [11].

Non-absorbed oral antibiotic therapy, unlike systemically available antibiotics, allows localized enteric targeting of pathogens and is associated with minimal risk of systemic toxicity or side effects [12]. Provided that non-absorbed antibiotics are as effective as systemically absorbed drugs for the target illness, their safety and tolerability profiles may render them more appropriate for certain patient groups, such as young children, pregnant or lactating women, and the elderly, among whom side effects are a particular concern. The restricted use of non-absorbed oral antibiotics only for enteric infections should also reduce the development of widespread resistance, a major limitation of current antibiotics for enteric infections [12].

Compared to systemic drugs, the number of poorly absorbed antimicrobials that would best target the GI tract is relatively small and almost completely limited to aminoglycosides. Indeed, oral vancomycin [13], teicoplanin [14], and bacitracin [15] are confined to the treatment of *Clostridium difficile* infection [16–18]. Ramoplanin, a glycolipodepsipeptide antibiotic [19], is being developed for the treatment of *C. difficile*-associated diarrhea [20] and vancomycin-resistant enterococcal infection in high-risk patients [21]. Paromomycin and neomycin represent therefore the most widely used compounds [22, 23]. Neomycin is often associated to bacitracin, which is highly active against Gram-positive microorganisms, in order to extend its antibacterial activity. However, even poorly absorbed aminoglycosides are not completely devoid of untoward effects. Indeed, both ototoxicity [24–26] and nephrotoxicity [27] have been reported after oral neomycin especially in patients with renal dysfunction. Such patients can in fact accumulate toxic levels of the antimicrobial since the kidneys represent the major route of drug excretion [28]. Ototoxicity has actually been reported after ototopic (i.e. ear drops) aminoglycoside administration [29].

In order to overcome the limitations of the above drugs, a series of rifamycin derivatives with improved pharmacokinetic (i.e. virtually absence of GI absorption) and pharmacodynamic (i.e. with broad spectrum of anti-bacterial activity) properties have been synthesized at Alfa Wassermann laboratories

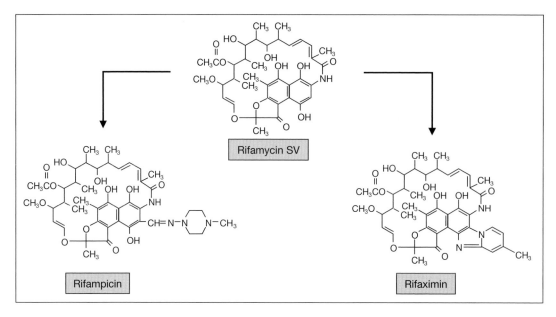

Fig. 1. Chemical structures of rifampicin and rifaximin as well as of their parent compound, rifamycin SV. The empirical formula of rifaximin is $C_{43}H_{51}N_3O_{11}$ [CAS Registry No.: 80621-81-4] and its molecular weight 785.9 daltons.

[30]. Amongst the different molecules, the compound marked L/105 (4-deoxy-4'-methylpyrido[1',2'-1,2]imidazo[5,4-c]rifamycin SV) and later named rifaximin was selected for further development (fig. 1). The antibiotic was first marketed in Italy and subsequently introduced in other European countries. Rifaximin was also licensed in some Northern African and Asian areas as well as in Mexico. The compound has recently been approved by the US FDA for the treatment of infectious diarrhea in the traveler [31].

The aim of this review is to summarize the available pharmacology and safety data on this non-systemic antibiotic.

Antimicrobial Activity

The in vitro antibacterial activity of rifaximin has been determined by using minimum inhibitory concentrations (MICs) against bacteria from clinical isolates or stock culture collections. It should be pointed out that – in the absence of known GI concentrations – interpretation of MIC values is difficult. It is likely, however, that the drug concentration achieved at the desired site of

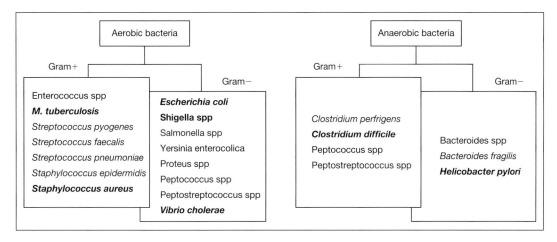

Aerobic bacteria				Anaerobic bacteria		
Gram+		Gram−		Gram+		Gram−
Enterococcus spp **M. tuberculosis** Streptococcus pyogenes Streptococcus faecalis Streptococcus pneumoniae Staphylococcus epidermidis **Staphylococcus aureus**		**Escherichia coli** **Shigella spp** Salmonella spp Yersinia enterocolica Proteus spp Peptococcus spp Peptostreptococcus spp **Vibrio cholerae**		Clostridium perfrigens **Clostridium difficile** Peptococcus spp Peptostreptococcus spp		Bacteroides spp Bacteroides fragilis **Helicobacter pylori**

Fig. 2. Rifaximin: spectrum of antimicrobial activity.

action, i.e. the GI tract, will largely exceed the reported MIC values. For instance, fecal levels after oral administration of the antibiotic range between 4,000 and 8,000 µg/g of stool, which are 160–250 times higher than the MIC_{90} for the various bacterial enteropathogens [32, 33].

Several in vitro studies, summarized by recent reviews [33–40], have shown that – like rifampicin – rifaximin displays an inhibitory activity against Gram-positive and Gram-negative, aerobic and anaerobic bacteria (fig. 2). Its activity against a wide variety of enteropathogens underlines the clinical efficacy of this antibiotic in GI infections [35, 36, 38] and other functional and organic GI diseases where gut flora has an important pathogenetic role [34, 37, 38]. When 427 enteropathogens isolated from patients with infectious diarrhea enrolled in clinical trials were tested in vitro, rifaximin was found to be active against *all* isolates [41]. The distribution of MICs by pathogen is shown in figure 3. In all cases, the MICs were substantially lower than the fecal concentrations of rifaximin achieved during clinical use [32].

Thorough microbiological studies have also shown that other clinically relevant anaerobic bacteria such as *C. difficile* [42–44] and also *H. pylori* [45–47] are very sensitive to this antibiotic and that its activity extends to *Vibrio cholerae* [48]. It is worthwhile mentioning that treatment with high-dose (600 mg, 3 times a day, for 14 days) rifaximin was also efficacious in resolving the clinical symptoms and clearing protozoan infections in HIV-1-infected patients with CD4 count ≥200/mm³, who presented enteric and systemic symptoms due to *Cryptosporidium parvum* or *Blastocystis hominis* associated with enteropathogens [49]. The favorable effects of this antibiotic on protozoal

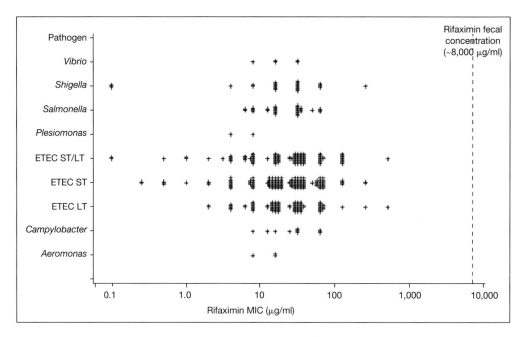

Fig. 3. Distribution of rifaximin MIC values by pathogen in clinical isolates from patients enrolled in three controlled trials of infectious diarrhea. Of the 427 enteropathogens, 298 came from the pre-treatment stool sample, and 129 came from the post-treatment stool sample. ETEC = Enterotoxigenic *E. coli* (from DuPont [41]).

diarrhea have also been reported in a recent multicenter study on patients with traveler's diarrhea (TD) [50]. Indeed, in patients with pretreatment stools positive for *Cryptosporidium* infections, the clinical improvement obtained with rifaximin was significantly superior to that observed in the placebo-treated subjects.

Like the other members of the rifamycin family [51, 52], rifaximin specifically inhibits RNA synthesis by binding the β-subunit of the bacterial DNA-dependent RNA polymerase [53, 54]. Very recent studies [55] using X-ray crystallography have actually shown that these antibiotics act by removing the catalytic magnesium ions from bacterial RNA polymerase and that the binding of structurally different rifamycins to the enzyme is different.

Development of resistance to rifaximin may be similar to that of rifampicin, which is primarily due to a chromosomal single-step alteration in the drug target, the DNA-dependent RNA polymerase [56, 57]. This differs from the plasmid-mediated resistance commonly acquired by bacteria to aminoglycoside antibiotics, such as neomycin or bacitracin [58]. The spread of resistance due to the chromosomal mechanism is however less frequent than that due to plasmid-mediated transfer [57, 59].

The development of resistance to rifaximin was studied in detail on several aerobic (Gram-negative and Gram-positive) and anaerobic strains. As expected, spontaneous selection of resistance was rare for the anaerobic bacteria; in fact, among these anaerobes only a few species showed the spontaneous emergence of resistant mutants [44, 60]. Rifaximin selected resistant aerobic Gram-positive cocci mutants more easily under aerobic conditions than in an anaerobic atmosphere [44, 60]. In comparison with Gram-positive microorganisms, drug-resistant Gram-negative bacilli were rarely detected [44, 60].

Spontaneously resistant mutants were more easily selected after preincubation of the test bacteria with sub-inhibitory concentrations of rifaximin rather than after exposing the microorganisms to high levels of the antibiotic. Taking into account that rifaximin is poorly absorbed (see below), the high amounts of the drug available within the digestive lumen compare better with suprarather than with sub-inhibitory concentrations of the drug. Furthermore, since the anaerobic atmosphere did hinder the selection of rifaximin-resistant enterobacteria, it is expected that – during antibiotic therapy with this drug – the selection of resistant mutants in the GI tract (a prevalently anaerobic environment) be very low. In summary, thanks to the high drug bioavailability in an oxygen-deficient milieu, the in vivo occurrence of bacterial resistance with rifaximin should be an infrequent phenomenon. The constant therapeutic efficacy of the antibiotic in the management of different GI infections [30, 35–40] clearly suggests that this is the case.

Repeated oral administration of an antibiotic that reaches very high concentrations within the GI lumen could have profound effects on intestinal flora [61, 62]. As expected, rifaximin markedly reduced fecal bacterial counts during oral intake, but the effect was short-lasting since the bacterial population recovered within 1–2 weeks from the end of treatment (table 2) [63]. Most importantly, fungal colonization occurred very rarely. Indeed, *Candida albicans*, which has been implicated in the pathogenesis of antibiotic-associated diarrhea [64], was isolated from the fecal samples of only 2 out of 10 patients given 1,200 mg of rifaximin daily [63] and in none of the volunteers taking 800 mg daily [65].

Antimicrobial resistance to rifamycins develops rapidly both in vitro and in vivo [56, 66, 67]. As a consequence, all the three members of the family (i.e. rifampicin, rifabutin and rifapentine) are used clinically as components of combination therapies [56, 68]. Being structurally related, rifaximin could share this potential. And indeed, resistance rates, recorded in fecal strains of Enterobacteriaceae, *Enterococcus, Bacteroides, Clostridium* and anaerobic cocci, ranged between 30 and 90% after short-term (5 days) antibiotic (800 mg daily) treatment [65]. A similar pattern was observed in 10 patients with hepatic

Table 2. Changes in fecal bacterial population after oral rifaximin administration in healthy volunteers (from Testa et al. [63])

Organisms		Weeks					
		0	1	2	4	8	12
Escherichia coli	$\cdot 10^8$	2.9	0.46	2.5	2.7	3.0	3.0
Other enterobacters	$\cdot 10^7$	1.0	0.09	1.0	1.2	1.1	1.2
Enterococci	$\cdot 10^7$	5.6	0.08	3.1	5.7	5.6	4.9
Bacteroides spp.	$\cdot 10^9$	6.0	0.10	5.4	6.1	6.2	5.6
Clostridium spp.	$\cdot 10^8$	1.1	0.04	1.0	1.1	1.0	0.9
Anaerobic cocci	$\cdot 10^7$	6.1	0.02	5.6	6.0	6.2	5.8

Rifaximin (800 mg) was given in two daily doses for 5 days after the first stool collection.

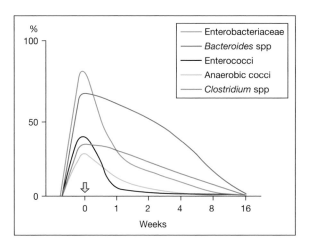

Fig. 4. Disappearance of rifaximin-resistant bacteria from human intestine after stopping the antibiotic treatment (week 0) (from De Leo et al. [65]).

encephalopathy after treatment with rifaximin 1,200 mg/day for 5 days [63]. Nevertheless, a rapid disappearance of resistant bacteria was observed after stopping the antibiotic treatment (fig. 4). Different kinetics of disappearance were however observed. The aerobic species showed a more rapid return to the baseline 'sensitive' status, whereas the anaerobic bacteria, especially the Gram-negative rods, regained sensitivity to rifaximin more slowly. In any case, 3 months after the end of treatment, resistant strains were no longer detectable in the feces [65]. These results support the cyclic use of rifaximin that has been adopted by the investigators in the treatment of hepatic encephalopathy [69] and colonic diverticular disease [70].

It is worth mentioning that the very-short-term use of the antibiotic, adopted to treat TD, is unlikely to induce any microbial resistance. Indeed, DuPont and Jiang [71], by studying changes in susceptibility of intestinal flora during a 3-day rifaximin course among US students with TD, failed to document the emergence of drug-resistant Gram-positive (e.g. enterococci) and Gram-negative (*Escherichia coli*) organisms during treatment.

Pharmacokinetics and Drug Interactions

Animal and Human Pharmacokinetics

The first pharmacokinetic investigations [72, 73] were performed in rats and dogs by using a microbiological assay (i.e. agar diffusion test and *Staphylococcus aureus* 209 P FDA as test organism). Conversely from rifampicin, whose serum levels were already detectable 30 min after the administration and still measurable after 48 h, only trace amounts (i.e. 0.2 µg/ml) of rifaximin were detected in serum of fed rats 4 h later. The amount of detectable antibiotic was reduced by 50% in fasted animals. Similar results have been obtained in dogs after oral administration of 25 mg/kg of both rifamycin derivatives [72, 73]. No detectable amount of rifaximin was found in serum at any time. The negligible intestinal absorption of rifaximin was subsequently confirmed with the use of the labeled drug [53, 74]. These isotope studies also showed that the greatest concentration of radioactivity is found in the GI tract [53, 74], that represents the therapeutic target organ. The radioactivity peak was reached at 0. 5 h in the stomach, at 2 h in the small intestine and at 7 h in the cecum and large intestine. Other than in the GI tract, radioactivity counts were generally low and only liver and kidney contained more than 0.01% of the dose administered, a finding consistent with the results obtained with unlabeled rifaximin measured by a microbiological assay [72].

Although theoretically safe, poorly absorbed antimicrobials could become 'absorbable' in the presence of mucosal inflammatory or ulcerative changes [75], like those occurring in inflammatory bowel disease (IBD) or when invasive bacteria colonize the intestine. To verify whether the presence of intestinal lesions would affect rifaximin absorption, the drug was given to rats with experimentally induced colitis [76]. The indomethacin-induced enteropathy did not affect intestinal absorption of rifaximin. However, under the same experimental conditions, systemic bioavailability of neomycin did increase [76].

The human pharmacokinetics of rifaximin after oral administration has been studied in healthy volunteers, in patients with IBD or hepatic encephalopathy

Table 3. Summary of the pharmacokinetic studies with rifaximin in humans

Study	Ref.	Subjects	Dose regimen	C_{max}, ng/ml	Urinary recovery, %
Descombe et al., 1994	77	Healthy volunteers	400 mg, single dose	1.56 ± 0.43	0.007 ± 0.001
FDA-driven study, 2004	31	Healthy volunteers	400 mg, ^{14}C single dose	4.30 ± 2.80	0.32
FDA-driven study, 2004	31	Healthy volunteers	400 mg, single dose	3.80 ± 1.32	0.023 ± 0.009
Rizzello et al., 1998	78	UC patients	400 mg, single dose	4.75 ± 2.11	0.009 ± 0.006
Campieri et al., unpubl. data	–	CD patients	400 mg, single dose	2.74 ± 0.88	0.007 ± 0.005
Gionchetti et al., 1999	80	Severe UC patients	800 mg daily for 10 days	ND*	0.008**
Taylor et al., 2003	97, 31	Healthy volunteers with exptl shigellosis	600 mg daily for 3 days	1.63 ± 0.86	NA
FDA-driven study, 2004	31	Patient with HE	600 mg daily for 7 days	2.69 ± 0.99	0.061 ± 0.015

CD = Crohn's disease; HE = hepatic encephalopathy; NA = not available; ND = not detectable; UC = ulcerative colitis. Each value represents the mean $\pm$ SEM. *Measured 12 h after the last dose. **Cumulative excretion.

and in experimentally induced shigellosis (table 3). The aim of these studies was to confirm the low, if any, systemic absorption of the drug; metabolism and excretion data are scant. In all these investigations a sensitive high-pressure liquid chromatographic method was used to measure rifaximin in body fluids.

After oral administration of 400 mg of rifaximin to fasted healthy volunteers, blood drug concentration was found to be lower than the detection limit of the analytical method (i.e. 2.5 ng/ml) in half of them [77]. In the remaining subjects, very low amounts were detected at some of the time intervals during the first 4 h after intake. Along the same lines, the urinary concentrations of the drug were very low and often undetectable. The effect of food on the absorption of the antibiotic was also evaluated [31] and a significant, albeit not clinically relevant, increase of bioavailability was observed after a high-fat breakfast.

Systemic absorption of rifaximin (200 mg three times daily) was also evaluated in 13 healthy subjects fed with *Shigella flexneri* 2a on days 1 and 3 of a 3-day course of treatment [31]. Rifaximin plasma concentrations were low and variable. There was no evidence of drug accumulation following repeated administration for 3 days (9 doses). Peak plasma rifaximin concentrations after 3 and 9 consecutive doses ranged from 0.81 to 3.4 ng/ml on day 1 and 0.68 to 2.26 ng/ml on day 3 [31]. Fecal excretion of the drug was also assessed in 39 patients with acute diarrhea after administration of 400 mg every 12 h for

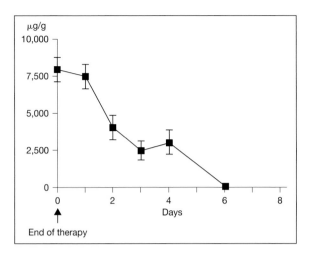

Fig. 5. Fecal concentration of rifaximin in patients with TD after treatment with 800 mg/day of the drug for 3 consecutive days. Each square refers to the mean of the values obtained from 39 subjects. Vertical bars are standard errors (from Jiang et al. [32]).

3 consecutive days [32]. As shown in figure 5, post-therapy stool rifaximin levels were high, decreasing gradually over a 5-day period. It is worthwhile mentioning that fecal drug concentrations largely exceeded the MIC values for the bacterial isolates obtained from patients with TD [32].

As IBD is one of the therapeutic indications of rifaximin, its absorption was carefully studied in patients with mild-to-moderate ulcerative colitis, after administration of two tablets (i.e. 400 mg) orally [78]. Rifaximin concentrations were below the detection limits in most plasma samples. Only in few patients was the drug detected during the first 8 h after administration. The total rifaximin amount recovered in the urine was only 0.009% of the dose. This figure fits well with the corresponding value (i.e. 0.007%) observed in healthy volunteers [77]. No correlation between disease activity and urinary concentrations was found after repeated drug administration [79].

It is worthwhile mentioning that, even after 15 days of therapy of patients with resistant pouchitis with a high dose (2 g daily) of rifaximin together with ciprofloxacin (1 g daily), no plasma level of the antibiotic was detectable in any patient [80].

Although the pharmacokinetics of rifaximin in patients with renal insufficiency has not been specifically studied, its very low renal excretion makes any dose adjustment unnecessary. The same holds true for patients with hepatic insufficiency. In fact, the mean peak drug plasma concentrations (i.e. 13.5 ng/ml) detected in subjects with hepatic encephalopathy patients given rifaximin 800 mg three times daily for 7 days [31, 81] was not dissimilar to that found in healthy subjects [77] and patients with IBD [78]. And indeed, in all the trials performed in this condition the drug has been well tolerated [69, 81, 82].

Finally, drug absorption and excretion have not been evaluated in pediatric or geriatric populations. However, here again the tolerability of rifaximin in childhood and in the elderly has found to be extremely good [34, 37].

Drug-to-Drug Interactions

As new classes of antimicrobial drugs have become available, pharmacokinetic drug interactions with antimicrobials have become more common. Macrolides, fluoroquinolones, rifamycins, azoles and other agents can interact adversely with commonly used drugs, usually by altering their hepatic metabolism [83]. The mechanisms by which antimicrobial agents alter the biotransformation of other drugs are increasingly understood to reflect inhibition or induction of specific cytochrome P_{450} enzymes. Rifampicin and rifabutin induce several cytochromes P_{450}, including CYP3A4, and hence can enhance the metabolism of many other drugs [83].

By using in vitro preparations of human enzymes it is possible to predict those antibiotics that will adversely affect the metabolism of other drugs [84]. Such studies have shown that rifaximin, at concentrations ranging from 2 to 200 ng/ml, did not inhibit human hepatic cytochrome P_{450} isoenzymes 1A2, 2A6, 2B6, 2C9, 2C19, 2D6, 2E1, and 3A4 [31]. In an in vitro hepatocyte induction model, rifaximin was shown to induce cytochrome P_{450} 3A4 (CYP3A4) [31], an isoenzyme which rifampicin is also known to induce [83].

Since rifampicin impairs oral contraceptives (OCs) effectiveness and pregnancies have been reported in women taking OCs and antibiotics [85], the interaction between an OC containing ethinyl estradiol and norgestimate and rifaximin was studied in 28 healthy female subjects given a short course of the drug [31]. The results of this study showed that the pharmacokinetics of single doses of ethinyl estradiol and norgestimate were not altered by concomitant antibiotic administration [86].

Midazolam and other benzodiazepines (e.g. alprazolam and triazolam) are selective substrates of CYP3A4 [84] and the concomitant administration of potent metabolic CYP3A4 inducers results in statistically significant pharmacokinetic changes and consequent loss of therapeutic efficacy [87]. To evaluate the possible midazolam-rifaximin interaction, an open-label, randomized, crossover trial was designed to assess the effect of oral rifaximin (200 mg three times daily for 3 or 7 days) on the pharmacokinetics of a single dose of midazolam, administered either intravenously (2 mg) or orally (6 mg) [31]. No significant difference was observed in all the pharmacokinetic parameters of midazolam or its major metabolite, 1'-hydroxy-midazolam, with or without simultaneous antibiotic therapy [88]. These results therefore show that rifaximin does not significantly affect intestinal or hepatic CYP3A4 activity.

The lack of any significant in vivo interaction between rifaximin and human cytochrome P_{450} is also consistent with the absence of any significant induction of drug metabolizing enzymes in the liver and the GI tract of rats given the antibiotic orally for 6 months [50]. When given for prevention or treatment of diarrhea in travelers (TD) [35, 38, 40], rifaximin should therefore not affect the pharmacokinetics (and consequently pharmacodynamics) of other prophylactic drugs (e.g. antimalarials) [50].

General Pharmacology

As the GI tract is the main therapeutic target of rifaximin, its potential effects on gastric secretion and GI motility have been investigated in rats and mice [53]. The antibiotic was given intraduodenally to pylorus-ligated rat (Shay rat) at doses ranging from 10 to 500 mg/kg, i.e. up to 50 times the therapeutic daily dose. No effect on pH and volume, of gastric juice as well as on acid output and pepsin activity was observed.

Gastric emptying was studied in rats by means of a liquid meal labeled with phenol red [Scarpignato, unpubl. observations], while intestinal transit was evaluated in mice by means of the charcoal test meal [53]. Here again, rifaximin was unable to influence either emptying rate or intestinal motility. The drug could however be capable of correcting the GI motility derangement often observed in the presence of small intestinal bacterial overgrowth (SIBO) [89]. This is the case of patients with diabetes [90] or Crohn's disease [91], in whom the delayed intestinal transit, detected together with SIBO, was accelerated by a short-course treatment with rifaximin.

The effect of rifaximin on cardiovascular and respiratory systems was investigated in anaesthetized rats and guinea pigs, respectively [53]. Rifaximin was given intraduodenally at doses up to 100 mg/kg and carotid pressure and flow as well as heart rate were continuously measured in rats, while respiration amplitude and frequency were monitored in guinea pigs. The rifamycin derivative did not affect any of the measured parameters at any time after its administration.

Clinical pharmacological studies to specifically address the effect of rifaximin on GI or cardiovascular and respiratory functions have been not performed. However, while the most frequently reported, albeit few, adverse events associated with rifaximin administration were gastrointestinal in nature, no untoward reactions involving the cardiovascular or respiratory systems have been described [30, 34, 37, 92].

It is worth mentioning that rifamycins inhibit human neutrophil functions and may therefore display an anti-inflammatory action [93, 94]. And indeed, intra-articular rifamycin has been successfully used in chronic arthritides, like juvenile rheumatoid arthritis and ankylosing spondylitis [95]. The fact that oral administration of another rifamycin derivative (namely rifampicin) was completely devoid of any therapeutic activity [96] suggests that this peculiar pharmacologic activity is a topical one. Provided an anti-inflammatory action of rifaximin be confirmed, it could represent an additional therapeutic mechanism underlying its efficacy in IBD and diverticular disease.

Clinical Use and Therapeutic Potential

Data from both experimental and clinical pharmacology clearly show that rifaximin is a non-systemic antibiotic with a broad spectrum of antibacterial action covering Gram-positive and Gram-negative organisms, both aerobes and anaerobes. Being virtually non-absorbed, its bioavailability within the GI tract is rather high with intraluminal and fecal drug concentrations that largely exceed the MIC values observed in vitro against a wide range of pathogenic organisms. The GI tract represents therefore the primary therapeutic target and GI infections the main indication [34–40]. Besides TD, where the antibiotic is being increasingly used [35, 39, 40], rifaximin proved to be effective in homeland infectious diarrhea [36, 38]. A recent clinical pharmacological study [97] has also shown its ability to prevent experimentally-induced shigellosis (fig. 6). The results of this study support the use of rifaximin in the *prevention* of infectious diarrhea in the traveler (TD). And indeed, DuPont et al. [98] have just reported that even once-daily administration of rifaximin is able to prevent TD.

Since gut bacteria play a pathogenic role in several GI disorders (like for instance IBD or irritable bowel syndrome (IBS)), the broad antimicrobial activity of rifaximin is of value also in these clinical conditions [34, 37, 38]. Thanks to the lack of transcutaneous absorption pointed out in both animal [99] and human [100] studies, its topical use in skin infections has also been investigated [101]. Finally, since rifaximin spectrum of antibacterial action includes many organisms (e.g. *Bacteroides bivius-disiens, Gardnerella vaginalis, Haemophilus ducreyi*, etc.) causing genital infections [60], including *Trichomonas vaginalis* [60] and *Chlamydia trachomatis* [102], its local application in the treatment of bacterial vaginosis has been attempted [101]. The growing list of therapeutic applications of rifaximin for which there are published clinical studies is shown in table 4. Amongst them, some are established indications for which the clinical trials so far performed have provided evidence for a substantial benefit of rifaximin. These include infectious diarrhea [35, 36, 38], hepatic encephalopathy

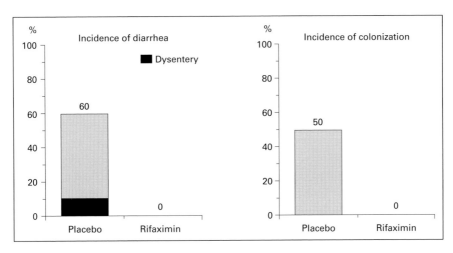

Fig. 6. Preventive effect of rifaximin on experimentally-induced shigellosis in humans. In this investigation, two groups of healthy volunteers pretreated with either the antibiotic (200 mg t.i.d. for 3 days) or placebo were challenged after the fourth drug dose with *S. flexneri* 2a (1,000–1,500 CFU). Rifaximin completely prevented both the bacterial colonization and the insurgence of diarrhea (p = 0.001 at Fisher's exact test; from Taylor et al. [97]).

Table 4. Established and potential clinical indications for rifaximin (from Scarpignato and Pelosini [34])

Established indications
Infectious diarrhea (including TD)
Hepatic encephalopathy
Small intestine bacterial overgrowth (SIBO)
Inflammatory bowel disease (IBD)
Colonic diverticular disease

Potential indications
IBS and chronic constipation
C. difficile infection
Bowel preparation before colorectal surgery
H. pylori infection
Selective bowel decontamination in acute pancreatitis
Prevention of spontaneous bacterial peritonitis in cirrhosis
Prevention of NSAID-induced intestinal injury
Extra-GI indications
  Skin infections
  Bacterial vaginosis
  Periodontal disease

[69, 82], SIBO [103], colonic diverticular disease [70] and IBD [104]. For each of these indications a summary of scientific rationale and of available data, which the reader is referred to, has recently been published [35, 69, 70, 82, 103, 104].

Safety and Tolerability

Animal Studies

Although rifaximin is poorly absorbed and therefore its systemic bioavailability, if any, is very low, thorough toxicological studies [summarized in 53] have shown that it is devoid of any acute and chronic toxicity in laboratory animals. In vitro and in vivo studies did also not reveal any genotoxic potential.

Despite the fact that reproductive studies have been unable to detect fetal anomalies definitely related to maternal treatment with rifaximin [34], the US FDA put rifaximin – like many other antimicrobial agents [105] – in the pregnancy category C[1] [31]. It is worthwhile mentioning that a population-based case-control study [106] showed that maternal exposure of anti-tuberculosis drugs during pregnancy does not show a detectable teratogenic risk to the fetus. It is therefore very unlikely that the minute amounts of absorbed rifaximin, which will never be taken throughout the full gestation period, affect fetal development in humans.

No studies evaluating the excretion of rifaximin into breast milk and its bioavailability to the infant have been performed. However, due to its very limited, if any, absorption from the GI tract and its physicochemical characteristics, any milk excretion of the drug is unlikely [107].

Tolerability Profile in Humans

An evaluation of rifaximin tolerability profile observed in almost 1,000 patients from 30 clinical trials was unable to identify a definite pattern of intolerance [34, 37]. Very few adverse events have been reported during short-term treatment with the drug, the most frequently reported being gastrointestinal in nature (e.g. flatulence, nausea, abdominal pain and vomiting). It is worthwhile to emphasize that the detection of GI adverse reactions could have been difficult in rifaximin trials since the symptoms of the underlying diseases were often similar to the GI complaints observed after drug treatment.

The safety of rifaximin, taken 200 mg three times daily, was evaluated more recently in 320 patients from two placebo-controlled clinical trials [31].

---

[1] Animal reproduction studies have shown an adverse effect on the fetus and there are no adequate and well-controlled studies in humans, but potential benefits may warrant use of the drug in pregnant women despite potential risks.

Table 5. Adverse events with an incidence ≥2% among patients with TD receiving rifaximin (600 mg daily) or placebo in placebo-controlled trials (from Rifaximin FDA label [31])

Symptoms (MedDRA-preferred term)	Percentage of patients	
	Rifaximin 600 mg/day (n = 320)	Placebo (n = 228)
Flatulence	11 ← p = 0.0071 →	20
Headache	10	9
Abdominal pain	7	10
Rectal tenesmus	7	9
Defecation urgency	6	9
Nausea	5	8
Constipation	4	4
Pyrexia	3	4
Vomiting	2	2

MedDRA = Medical Dictionary for Regulatory Activities.

All the adverse events for either rifaximin or placebo that occurred at a frequency ≥2% are shown in table 5. With the exception of flatulence, which was significantly ($p = 0.0071$) less after drug treatment, the adverse event profile of rifaximin overlapped that of placebo. When the drug was given to *healthy* students traveling to Mexico in order to prevent the occurrence of TD [98], the incidence of adverse events was remarkably low, again overlapping those observed with placebo (table 6). These findings confirm that the GI complaints observed after drug treatment in therapeutic trials did represent symptoms of the underlying disease (i.e. TD) rather than being rifaximin-related.

Prolonged therapy with high doses of the antibiotic has been associated with infrequent urticarial skin reactions [34]. A significant increase in serum potassium and sodium concentrations, although within the physiological range, has been observed after the drug. Since rifaximin was employed mainly for the treatment of diarrheal diseases, this finding could likely be connected to the electrolyte disturbances of underlying conditions.

Post-Marketing Surveillance

The excellent safety profile observed in clinical trials has been confirmed by the post-marketing surveillance program [92]. More than 8.5 million patients have been treated in Italy and abroad with rifaximin since its introduction in

Table 6. Reported signs and symptoms not associated with TD that occurred over a 2-week treatment with rifaximin in healthy subjects and were considered possible adverse events (from DuPont et al. [98])

Symptom	Study group			
	Rifaximin, once daily (n = 50), %	Rifaximin, twice daily (n = 52), %	Rifaximin, 3 times daily (n = 54), %	Placebo (n = 54), %
Headache	6 (12.00)	0	0	1 (1.85)
Migraine	0	0	0	1 (1.85)
Dizziness	0	0	1 (1.85)	0
Body aches	0	0	1 (1.85)	0
Sore throat	2 (4.00)	0	0	0
Keratitis from foreign body	1 (2.00)	0	0	0
Fever (subjective)	0	0	2 (3.70)	0
Runny nose	1 (2.00)	0	0	0
Congestion	0	3 (5.77)	0	0
Heartburn	0	0	0	1 (1.85)
Constipation	0	0	1 (1.85)	0
Increase in leukocyte count	4 (8.00)	2 (3.85)	2 (3.70)	3 (5.56)
Increase in serum aminotransferase level[1]	5 (10.00)	11 (21.15)	6 (11.11)	10 (18.52)

Each rifaximin dose was 200 mg.
[1]Normal value <35 U/I (abnormal values identified as 36–70 U/I).

the market. During the overall post-marketing period, 26 adverse reactions (17 patients' cases) were reported to the manufacturer, of which only 4 were judged to be serious. They consisted in 1 case of angioneurotic edema, 1 of cutaneous rash and 2 of urticaria.

In summary, rifaximin appears to be extremely safe with a very favorable risk-to-benefit ratio.

Summary and Conclusions

Rifaximin was first described in 1982 and was introduced into the Italian market 5 years later. Taking into account its excellent activity against a broad range of enteropathogens, the first 'logical' indication for this GI-targeted antibiotic was the treatment of infectious diarrhea in both adults and children. However, the appreciation of the pathogenic role of gut bacteria in several organic and functional GI diseases [28, 29] has increasingly broadened its clinical use.

Table 7. Main pharmacokinetic and pharmacodynamic differences between poorly absorbed antibiotics: rifaximin vs. aminoglycosides

	Aminoglycosides	Rifaximin
Systemic absorption	3–5%	<1%
Untoward effects	Oto- or nephrotoxicity	Absent
Activity against Gram-positive bacteria	++	+++
Activity against anaerobic bacteria	0	+++
Resistance (type/frequency)	Plasmidic/high	Chromosomic/low

A careful review of its pharmacokinetic and antimicrobial properties reveals that rifaximin displays some distinct advantages, either in terms of safety and efficacy, over aminoglycosides currently used as poorly absorbed antibiotics (table 7). Being virtually unabsorbed, this antimicrobial has little value outside the area of enteric infections, thus minimizing both antimicrobial resistance and systemic adverse events. It proved to be safe in all patient populations, including young children. Although pregnant women were purportedly excluded from controlled trials, clinical experience does suggest that the use of a non-absorbable antibiotic, when strictly needed, represents the safest choice in this physiological condition. In this connection, it was shown that treatment with oral neomycin, a poorly absorbed aminoglucoside, during pregnancy presents no detectable teratogenic risk to the human fetus [108]. Rifaximin therefore possesses almost all the characteristics of the 'ideal' antibiotic targeted at the GI tract [109].

As shown in table 4, there are established and potential clinical indications for this peculiar drug. In all these conditions, many of which share SIBO as a common feature, gut bacteria represent the specific target of rifaximin. The drug can be used alone (like, for instance, in the treatment of infectious diarrhea) or as an add-on medication (as in the management of IBD) and given short term (single course of treatment) or long term (repeated courses of therapy, i.e. cyclically).

Although rifaximin has stood the test of time, it still attracts the attention of both basic scientists and clinicians as attested by the regular number of publications which appear every year in the medical literature [34]. As a matter of fact, with the advancement of the knowledge on microbial-gut interactions in health and disease, novel indications and new drug regimens are being explored. All this ongoing research clearly indicates that the final chapter on this interesting antibiotic has not yet been written.

References

1 WHO Progress Report 2002: Global defence against the infectious disease threat. http://www.who.int/infectious-disease-news/cds 2002/index.html

2 CDC's Global Infectious Disease Strategy: Protecting the Nation's health in an era of globalization. http://www.cdc.gov/globalidplan/ request.htm

3 Procop GW: Gastrointestinal infections. Infect Dis Clin North Am 2001;15:1073–1108.

4 Pithie AD, Ellis CJ: Review article: antibiotics and the gut. Aliment Pharmacol Ther 1989;3: 321–332.

5 Li E, Stanley SL Jr: The role of newer antibiotics in gastroenterology. Gastroenterol Clin North Am 1992;21:613–629.

6 Renner F, Mittermayer H, Hafner M, Schofl R: Prophylaxis with antibiotics in gastrointestinal endoscopy. Z Gastroenterol 2002;40: 1–7.

7 Guerrant RL, Van Gilder T, Steiner TS, Thielman NM, Slutsker L, Tauxe RV, Hennessy T, Griffin PM, DuPont H, Sack RB, Tarr P, Neill M, Nachamkin I, Reller LB, Osterholm MT, Bennish ML, Pickering LK: Infectious Diseases Society of America: practice guidelines for the management of infectious diarrhea. Clin Infect Dis 2001;32:331–350.

8 Pickering LK, Cleary TG: Therapy for diarrheal illness in children; in Blaser MJ, Smith PD, Ravdin JI, Greenburg HB, Guerrant RL (eds): Infections of the Gastrointestinal Tract, ed 2. New York, Raven Press, 2002, pp 1223–1240.

9 Pickering LK: Limitations of antimicrobial therapy for enteric infections. Clin Update Infect Dis 2003;6(3). http://www.nfid.org/publications/clinicalupdates/id/

10 Norrby SR: Principles for targeted antibiotic use in urinary tract and enteric infections: a review with special emphasis on norfloxacin. Scand J Infect Dis 1986;18(suppl 48):7–19.

11 Van den Hazel SJ, Speelman P, Tytgat GNJ, Dankert J, Van Leeuwen DJ: Role of antibiotics in the treatment and prevention of acute and recurrent cholangitis. Clin Infect Dis 1994;19:279–286.

12 DuPont HL: Community-acquired diarrheal disease in western countries: applications of nonabsorbable oral antibiotic therapy. Adv Stud Med 2003;3(suppl A):S945–S950.

13 Cheung RP, DiPiro JT: Vancomycin: an update. Pharmacotherapy 1986;6:153–169.

14 Brogden RN, Peters DH: Teicoplanin. A reappraisal of its antimicrobial activity, pharmacokinetic properties and therapeutic efficacy. Drugs 1994;47:823–854.

15 Toscano WA Jr, Storm DR: Bacitracin. Pharmacol Ther 1982;16:199–210.

16 Zimmerman MJ, Bak A, Sutherland LR: Review article: treatment of *Clostridium difficile* infection. Aliment Pharmacol Ther 1997;11:1003–1012.

17 Surawicz CM, McFarland LV: Pseudomembranous colitis: causes and cures. Digestion 1999;60: 91–100.

18 Poutanen SM, Simor AE: *Clostridium difficile*-associated diarrhea in adults. CMAJ 2004;171: 51–58.

19 McCafferty DG, Cudic P, Frankel BA, Barkallah S, Kruger RG, Li W: Chemistry and biology of the ramoplanin family of peptide antibiotics. Biopolymers 2002;66:261–284.

20 Anonymous: Ramoplanin. A 16686, a 16686a, MDL 62198. Drugs R&D 2002;3:61–64.

21 Montecalvo MA: Ramoplanin: a novel antimicrobial agent with the potential to prevent vancomycin-resistant enterococcal infection in high-risk patients. J Antimicrob Chemother 2003; 51(suppl 3):31–35.

22 Simon HJ: Streptomycin, kanamycin, neomycin and paromomycin. Pediatr Clin North Am 1968;15:73–83.

23 Wright GD, Berghuis AM, Mobashery S: Aminoglycoside antibiotics. Structures, functions, and resistance. Adv Exp Med Biol 1998;456:27–69.

24 Berk DP, Chalmers T: Deafness complicating antibiotic therapy of hepatic encephalopathy. Ann Intern Med 1970;73:393–396.

25 Lerner SA, Matz GJ: Aminoglycoside ototoxicity. Am J Otolaryngol 1980;1:169–179.

26 Kavanagh KT, McCabe BF: Ototoxicity of oral neomycin and vancomycin. Laryngoscope 1983;93:649–653.

27 Appel GB, Neu HC: The nephrotoxicity of antimicrobial agents. 2. N Engl J Med 1977;296: 722–728.

28 Kunin CM, Chalmers TC, Leevy CM, Sebastyen SC, Lieber CS, Finland M: Absorption of orally administered neomycin and kanamycin with special reference to patients with severe hepatic and renal disease. N Engl J Med 1960;262:380–385.

29 Stockwell M: Gentamicin ear drops and ototoxicity: update. CMAJ 2001;164:93–94.

30 Marchi E, Montecchi L, Venturini AP, Mascellani G, Brufani M, Cellai L: 4-Deoxypyrido [1′,2′:1,2]imidazo[5,4-c]rifamycin SV derivatives. A new series of semisynthetic rifamycins with high antibacterial activity and low gastroenteric absorption. J Med Chem 1985;28:960–963.

31 Rifaximin label approved on 05/25/2004. http://www.fda.gov/cder/foi/label/2004/21361_ xifaxan_lbl.pdf

32 Jiang ZD, Ke S, Palazzini E, Riopel L, Dupont H: In vitro activity and fecal concentration of rifaximin after oral administration. Antimicrob Agents Chemother 2000;44:2205–2206.

33 Jiang ZD, DuPont HL: Rifaximin: in vitro and in vivo antibacterial activity. A review. Chemotherapy 2005;51(suppl 1):67–72.

34 Scarpignato C, Pelosini I: Rifaximin, a poorly absorbed antibiotic: pharmacology and clinical potential. Chemotherapy 2005;51(suppl):36–66.

35 Ericsson CD, DuPont HL: Rifaximin in the treatment of infectious diarrhea. Chemotherapy 2005;51(suppl 1):73–80.

36 Gerard L, Garey KW, DuPont HL: Rifaximin: a nonabsorbable rifamycin antibiotic for use in nonsystemic gastrointestinal infections. Expert Rev Anti Infect Ther 2005;3:201–211.

37 Baker DE: Rifaximin: a nonabsorbed oral antibiotic. Rev Gastroenterol Disord 2005;5:19–30.

38 Huang DB, DuPont HL: Rifaximin – a novel antimicrobial for enteric infections. J Infect 2005;50: 97–106.

39 Al-Abri SS, Beeching NJ, Nye FJ: Traveller's diarrhoea. Lancet Infect Dis 2005;5:349–360.

40 Robins GW, Wellington K: Rifaximin. A review of its use in the management of traveller's diarrhoea. Drugs 2005;65:1697–1713.

41 DuPont HL: New antibacterial agents in the management of acute infectious diarrhea. Clin Update in Infect Dis 2004;7(2). http://www.nfid.org/publications/clinicalupdates/id/

42 Lamanna A, Orsi A: In vitro activity of rifaximin and rifampicin against some anaerobic bacteria. Chemioterapia (Florence) 1984;3:365–367.

43 Ripa S, Mignini F, Prenna M, Falcioni E: In vitro antibacterial activity of rifaximin against Clostridium difficile, Campylobacter jejunii and Yersinia spp. Drugs Exp Clin Res 1987;13: 483–488.

44 Marchese A, Salerno A, Pesce A, Debbia EA, Schito GC: In vitro activity of rifaximin, metronidazole and vancomycin against Clostridium difficile and the rate of selection of spontaneously resistant mutants against representative anaerobic and aerobic bacteria, including ammonia-producing species. Chemotherapy 2000;46:253–266.

45 Mégraud F, Bouffant F, Camou JC: In vitro activity of rifaximin against Helicobacter pylori. Eur J Clin Microbiol Infect Dis 1994;13:184–186.

46 Holton J, Vaira D, Menegatti M, Barbara L: The susceptibility of Helicobacter pylori to the rifamycin, rifaximin. J Antimicrob Chemother 1995;35:545–549.

47 Quesada M, Sanfeliu I, Junquera F, Segura F, Calvet X: Evaluation of Helicobacter pylori susceptibility to rifaximin (in Spanish). Gastroenterol Hepatol 2004;27:393–396.

48 Scrascia M, Forcillo M, Maimone F, Pazzani C: Susceptibility to rifaximin of Vibrio cholerae strains from different geographical areas. J Antimicrob Chemother 2003;52:303–305.

49 Amenta M, Dalle Nogare ER, Colomba C, Prestileo TS, Di Lorenzo F, Fundaro S, Colomba A, Ferrieri A: Intestinal protozoa in HIV-infected patients: effect of rifaximin in Cryptosporidium parvum and Blastocystis hominis infections. J Chemother 1999;11:391–395.

50 Steffen R, Sack DA, Riopel L, Jiang ZD, Sturchler M, Ericsson CD, Lowe B, Waiyaki P, White M, DuPont HL: Therapy of travelers' diarrhea with rifaximin on various continents. Am J Gastroenterol 2003;98:1073–1078.

51 Burman WJ, Gallicano K, Peloquin C: Comparative pharmacokinetics and pharmacodynamics of the rifamycin antibiotics. Clin Pharmacokinet 2001;40:327–341.

52 Lancini GC, Sartori G: Rifamycins LXI: in vivo inhibition of RNA synthesis of rifamycins. Experientia 1968;24:1105–1106.

53 Dayan AD: Rifaximin (Normix®) Preclinical Expert Report. London 1997.

54 Umezawa H, Mizuno S, Yamazaki H, Nitta K: Inhibition of DNA-dependent RNA synthesis by rifamycins. J Antibiot (Tokyo) 1968;21:234–236.

55 Artsimovitch I, Vassylyeva MN, Svetlov D, Svetlov V, Perederina A, Igarashi N, Matsugaki N, Wakatsuki S, Tahirov TH, Vassylyev DG: Allosteric modulation of the RNA polymerase catalytic reaction is an essential component of transcription control by rifamycins. Cell 2005;122: 351–363.

56 Al-Orainey IO: Drug resistance in tuberculosis. J Chemother 1990;2:147–151.

57 Spratt BG: Resistance to antibiotics mediated by target alterations. Science 1994;264:388–393.

58 Smith CA, Baker EN: Aminoglycoside antibiotic resistance by enzymatic deactivation. Curr Drug Targets Infect Disord 2002;2:143–160.

59 Collignon PJ: Antibiotic resistance. MJA 2002;177:325–329.

60 Hoover WW, Gerlach EH, Hoban DJ, Eliopoulos GM, Pfaller MA, Jones RN: Antimicrobial activity and spectrum of rifaximin, a new topical rifamycin derivative. Diagn Microbiol Infect Dis 1993;16:111–118.

61 Hart AL, Stagg AJ, Frame M, Graffner H, Glise H, Falk P, Kamm MA: Review article: the role of the gut flora in health and disease, and its modification as therapy. Aliment Pharmacol Ther 2002;16:1383–1393.

62 Guarner F, Malagelada JR: Gut flora in health and disease. Lancet 2003;361:512–519.

63 Testa R, Eftimiadi C, Sukkar GS, De Leo C, Rovida S, Schito GC, Celle G: A non-absorbable rifamycin for treatment of hepatic encephalopathy. Drugs Exp Clin Res 1985;11: 387–392.

64 Lacour M, Zunder T, Huber R, Sander A, Daschner F, Frank U: The pathogenetic significance of intestinal *Candida* colonization – A systematic review from an interdisciplinary and environmental medical point of view. Int J Hyg Environ Health 2002;205:257–268.

65 De Leo C, Eftimiadi C, Schito GC: Rapid disappearance from the intestinal tract of bacteria resistant to rifaximin. Drugs Exp Clin Res 1986;12:979–981.

66 Gillespie SH: Evolution of drug resistance in *Mycobacterium tuberculosis*: clinical and molecular perspective. Antimicrob Agents Chemother 2002;46:267–274.

67 Kapusnik JE, Parenti F, Sande MA: The use of rifampicin in staphylococcal infections – a review. J Antimicrob Chemother 1984;13(suppl C):61–66.

68 Frieden TR, Sterling TR, Munsiff SS, Watt CJ, Dye C: Tuberculosis. Lancet 2003;362:887–899.

69 Zeneroli ML, Avallone R, Corsi L, Venturini I, Baraldi C, Baraldi M: Management of hepatic encephalopathy: role of rifaximin. Chemotherapy 2005;51(suppl 1):90–95.

70 Papi C, Koch M, Capurso L: Management of diverticular disease: is there room for rifaximin? Chemotherapy 2005;51(suppl 1):110–114.

71 DuPont HL, Jiang ZD: Influence of rifaximin treatment on the susceptibility of intestinal Gram-negative flora and enterococci. Clin Microbiol Infect 2004;10:1009–1011.

72 Venturini AP: Pharmacokinetics of L/105, a new rifamycin, in rats and dogs, after oral administration. Chemotherapy (Basel) 1983;29:1–3.

73 Venturini AP: L/105: report on pharmacokinetics in rats, dogs after oral administration and adverse reactions. Chemioterapia (Florence) 1983;2(suppl 5):162–163.

74 Cellai L, Colosimo M, Marchi E, Venturini AP, Zanolo G: Rifaximin (L/105), a new topical intestinal antibiotic: pharmacokinetic study after single oral administration of ^{3}H-rifaximin to rats. Chemioterapia (Florence) 1984;3:373–377.

75 Breen KJ, Bryant RE, Levinson JD, Schemker S: Neomycin absorption in man: studies of oral and enema administration and effect of intestinal ulceration. Ann Intern Med 1972;76:211–218.

76 Venturini AP: Gastrointestinal absorption of rifaximin (L/105) in experimentally-induced colitis in the rat (in Italian). Riv Tossicol Sper Clin (Rome) 1986;16:119A.

77 Descombe JJ, Dubourg D, Picard M, Palazzini E: Pharmacokinetic study of rifaximin after oral administration in healthy volunteers. Int J Clin Pharmacol Res 1994;14:51–56.

78 Rizzello F, Gionchetti P, Venturi A, Ferretti M, Peruzzo S, Raspanti X, Picard M, Canova N, Palazzini E, Campieri M: Rifaximin systemic absorption in patients with ulcerative colitis. Eur J Clin Pharmacol 1998;54:91–93.

79 Gionchetti P, Rizzello F, Ferrieri A, Venturi A, Brignola C, Ferretti M, Peruzzo S, Miglioli M, Campieri M: Rifaximin in patients with moderate or severe ulcerative colitis refractory to steroid-treatment: a double-blind, placebo-controlled trial. Dig Dis Sci 1999;44:1220–1221.

80   Gionchetti P, Rizzello F, Venturi A, Ugolini F, Rossi M, Brigidi P, Johansson R, Ferrieri A, Poggioli G, Campieri M: Antibiotic combination therapy in patients with chronic, treatment-resistant pouchitis. Aliment Pharmacol Ther 1999;13:713–718.

81   Williams R, James OF, Warnes TW, Morgan MY: Evaluation of the efficacy and safety of rifaximin in the treatment of hepatic encephalopathy: a double-blind, randomized, dosefinding multi-centre study. Eur J Gastroenterol Hepatol 2000;12:203–208.

82   Williams R, Bass N: Rifaximin, a nonabsorbed oral antibiotic, in the treatment of hepatic encephalopathy: antimicrobial activity, efficacy, and safety. Rev Gastroenterol Disord 2005; 5(suppl 1):10–18.

83   Gillum JG, Israel DS, Polk RE: Pharmacokinetic drug interactions with antimicrobial agents. Clin Pharmacokinet 1993;25:450–482.

84   Fry RF: Probing the world of cytochrome P_{450} enzymes. Mol Interv 2004;4:157–162.

85   Dickinson BD, Altman RD, Nielsen NH, Sterling ML, Council on Scientific Affairs, American Medical Association: Drug interactions between oral contraceptives and antibiotics. Obstet Gynecol 2001;98:853–860.

86   King A, Marshall O, Connolly M, Kamm A, Boxenbaum H, Kastrissios H, Trapnell C: The effect of rifaximin on the pharmacokinetics of a single dose of ethinyl estardiol and norgestimate in healthy female volunteers. Clin Pharmacol Ther 2004;75:P96.

87   Yuan R, Flockhart DA, Balian JD: Pharmacokinetic and pharmacodynamic consequences of metabolism-based drug interactions with alprazolam, midazolam, and triazolam. J Clin Pharmacol 1999;39:1109–1125.

88   King A, Laurie R, Connolly M, Kamm A, Boxenbaum H, Kastrissios H, Trapnell C: The effect of rifaximin on the pharmacokinetics of single doses of intravenous and oral midazolam in healthy volunteers. Clin Pharmacol Ther 2004;75:P66.

89   Husebye E: The pathogenesis of gastrointestinal bacterial overgrowth. Chemotherapy 2005; 51(suppl 1):1–22.

90   Cuoco L, Montalto M, Jorizzo RA, Santarelli L, Arancio F, Cammarota G, Gasbarrini G: Eradication of small intestinal bacterial overgrowth and orocecal transit in diabetics. Hepatogastroenterology 2002;49:1582–1586.

91   Tursi A, Brandimarte G, Giorgetti G, Nasi G: Assessment of orocaecal transit time in different localization of Crohn's disease and its possible influence on clinical response to therapy. Eur J Gastroenterol Hepatol 2003;15:69–74.

92   Palazzini E: Periodic Safety Update Report for Rixamin (January 1987–December 2003). Bologna, Alfa Wassermann, 2004.

93   Spisani S, Traniello S, Martuccio C, Rizzuti O, Cellai L: Rifamycins inhibit human neutrophil functions: new derivatives with potential anti-inflammatory activity. Inflammation 1997;21:391–400.

94   Spisani S, Traniello S, Onori AM, Rizzuti O, Martuccio C, Cellai L: 3-(Carboxyalkylthio)rifamycin S and SV derivatives inhibit human neutrophil functions. Infl ammation 1998;22:459–469.

95   Caruso I: Twenty years of experience with intra-articular rifamycin for chronic arthritides. J Int Med Res 1997;25:307–317.

96   Caruso I, Cazzola M, Santandrea S: Clinical improvement in ankylosing spondylitis with rifamycin SV infiltrations of peripheral joints. J Int Med Res 1992;20:171–181.

97   Taylor DN, MacKenzie R, Durbin A, Carpenter C, Atzinger CB, Haake R, Bourgeois AL: Double-blind, placebo-controlled trial to evaluate the use of rifaximin (200 mg tid) to prevent diarrhea in volunteers challenged with *Shigella flexneri* 2a (2457T). Am J Trop Med Hyg 2004;71(suppl 4): 1–303, abstr 2079.

98   DuPont HL, Jiang ZD, Okhuysen PC, Ericsson CD, de la Cabada FJ, Ke S, DuPont MW, Martinez-Sandoval F: A randomized, double-blind, placebo-controlled trial of rifaximin to prevent travelers' diarrhea. Ann Intern Med 2005;142:805–812.

99   Venturini AP, Bertoli D, Marchi E: Transcutaneous absorption of a topical rifamycin preparation: rifaximin (L/105). Drugs Exp Clin Res 1987;13:231–232.

100 Berlo JA, Debruyne HJ, Gortz JP: A prospective study in healthy volunteers of the topical absorption of a 5% rifaximin cream. Drugs Exp Clin Res 1994;20:205–208.

101 Pelosini I, Scarpignato C: Rifaximin, a peculiar rifamycin derivative: clinical use outside the gastrointestinal tract. Chemotherapy 2005;51(suppl 1):122–130.

102 Prasad ES, Wenman WM: In vitro activity of rifaximin, a topical rifamycin derivative, against *Chlamydia trachomatis*. Diagn Microbiol Infect Dis 1993;16:135–136.

103 Di Stefano M, Corazza GR: Treatment of small intestinal bacterial overgrowth and related symptoms by rifaximin. Chemotherapy 2005;51(suppl 1):103–109.

104 Gionchetti P, Rizzello F, Morselli C, Romagnoli R, Campieri M: Inflammatory bowel disease: does rifaximin offer any promise? Chemotherapy 2005;51(suppl 1):96–102.

105 Physicians' Desk Reference: Use-in-Pregnancy Ratings, ed 58. Montvale, Medical Economics Co, 2004.

106 Czeizel AE, Rockenbauer M, Olsen J, Sorensen HT: A population-based case-control study of the safety of oral anti-tuberculosis drug treatment during pregnancy. Int J Tuberc Lung Dis 2001;5:564–568.

107 Ito S, Lee A: Drug excretion into breast milk – overview. Adv Drug Deliv Rev 2003;55: 617–627.

108 Czeizel AE, Rockenbauer M, Olsen J, Sorensen HT: A teratological study of aminoglycoside antibiotic treatment during pregnancy. Scand J Infect Dis 2000;32:309–313.

109 DuPont HL, Ericsson CD: Prevention and treatment of traveler's diarrhea. N Engl J Med 1993;328:1821–1827.

Note Added in Proof

A recent prospective open label study [1] did confirm the effectiveness of rifaximin in controlling cryptosporidial diarrhea in patients with AIDS. The administration of this rifamycin derivative (400 mg b.i.d.) was associated with a rapid (within 1 week) and durable symptomatic control and eradication of the microorganism despite profound immunosuppression (CD4 count $<50/mm^3$) in the majority of patients. In addition, an interesting case report [2] de-scribed long-lasting albeit intermittent abdominal pain and diarrhea in a patient with kidney-pancreas transplant on immuno-suppressive therapy, which proved to be due to *Cryptosporidium parvum* infection. After the diagnosis, high dose (600 mg thrice daily) rifaximin treatment achieved complete symptom resolution within 1 week.

Recent in vitro [3] and in vivo [4] studies, presented at the last *Annual Interscience Conference on Antimicrobial Agents and Chemotherapy* in Washington, D.C., did confirm the activity of rifaximin against *C. difficile*. In an experimental model of *C. difficile*-associated diarrhea (CDAD) [4] the efficacy of the rifamycin derivative was comparable to that of vancomycin. However, after stopping antibiotic treatment, 75% of the vancomycin-treated animals developed recurrent infection while none of the rifaximin-treated ones relapsed. These results suggest that rifaximin may be superior to vancomycin for the eradication of *C. difficile* infection. Since recurrent CDAD is a common clinical problem, specifically designed clinical trials are worthwhile to confirm this hypothesis.

References

1   Gathe J, Smith K, Mayberry C, Clemmons J, Nemecek J: Cure of severe cryptosporidial diarrhea with rifaximin in patients with AIDS; in Abstract Book of the 10th European AIDS Conference/ (EACS), Dublin, November 17–20, 2005, abstract #A-007-0087-00253.
2   Burdese M, Veglio V, Consiglio V, Soragna G, Mezza E, Bergamo D, Tattoli F, Rossetti M, Jeantet A, Segoloni GP, Piccoli GB: A dance teacher with kidney-pancreas transplant and diarrhoea: what is the cause? Nephrol Dial Transplant 2005;20:1759–1761.
3   Gerding DN, Johnson S, Osmolski JR, Sambol SP, Hecht DW: In vitro activity of ramoplanin, rifalazil, rifaximin, metronidazole, and vancomycin against 110 unique toxigenic *Clostridium difficile* clinical isolates; in Abstracts presented at 45th Annual Interscience Conference on Antimicrobial Agents and Chemotherapy, Washington, DC, December 16–19, 2005 [http://www. abstractsonline. com/viewer/?mkey= %7B932BDC66%2D9511%2D42FD%2DA9D5%2DB 222E1D5236 B%7D%20].
4   Kokkotou E, Mustafa N, O'Brien M, Pothoulakis C, Kelly CP: Rifaximin: a novel nonabsorbed antibiotic therapy for *Clostridium difficile*-associated diarrhea (CDAD); in Abstracts presented at 45th Annual Interscience Conference on Antimicrobial Agents and Chemotherapy, Washington, DC, December 16–19, 2005 [http://www.abstractsonline. com/viewer/?mkey =%7B932BDC66% 2D9511%2D42FD%2DA9D5%2DB222E1D5236B%7D%20].

Prof. Carmelo Scarpignato, MD, DSc, PharmD, FRCP, FCP, FACG
Laboratory of Clinical Pharmacology, School of Medicine and Dentistry
University of Parma, Via Volturno, 39 IT–43100 Parma (Italy)
Tel. +39 0521 903 863, eFax +1 603 843 5621, E-Mail scarpi@tin.it

This chapter should be cited as follows:

Scarpignato C, Pelosini I: Experimental and Clinical Pharmacology of Rifaximin, a Gastrointestinal Selective Antibiotic. Digestion 2006;73(suppl 1):13–27.

Scarpignato C, Lanas Á (eds): Bacterial Flora in Digestive Disease.
Focus on Rifaximin.

....

Pharmacological Treatment of the Irritable Bowel Syndrome and Other Functional Bowel Disorders

Fermín Mearin

Institute of Functional and Motor Digestive Disorders, Centro Médico Teknon,
Barcelona, Spain

Abstract

Functional digestive disorders constitute one of the main causes of consultation in gastroenterology and primary health care. Is still unclear whether therapy has to be aimed to the gut, to the neural pathways controlling bowel motility and perception, or to the processing mechanisms of symptoms and disease behaviour. It is conceivable that in the next future better understanding of functional bowel disorders pathophysiology will help us to tailor treatment for different patients. At the moment, subclassification of the diverse patterns of symptomatology allows to adjust new treatments for irritable bowel syndrome (IBS) according to the clinical predominance for each patient. The knowledge of motor and sensorial response to different stimuli in IBS patients and the pathways to the central nervous system is an important source of information for the development of new molecules. Fiber-enriched diet is frequently given for constipation-predominant IBS. Loperamide, antispasmodic drugs and tricyclic antidepressants are nowadays the basis for pharmacological treatment of diarrhea-predominant IBS. The scientific evidence supporting this therapeutical approach is however limited. Visceral analgesics and serotonin agonists and antagonists may play an important therapeutical role in the near future. However, it is not likely that one single treatment will help every functional bowel disorder patient and many of them will need a more complex approach with a multidisciplinary therapy (diet, psychotherapy, medications).

Magnitude of the Problem: How Relevant Are Functional Digestive Disorders?

Functional digestive disorders globally constitute one of the main causes of consultation in gastroenterology and primary health care. In fact, patients with the two most frequent functional disorders – irritable bowel syndrome (IBS) and functional dyspepsia – account for 35% of all gastroenterological visits according to Spanish data [1]. These diseases also represent an important percentage of consultations in primary care (approx. 5% of all visits) [2, 3]. This large number of patients implies important direct and indirect economical costs [4]; it has been calculated that in the eight most industrialized countries, functional digestive disorders generate a total cost of over 40 billion US dollars [5]. In addition to this important sociosanitary impact, functional digestive disorders also cause notorious deterioration in patient health-related quality of life [6].

The diagnosis of functional digestive disorders is clinical, and has been based fundamentally on exclusion criteria. More recently, in an attempt to unify the clinical diagnosis of functional digestive disorders, a series of criteria have been developed, grouping the different symptoms, with the purpose of establishing a definitive positive diagnosis of these disorders. Several clinical diagnostic criteria have been developed, the most widely used being Manning criteria [7] , Rome I criteria and Rome II criteria [8]. The diagnostic criteria currently used since 1999 are referred to as the Rome II criteria [9, 10].

The prevalence of functional digestive disorders is high all over the world. More than 10 years ago, Drossman et al. [11] evaluated the prevalence of functional gastrointestinal disorders in the US householder population. They assessed the prevalence of 20 functional gastrointestinal syndromes based on fulfilment of Rome I criteria. For this sample, 69% reported having at least one of 20 functional gastrointestinal syndromes in the previous 3 months. The symptoms were attributed to four major anatomic regions: oesophageal (42%), gastroduodenal (26%), bowel (44%), and anorectal (26%), with considerable overlap. More recently, in a random sample of subjects representative of the Australian population, the prevalence of any functional gastrointestinal disorder was 34.6%, and there was considerable overlap among different ones (19.2% had more than two disorders) [12].

By applying the Rome I and Rome II diagnostic criteria and analyzing the studies conducted in western countries in the general population, the prevalence of IBS is seen to vary between 3.3 and 13.6% [13–16]. Functional abdominal bloating occurs in approximately 15% of community-based populations [11, 17], and appears to be more frequent in females than males. Functional constipation and functional diarrhea prevalences in the general population are about 20 and 4%, respectively [11, 18–20].

Estimated IBS prevalence depends very much on the diagnostic criteria applied to define the syndrome [14] (fig. 1). It has been observed that Rome II criteria are too restrictive in clinical practice though useful to select patients for clinical trials. In our own experience, more than two thirds of subjects meeting

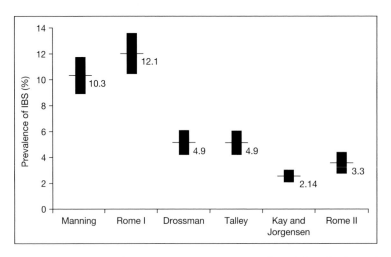

Fig. 1. IBS prevalence varies enormously depending of the criteria employed for diagnosis (from Mearin et al. [14]).

Manning or Rome I criteria would not be diagnosed as having IBS if Rome II criteria were employed [14].

Patients with functional digestive disorders frequently have some other co-morbid conditions. Thus, many IBS suffers also have heartburn and other upper gastrointestinal symptoms, fibromyalgia, headache, backache, genitourinary symptoms, and psychosocial dysfunction. Some authors have hypothesized that multiple co-morbid disorders are associated with psychological factors [21]. Moreover, incorrect diagnosis can result in hospitalization and surgery, especially cholecystectomy, appendectomy and hysterectomy [22].

Definition of the Problem: How to Identify Functional Bowel Disorder?

A functional bowel disorder (FBD) is a functional gastrointestinal disorder with symptoms attributable to the mid or lower gastrointestinal tract. FBDs include the IBS, functional abdominal bloating, functional constipation, functional diarrhea and unspecified FBD [7]. Subjects with FBD may be divided into the following groups: (1) *non-patients*: those who have never sought health care for the FBD, and (2) *patients*: those who have sought health care for the FBD.

According to Rome II criteria, and having in mind the absence of structural or metabolic abnormalities to explain the symptoms, FBDs are defined as follows:

Irritable Bowel Syndrome. Twelve or more weeks (not necessarily consecutive) in the past 12 months of abdominal discomfort or pain that has two out of three features: (a) relieved with defecation; (b) onset associated with a change in frequency of stool, and (c) onset associated with a change in form (appearance) of stool.

Some other symptoms, not essential for the diagnosis, are usually present and may be helpful be to identify sub-types of IBS according to bowel habit: (1) fewer than three bowel movements a week; (2) more than three bowel movements a day; (3) hard or lumpy stools; (4) loose (mushy) or watery stools; (5) straining during a bowel movement; (6) urgency; (7) feeling of incomplete bowel movement; (8) passing mucus during a bowel movement; (9) abdominal fullness, bloating, or swelling. A given subject is considered to have diarrhea-predominant IBS subtype if one or more of 2, 4, or 6 are present and none of 1, 3, or 5. Constipation-predominant IBS subtype is established if one or more of 1, 3, or 5 were present and none of 2, 4, or 6. Alternating IBS subtype is defined as the presence in the same patient of at least one diarrhea criterion and one constipation criterion [23].

Functional Abdominal Bloating. It comprises a group of FBDs which are dominated by a feeling of abdominal fullness or bloating, without sufficient criteria for another functional gastrointestinal disorder. Diagnosis of functional abdominal bloating requires the presence during 12 or more weeks in the past 12 months of: (1) feeling of abdominal fullness, bloating, or visible distension, and (2) insufficient criteria for a diagnosis of functional dyspepsia, IBS or other functional disorder.

Functional Constipation. It comprises a group of functional disorders which present as persistent difficult, infrequent or seemingly incomplete defecation. For diagnosis it is required to have been present during 12 or more weeks in the past 12 months of two or more of: (1) straining $>1/4$ of defecations; (2) lumpy or hard stools $>1/4$ of defecations; (3) sensation of incomplete evacuation $>1/4$ of defecations; (4) sensation of anorectal obstruction/blockage $>1/4$ of defecations; (5) manual manoeuvres to facilitate $>1/4$ of defecations (e.g. digital evacuation, support of the pelvic floor), and (6) <3 defecations per week. In addition, loose stools have not to be present, and criteria for IBS not to be fulfil.

Functional Diarrhea. It is defined as continuous or recurrent passage of loose (mushy) or watery stools without abdominal pain. Diagnosis requires 12 or more weeks in the past 12 months of: (1) loose (mushy) or watery stools present $>3/4$ of the time, and (2) no abdominal pain.

An unspecified FBD is defined as functional bowel symptoms that do not meet criteria for the previously defined categories.

Towards a Solution of the Problem: Treatment of Functional Bowel Disorder

At the beginning of this century it was thought that there are four main mechanisms implicated in the pathophysiology of FBD: altered intestinal motility, increased visceral sensitivity, disturbed intestinal reflexes (intrinsic and extrinsic), and psychological disorders; digestive infections have also been postulated as putative pathophysiological causes of some FBDs. The predominance and combination of these mechanisms are most probably responsible for the different clinical manifestations of FBD.

Treating Irritable Bowel Syndrome

General Measurements

Explaining the syndrome and reassuring the patient are very important physician's therapeutic tools. Fear of cancer is a major concern in many IBS patients. Therefore, a confident diagnosis is basic to establish a good patient-physician relation. However, repeated or inappropriate tests communicate physician insecurity and breed fear and uncertainty in the patient.

Dietary modifications are frequently recommended as a first step in the management of IBS patients. Avoidance of nutrients that will probably induce symptoms seems to be logical (i.e. voluminous meals, fat, non-absorbable carbohydrates, coffee, tea, lactose); however, there is no scientific evidence supporting this approach, and severe limitations of usual dietary habits may impair even more IBS patients quality of life. Clinical trials evaluating diet modifications have been centred on pain relief and changes of stool characteristics. Most placebo-controlled trials were performed with fiber. A fiber-enriched diet (20–30 g/day) improves constipation, accelerates intestinal transit and may reduce intracolonic pressure. Nevertheless, patients with IBS do not have less fiber intake than asymptomatic control subjects [24]. In addition, clinical trials have not found any significant benefit of a fiber-enriched diet compared to placebo [25]. Moreover, fiber therapy may aggravate IBS symptoms by decreasing pain threshold secondary to distension and by inducing colon distension through gas formation from bacterial fermentation [26]. Therefore, there is no scientific evidence supporting that standard changes of dietary habits or lifestyle improve symptomatology of IBS. Diet with fiber supplementation could improve constipation in constipation-predominant IBS, but the appearance or worsening of symptoms related to gas formation limits the clinical utility of this approach.

A recent systematic review has evaluated the role of different types of fiber in the treatment of IBS [27]. It was concluded that soluble and insoluble fiber have different effects on IBS symptoms: soluble fiber is beneficial to global symptom improvement, though the effect on pain is controversial, whereas insoluble fiber is not more effective than placebo and may, in some patients, worsen symptoms when compared with a normal diet.

Antidiarrheal Drugs

Loperamide is the most widely used drug for diarrhea-predominant IBS. Most of the trials with loperamide on diarrhea-predominant IBS proved a benefit compared to placebo. In a 13-week, double-blind, placebo-controlled trial, loperamide significantly improved stool frequency, consistency and urgency [28]. Another, more recent, double-blind study confirmed these results but also revealed an increase in nocturnal pain in patients treated with loperamide [29]. However, the clinical relevance of both trials is limited by the high proportion of dropouts (19 and 30%, respectively). Thus, scientific evidence of loperamide efficacy for the treatment of IBS is limited and further trials are required.

Antispasmodics

Antispasmodics are frequently used in the management of IBS. Several drugs have been evaluated but most trials underwent strong criticisms because of methodological limitations (i.e., scarce number of patients, large amount of dropouts, short duration of the trials, etc.). In fact, among 36 placebo-controlled, double-blind, randomized clinical trials with antispasmodics lasting for more than 2 weeks, only 15 evaluated pain or general symptomatic improvement as end point. Furthermore, the proportion of dropouts was as high as up to 59%. Nevertheless, among the trials mentioned above, 26 were comparable from a methodological point of view and were included by Poynard et al. [30] in a meta-analysis. As a result of this analysis, antispasmodics resulted to be superior to placebo in terms of global improvement (62 vs. 35%, p < 0.01) and abdominal pain relief (64 vs. 45%, p < 0.01). These positive results were obtained with five different drugs: cimetropium bromide, pinaverium bromide, octylonium bromide, trimebutine and mebeverine [25]. Another meta-analysis, performed some years later also by Poynard et al. [31], again showed smooth muscle relaxants and anticholinergics to be better than placebo for some IBS symptoms (fig. 2). In a systematic review including 13 studies, 7 considered as high-quality trials, it was concluded that antispasmodics were effective for abdominal pain in IBS patients [32].

In conclusion, and bearing in mind some methodological limitations of published clinical trials, the available scientific evidence suggests antispasmodics to be useful in IBS, although new and more conclusive investigations are required. Furthermore, these drugs are not available in every country.

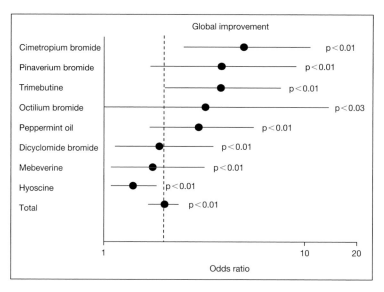

Fig. 2. Meta-analysis of smooth muscle relaxant in the treatment of IBS (from Poynard et al. [31]).

Antidepressants

Tricyclic antidepressants have an analgesic effect that is obtained at lower doses than that required for depression therapy. Best results are obtained in pain relief in diarrhea-predominant IBS. A trial with desipramine demonstrated a significant decrease in stool frequency, abdominal pain and depression, compared to placebo and atropine [33]. Similar results were obtained in another study using trimipramine [34].

A meta-analysis of 11 randomized controlled trials using antidepressants for functional gastrointestinal disorders, including 8 that evaluated IBS, found that 1 of every 3 treated patients improved (fig. 3) [35]. However, it must be taken into account that these drugs may have side effects (urinary retention, xerostomy, etc.) that can limit its use in many patients. Desipramine and nortriptyline cause fewer side effects than imipramine and amitriptyline.

In conclusion, patients with IBS may benefit from antidepressant drugs, especially tricyclic antidepressants, at low doses. This is especially true in patients with severe pain who do not respond to first-line therapies, with intense limitations of day life activities, with diarrhea predominance and/or with depression linked to the IBS.

Mearin

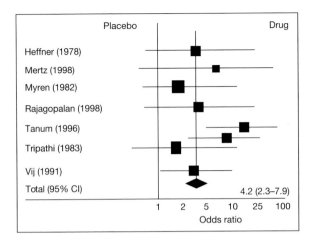

Fig. 3. Meta-analysis of antidepressant medications in the treatment of IBS (from Jackson et al. [35]).

Visceral Analgesics

Based on the concept that visceral hypersensitivity seems to play a key role in IBS pathophysiology, therapeutical research has also focused on new molecules able to modulate visceral perception of the gastrointestinal tract. Fedotozine, an opioid analogue with selective κ receptors affinity, was evaluated in the treatment of IBS patients. A trial performed with fedotozine (3.5, 15 and 30 mg) revealed that the 30-mg group was significantly superior to placebo in controlling abdominal pain, abdominal bloating and global severity of the disease [36]. Nevertheless, due to its marginal clinical benefit and putative secondary effects, fedotozine never was available for clinical use.

Some other drugs such as octreotide (a somatostatin analogue) and leuprolide (a GRH analogue) might also improve abdominal pain in some IBS patients. Clonidine, an α_2-adrenergic agonist, decreases pain sensation during colonic distension and increases rectal compliance in healthy controls and IBS patients. However, several problems (i.e., administration route, secondary effects) preclude its clinical application.

Serotonin: The Queen of the Gut

Over the last decade there has been an increased interest in treating patients with IBS according to pathophysiological mechanisms and not only to clinical complaints. In this context, the role of serotonin (5-HT) in the enteric nervous system has become one of the most important research areas. It is important to note that around 95% of 5-HT is located in the gastrointestinal tract and only 5% in the central nervous system. Two different 5-HT pathways exist in the enteric nervous system, having different responses after stimulation. The intrinsic pathway (mainly mediated through 5-HT$_4$ receptors) is involved in the peristaltic reflexes and water and ions secretion. The extrinsic pathway (mainly mediated by 5-HT$_3$ receptors) is associated to visceral sensations. Thus, 5-HT plays a key role in at least two of the most important mechanisms implicated in IBS manifestations: abnormal gut motility and visceral hypersensitivity.

5-HT$_3$ Antagonists

The most evaluated 5-HT$_3$-selective antagonist in IBS has been alosetron, which proved its capacity to decrease colonic transit and to increase jejunal absorption of water and sodium. A trial performed in 647 non-constipated women with IBS, focusing on abdominal pain, showed improvement in 41% of patients receiving alosetron vs. 29% receiving placebo [37]. A similar study with 462 patients had equivalent results with significant differences for alosetron vs. placebo in decreasing the score for diarrhea and increasing the number of days free from pain [38]. It has also been demonstrated that alosetron significantly improves health-related quality of life in women with diarrhea-predominant IBS [39]. A comparison of alosetron with two antispasmodic drugs (mebeverine and trimebutine) also showed significant differences in favour of alosetron in controlling IBS-related symptomatology [40]. These findings made alosetron the first Food and Drug Administration-approved agent for diarrhea-predominant IBS. A meta-analysis published in 2003 reported a pooled odds ratio for adequate relief of pain or global symptom improvement of 1.81 (95% confidence interval: 1.57–2.10) [41] (fig. 4). However, significant side effects were observed after launching this drug, including severe constipation and ischemic colitis [42]. For these reasons, alosetron was withdrawn from the market in March 2001, but it was reintroduced in the United States in November 2002. A number of restrictions have been imposed: indicated only in women with severe diarrhea-predominant IBS for whom conventional treatments have failed; mandatory doctor training and certification; patient signed consent, and cautious monitoring of severe constipation or ischemic colitis.

Cilansetron is another highly specific and selective 5-HT$_3$ receptor antagonist that is significantly superior to placebo in relieving symptoms and improving quality of life in men and women with diarrhea-predominant IBS [43–45].

5-HT$_4$ Agonists

Tegaserod is a partial agonist of 5-HT$_4$ receptors with prokinetic effect on gastric emptying and able to increase colonic and bowel transit. It stimulates intestinal secretion of water and Cl$^-$, and decreases the nociceptive response to

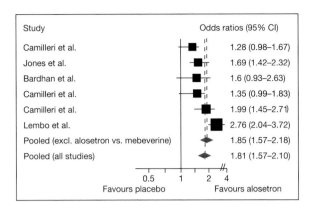

Fig. 4. Meta-analysis of the efficacy of alosetron in the treatment of IBS; pooled data are shown excluding and including the Jones study that used mebeverine as the control treatment (from Cremonini et al. [41]).

rectal distension [46]. Tegaserod efficacy has been evaluated in several large, multicentre, randomized, double-blind trials [47–49]. It has been shown to improve abdominal pain and bloating, and increase bowel movement frequency in women with constipation-predominant IBS. A Cochrane Database systematic review found that the relative risk of being a responder in terms of global relief of gastrointestinal symptoms was significantly higher with tegaserod 12 mg than with placebo (1.19; 95% confidence interval: 1.09–1.29) (Table 1) [50]. Tegaserod is well tolerated, with diarrhea and headache being the most frequently reported adverse events; diarrhea is usually mild and transit.

Treatment of Bacterial Overgrowth

In the past years some authors, especially Pimentel et al. [51], have defended that bacterial overgrowth is a key factor in IBS. They described that 78% of IBS patients had small intestinal bacterial overgrowth diagnosed by lactulose hydrogen breath test and that overgrowth treatment eliminated IBS symptoms in 48%. Nevertheless, this has been a very controversial report [52]. Subsequently the same group performed a double-blind, placebo-controlled randomized study using neomycin leading to a significant reduction in IBS symptoms: 75% of patients when the antibiotic was successful in eliminating the overgrowth [53]. Rifaximin could be an interesting treatment option in cases of bacterial overgrowth associated to IBS due to its excellent efficacy/safety profile [54].

Probiotics

Several probiotics have been tried in the treatment of IBS but most trials have included few patients and had methodological pitfalls; results have been

Table 1. Meta-analysis of the efficacy of tegaserod 12 mg/day vs. placebo in global relief of symptoms in patients with IBS (from Evans et al. [50])

Study	Tegaserod 12 mg, n/N	Placebo n/N	Relative risk (fixed) 95% CI	Weight	Relative risk (fixed) 95% CI
B307	116/275	105/284		18.0	1.14 [0.93, 1.40]
Lefkowitz, 1999	122/267	89/267		15.5	1.37 [1.11, 1.70]
Muller-Lissner, 2001	113/294	87/288		15.3	1.27 [1.01, 1.60]
Novick, 2002	334/767	292/752		51.3	1.12 [0.99, 1.27]
Total (95% CI)	1,603	1,591		100.0	1.19 [1.09, 1.29]

Total events 685 (tegaserod 12 mg), 573 (placebo).
Test for heterogeneity: χ^2 = 3.09, d.f. = 3, p = 0.38, p = 2.8%.
Test for overall effect: z = 3.88, p = 0.0001.

0.5   0.7   1   1.5   2

Favours placebo   Favours tegaserod

inconsistent [55]. However, a recently published clinical trial has demonstrated that *Bifidobacterium infantis* 35,624 alleviates symptoms in IBS; this symptomatic response was associated with normalization of the ratio of an anti-inflammatory to a proinflammatory cytokine, suggesting an immune-modulating role for this organism, in this disorder [56].

Treating Other Functional Bowel Disorders

Functional Abdominal Bloating
No treatment is completely effective in patients with abdominal bloating. Some diet modification might be helpful; avoidance of lactose-containing foods or vegetables that promote flatus should be advice, although their exclusion does not guarantee improvement [57]. Simethicone, a surfactant agent, is frequently prescribed, but its efficacy is more than controversial [58, 59]. Pancreatic enzymes reduced bloating after a high-fat meal and until bedtime in healthy subjects [60], but there are no solid data to this respect in patients with FBD. Antibiotics are not always effective, but it has been shown that the non-absorbable antibiotic rifaximin is able to reduce gas-related symptoms [61]. Regarding probiotics, it is to mention that the administration of *Lactobacillus plantarum* was followed by an improvement in bloating and reduction of abdominal girth in patients with IBS [62]. Tegaserod also improves bloating in

IBS subjects with constipation, but no data in patients with functional abdominal bloating have been published.

Functional Constipation

Reviewing treatment of constipation is out of the focus of this chapter; excellent revisions have been recently published, including one of the American Gastroenterology Association [63].

For patients with mild to moderate constipation, increasing the amount of dietary fiber often improves gut transit, stool frequency and consistency. However, compliance is frequently poor and many patients complain of flatulence, distension and bloating. Laxatives are used (and abused) in more severe cases. Unabsorbed monoand disaccharides, such as lactulose, lactitol, mannitol or sorbitol, are osmotic agents able to increase intraluminal bulk and stimulate colonic peristalsis [64]. Low doses of polyethylene glycol have also been used to successfully treat patients with slow-transit constipation [65, 66].

Saline laxatives, such as magnesium citrate, sodium phosphate or magnesium sulphate, induce a net osmotic flux of water into the small intestine and colon, making faeces softer. Stimulant laxatives include diphenylmethane derivatives, such as phenolphthalein, bisacodyl and sodium picosulfate, and conjugated anthraquinone derivatives such as cascara sagrada, aloin and senna. These drugs have both antiabsorptive-secretagogue and prokinetic effects; many constipated patients abuse of these laxatives.

Prokinetic agents should be helpful in patients with slow-transit constipation. In fact, cisapride improved mild to moderate constipation [67] but unfortunately is no longer available in the market. Tegaserod, another 5-HT$_4$ receptor agonist, was superior to placebo for the treatment of patients with chronic constipation in a large, randomized, double-blind, controlled trial [68].

Other drugs used in patients with constipation not responding to standard medications are: prostaglandin E$_1$ analogue, misoprostol [69], and microtubule formation inhibitor, colchicines [70]. It is important to remember that misoprostol cannot be used during pregnancy and should be used cautiously in reproductive age women who could become pregnant because of effects on uterine contractility and risk of abortion.

Functional Diarrhea

Dietary measures have never been formally assessed but, according to clinical experience, a low-residue diet may be helpful. Excessive coffee and other stimulant drinks should be restricted, as well as other drinks containing sorbitol or mannitol and non-calorie sweeteners, since these sugars cause acceleration of intestinal transit and diarrhea. Temporal exclusion of lactose and fructose might be helpful in some cases to determine a causal relation with diarrhea.

Pharmacological treatment has been based mainly on opiates, mainly loperamide. Randomized control trials have shown it to control diarrhea and reduce defecatory urgency [71]. Alosetron and cilansetron, 5-HT$_3$ antagonists, also improve diarrhea but have been tested only in IBS subjects. Cholestyramine is an ion-exchange resin that binds bile acids and renders them biologically inactive in the colon. A therapeutic trial with cholestyramine may be tried in patients not responding to other treatments.

When depression is prominent, tricyclic antidepressants are reasonable to try due also to their intrinsic constipating effect.

References

1   Bixquert M: Epidemiología de la dispepsia funcional: importancia sanitaria, social y económica; in Mearin F (ed): Dispepsia funcional: tan desconocida como frecuente. Barcelona, Doyma, 1997, pp 11–18.
2   Thompson WG, Heaton KW, Smyth GT, Smyth C: Irritable bowel syndrome in general practice: prevalence, characteristics, and referral. Gut 2000;46:78–82.
3   Knill-Jones RP: Geographical differences in the prevalence of dyspepsia. Scand J Gastroenterol 1991;182(suppl):17–24.
4   Badia X, Mearin F, Balboa A, Baró E, Caldwell E, Cucala M, Díaz-Rubio M, Fueyo A, Ponce J, Roset M, Talley NJ: Burden of illness in irritable bowel syndrome. Comparing Rome I and Rome II criteria. Pharmacoeconomics 2002;20:749–758.
5   Fullerton S: Functional digestive disorders in the year 2000. Economic impact. Eur J Surg 1998;582(suppl):62–64.
6   Koloski NA, Talley NJ, Boyce PM: The impact of funcional gastrointestinal disorders on quality of life. Am J Gastroenterol 2000;95:67–71.
7   Manning AP, Thompson WG, Heaton KW, Morris AF: Towards a positive diagnosis of the irritable bowel. BMJ 1978;2:653–654.
8   Thompson WG, Dotevall G, Drossman DA, Heaton KW, Kruis W: Irritable bowel syndrome: guidelines for the diagnosis. Gastroenterol Int 1989;2:92–95.
9   Thompson WG, Longstreth G, Drossman DA, Heaton K, Irvine EJ, Muller-Lissner S: Functional bowel disorders and functional abdominal pain; in Drossman DA, Corazziari E, Talley NJ, Thompson WG, Whitehead WE (eds): Rome II. The Functional Gastrointestinal Disorders, ed 2. McLean/Va, Degnon Assoc, 2000, pp 351–432.
10 Talley NJ, Stanghellini V, Heading RC, Koch KL, Malagelada JR, Tytgat GNJ: Functional gastro-duodenal disorders; in Drossman DA, Corazziari E, Talley NJ, Thompson WG, Whitehead WE (eds): Rome II. The Functional Gastrointestinal Disorders, ed 2. McLean/Va, Degnon Assoc, 2000, pp 299–350.
11 Drossman DA, Li Z, Andruzzi E, Temple RD, Talley NJ, Thompson WG, Whitehead WE, Janssens J, Funch-Jensen P, Corazziari E, et al: US householder survey of functional gastrointestinal disorders. Prevalence, sociodemography, and health impact. Dig Dis Sci 1993;38: 1569–1580.
12 Koloski NA, Talley NJ, Boyce PM: Epidemiology and health care seeking in the functional gastrointestinal disorders: a population-based study. Am J Gastroenterol 2002;97:2290–2299.
13 Balboa A, Mearin F: Características epidemiológicas e importancia socioeconómica del síndrome del intestino irritable. Rev Esp Enferm Dig 2000;92:806–812.
14 Mearin F, Badía X, Balboa A, Baró E, Caldwell E, Cucala M, et al: Irritable bowel syndrome prevalence varies enormously depending on the employed diagnostic criteria: comparison of Rome II versus previous criteria in a general population. Scand J Gastroenterol 2001;36: 1155–1161.

15 Hungin AP, Whorwell PJ, Tack J, Mearin F: The prevalence, patterns and impact of irritable bowel síndrome: an international survey on 40,000 subjects. Aliment Pharmacol Ther 2003;17: 643–650.

16 Mearin F, Ponce J, Badía X, Balboa A, Baró E, Caldwell E, Cucala M, Díaz-Rubio M, Fueyo A, Roset M, Talley NJ: Splitting irritable bowel syndrome: from original Rome to Rome II criteria. Am J Gastroenterol 2004;99:122–130.

17 Johnsen R, Jacobsen BK, Forde OH: Association between symptoms of irritable colon and psychological and social conditions and lifestyle. Br Med J 1986;292:1633–1635.

18 Heaton KW, Radvan J, Cripps H, Mountford RA, Braddon FEM, Hughes AO: Defecation frequency and timing, and stool form in the general population – a prospective study. Gut 1992;33: 818–824.

19 Everhart JE, Go VL, Johannes RS, Fitzsimmons SC, Roth HP, White LR: A longitudinal survey of self-reported bowel habits in the United States. Dig Dis Sci 1989;34:1153–1162.

20 Sonnenberg A, Koch TR: Physician visits in the United States for constipation: 1958–1986. Dig Dis Sci 1989;34:606–611.

21 Whitehead WE, Paulsson O, Jones KR: Systematic review of the comorbidity or irritable bowel syndrome with other disorders: what are the causes and implications? Gastroent 2002;122: 1140–1156.

22 Longstreth GF, Yao JF: Irritable bowel syndrome and surgery: a multivariable analysis. Gastroenterology 2004;126:1665–1673.

23 Mearin F, Balboa A, Badía X, Baró E, Caldwell E, Cucala M, Díaz-Rubio M, Fueyo A, Ponce J, Roset M, Talley NJ: Irritable bowel syndrome subtypes according to bowel habit: revisiting the alternating subtype. Eur J Gastroenterol Hepatol 2003;15:165–172.

24 Cann PA, Read NM, Holdsworth CD: What is the benefit of coarse wheat bran in patients with irritable bowel syndrome? Gut 1984;25:168–173.

25 Lucey MR, Clarck ML, Lowndes J, Dawson AM: Is bran efficacious in irritable bowel syndrome? A double-blind, placebo-controlled crossover study. Gut 1987;28:221–225.

26 Haderstorfer B, Psycholgin D, Whitehead WE, Schuster MM: Intestinal gas production from bacterial fermentation of indigested carbohydrate in irritable bowel syndrome. Am J Gastroenterol 1989;84:375–378.

27 Bijkerk CJ, Muris JW, Knottnerus JA, Hoes AW, de Wit NJ: Systematic review: the role of different types of fibre in the treatment of irritable bowel syndrome. Aliment Pharmacol Ther 2004;19:245–251.

28 Lavo B, Stenstam M, Nielsen AL: Loperamide in treatment of irritable bowel syndrome, a double-blind, placebo-controlled study. Scand J Gastroenterol 1987;130:77–80.

29 Efskind PS, Bernklev T, Vatn MH: A double-blind, placebo-controlled trial with loperamide in irritable bowel syndrome. Scand J Gastroenterol 1996;31:463–468.

30 Poynard T, Naveau S, Mory B, Chaput JC: Meta-analysis of smooth muscle relaxant in the treatment of irritable bowel syndrome. Aliment Pharmacol Ther 1994;8:499–510.

31 Poynard T, Regimbeau C, Benhamou Y: Meta-analysis of smooth muscle relaxant in the treatment of irritable bowel syndrome. Aliment Pharmacol Ther 2001;15:355–361.

32 Jailwala J, Imperiale TF, Kroenke K: Pharmacologic treatment of the irritable bowel syndrome: a systematic review of randomized, controlled trials. Ann Intern Med 2000;133:136–147.

33 Greenbaum DS, Mayle JE, Vanegeren LE, Jerome JA, Mayor JW, Greenbaum RB, Matson RW, Stein GE, Dean HA, Halvorsen NA, Rosen LW: The effects of desipramine on IBS compared with atropine and placebo. Dig Dis Sci 1987;32:257–266.

34 Myren J, Lovland B, Larssen SE, Larsen S: A double-blind study of the effect of trimipramine in patients with the irritable bowel syndrome. Scand J Gastroenterol 1984;19:835–843.

35 Jackson AL, O'Malley PG, Tomkins G, Balden E, Santoro MJ, Kroenke K: Treatment of functional gastrointestinal disorders with antidepressant medications: a meta-analysis. Am J Med 2000;108:65–72.

36 Dapoigny M, Abitbol JL, Fraitag B: Efficacy of peripheral κ agonist, fedotozine vs. placebo in treatment of irritable bowel syndrome: a multicenter dose-response study. Dig Dis Sci 1995;40: 2244–2249.

37 Camilleri M, Northcutt AR, Kong S, Dukes GE, McSorley D, Mangel AW: Efficacy and safety of alosetron in women with irritable bowel syndrome: a randomised, placebo-controlled trial. Lancet 2000;355:1035–1040.

38 Bardhan KD, Bodemar G, Geldof H, Schutz E, Heath A, Mills JG, Jacques LA: A double-blind, randomized, placebo-controlled dose-ranging study to evaluate the efficacy of alosetron in the treatment of irritable bowel syndrome. Aliment Pharmacol Ther 2000:14;23–34.

39 Watson ME, Lacey L, Kong S, Northcutt AR, McSorley D, Hahn B, Mangel AW: Alosetron improves quality of life in women with diarrhea-predominant irritable bowel syndrome. Am J Gastroenterol 2001;96:455–459.

40 Jones RH, Holtmann G, Rodrigo L, Ehsanullah RS, Crompton PM, Jacques LA, Mills JG: Alosetron relieves pain and improves bowel function compared with mebeverine in female nonconstipated irritable bowel syndrome patients. Aliment Pharcacol Ther 1999;13:1419–1427.

41 Cremonini F, Delgado-Aros S, Camilleri M: Efficacy of alosetron in irritable bowel syndrome: a meta-analysis of randomized controlled trials. Neurogastroenterol Motil 2003;15:79–86.

42 Friedel D, Thomas R, Fisher RS: Ischemic colitis during treatment with alosetron. Gastroenterology 2001;120:557–560.

43 Caras S, Borel R, Krause G, Biesheuvel E, Steinborn C: Cilansetron shows efficacy in male and female non-constipated IBS subjects in a US study. Gastroenterology 2001;120(suppl 1):A217.

44 Bradette M, Moennikes H, Carter F, Krause G, Caras S, Steinborn C: Cilansetron in irritable bowel syndrome with diarrhea predominance (IBS-D): efficacy and safety in a 6-month global study. Gastroenterology 2004;126(suppl 2):A42.

45 Coremans G, Clouse RE, Carter F, Krause G, Caras S, Steinborn C: Cilansetron, a novel 5-HT[3] antagonist, demonstrated efficacy in males with irritable bowel syndrome with diarrhea-predominance (IBS-D). Gastroenterology 2004;126(suppl2):A643.

46 Prather CM, Camilleri M, Zinsmeister AR, McKinzie S, Thomforde G: Tegaserod accelerates orocecal transit in patients with constipation-predominant irritable bowel syndrome. Gastroenterology 2000;118:463–468.

47 Kellow JE, Lee OY, Chang FY, et al: An Asia-Pacific, double-blind, placebo-controlled, randomised study to evaluate the efficacy, safety, and tolerability of tegaserod in patient with irritable bowel syndrome. Gut 2003;52:671–676.

48 Muller-Lissner SA, Fumagalli I, Bardhan KD, Pace F, Pecher E, Nault B, Ruegg P: Tegaserod, a 5-HT[4] receptor agonist, relieves symptoms in irritable bowel syndrome patients with abdominal pain, bloating and constipation. Aliment Pharmacol Ther 1999;15:1655–1666.

49 Novick J, Miner P, Krause R, Glebas K, Bliesath H, Ligozio G, Ruegg P, Lefkowitch J: A randomized, double-blind, placebo-controlled trial of tegaserod in female patients suffering with irritable bowel syndrome with constipation. Aliment Pharmacol Ther 2002;16:1877–1888.

50 Evans BW, Clark WK, Moore DJ, Whorwell PJ: Tegaserod for the treatment of irritable bowel syndrome. Cochrane Database Syst Rev 2004;(1):CD003960.

51 Pimentel M, Chow EJ, Lin HC: Eradication of small intestinal bacterial overgrowth reduces symptoms of irritable bowel syndrome. Am J Gastroenterol 2000;95:3503–3506.

52 Hasler WL: Lactulose breath testing, bacterial overgrowth, and IBS: just a lot of hot air? Gastroenterology 2003;125:1898–1900.

53 Pimentel M, Chow EJ, Lin HC: Normalization of lactulose breath testing correlates with symptom improvement in irritable bowel syndrome: a double-blind, randomized, placebo-controlled study. Am J Gastroenterol 2003;98:412–419.

54 Scarpignato C, Pelosini I: Rifaximin, a poorly absorbed antibiotic: pharmacology and clinical potential. Chemotherapy 2005;51(suppl):36–66.

55 Spanier JA, Howden CW, Jones MP: A systematic review of alternative therapies in the irritable bowel syndrome. Arch Intern Med 2003;163:265–274.

56 O'Mahony L, McCarthy J, Kelly P, Hurley G, Luo F, Chen K, O'Sullivan GC, Kiely B, Collins JK, Shanahan F, Quigley EM: Lactobacillus and bifidobacterium in irritable bowel syndrome: symptom responses and relationship to cytokine profiles. Gastroenterology 2005;128:541–551.

57 Tolliver BA, et al: Does lactose maldigestion really play a role in the irritable bowel syndrome? J Clin Gastroenterol 1996;23:15–17.

58 Friis H, Bode S, Rumessen JJ, Gudmand-Hoyer E: Effect of simethicone on lactulose-induced H[2] production and gastrointestinal symptoms. Digestion 1991;49:227–230.

59 Holtmann G, Gschossmann J, Karaus M, Fischer T, Becker B, Mayr P, Gerken G: Randomised double-blind comparison of simethicone with cisapride in functional dyspepsia. Aliment Pharmacol Ther 1999;13:1459–1465.

60 Suarez F, Levitt MD, Adshead J, Barkin JS: Pancreatic supplements reduce symptomatic response of healthy subjects to a high fat meal. Dig Dis Sci 1999;44:1317–1321.

61 Di Stefano M, Strocchi A, Malservisi S, Veneto G, Ferrieri A, Corazza GR: Non-absorbable antibiotics for managing intestinal gas production and gas-related symptoms. Aliment Pharmacol Ther 2000;14:1001–1008.

62 Nobaek S, Johanssen ML, Molin G, Ahrne S, Jeppsson B: Alteration of intestinal microflora is associated with reduction of abdominal bloating and pain in patients with irritable bowel syndrome. Am J Gastroenterol 2000;95:1231–1238.

63 American Gastroenterological Association technical review on constipation. Gastroenterology 2000;119:1766–1778.

64 Bass P, Dennis S: The laxative effects of lactulose in normal and constipated subjects. J Clin Gastroenterol 1981;3(suppl 1):23–28.

65 Chaussade S, Minic M: Comparison of efficacy and safety of two doses of two different polyethylene glycol-based laxatives in the treatment of constipation. Aliment Pharmacol Ther 2003;17:165–172.

66 Corazziari E, Badiali D, Bazzocchi G, Bassotti G, Roselli P, Mastropaolo G, Luca MG, Galeazzi R, Peruzzi E: Long term efficacy, safety, and tolerability of low daily doses of isosmotic polyethylene glycol electrolyte balanced solution (PMF-100) in the treatment of functional chronic constipation. Gut 2000;46:522–526.

67 Van Outryve M, Milo R, Toussaint J, Van Eeghem P: Prokinetic treatment of constipation-predominant irritable bowel syndrome: a placebo-controlled study of cisapride. J Clin Gastroenterol 1991;13:49–57.

68 Johansen JF, Tougas G, Chey WD, Novick JS, Lembo A, Fordham F, Guella MP, Nault B: Tegaserod provides rapid and sustained relief of constipation, abdominal bloating/distension, and abdominal discomfort/pain in patients with chronic constipation. Gastroenterology 2003;124:A47.

69 Soffer EE, Metcalf A, Launspach J: Misoprostol is effective treatment for patients with severe chronic constipation. Dig Dis Sci 1994;39:929–933.

70 Sninsky CA, Verne GN, Gordon JM, Eaker EY, Davis RH: Double-blind, placebo-controlled, cross-over study evaluating the effectiveness of colchicine in the treatment of severe constipation. Gastroenterology 1998;114: A839.

71 Palmer KR, Corbett CL, Holdsworth CD: Double-blind, cross-over study comparing loperamide, codeine and diphenoxylate in chronic diarrhea. Gastroenterology 1980;79:1272–1275.

Fermín Mearin, MD, PhD
Institute of Functional and Motor Digestive Disorders, Centro Médico Teknon
Vilana 12, ES–08022 Barcelona (Spain)
Tel. +34 93 393 3143, Fax +34 93 393 3062
E-mail mearin@dr.teknon.es

This chapter should be cited as follows:

Mearin F: Pharmacological Treatment of the Irritable Bowel Syndrome and Other Functional Bowel Disorders. Digestion 2006;73(suppl 1):28–37.

••••••••••••••••••••••••

Treatment of Functional Bowel Disorders: Is There Room for Antibiotics?

Gino Roberto Corazza[a], *Michele Di Stefano*[a], *Carmelo Scarpignato*[b]

[a]First Department of Internal Medicine, School of Medicine and Dentistry, University of Pavia, Pavia, [b]Laboratory of Clinical Pharmacology, Department of Anatomy, Pharmacology and Forensic Sciences, University of Parma, Parma, Italy

Abstract

Small bowel bacterial overgrowth is a syndrome associated with a broad range of predisposing conditions, characterized by the presence of pathological amounts or types of bacteria at the level of the small bowel, clinically evident with a spectrum of symptoms such as diarrhea, flatulence, abdominal pain and bloating. Some of these symptoms are very common complaints in patients suffering from functional bowel disorders (FBDs). Although the pathophysiological mechanisms responsible for FBDs are certainly multifactorial and not yet completely understood, several pieces of evidence suggest that an increased metabolic activity of intestinal bacteria is responsible for gas-related intestinal symptoms in a large subgroup of patients. In addition, byproducts of colonic fermentation might be able to trigger symptoms in those patients displaying visceral hyper-sensitivity. Targeting enteric bacteria with antibiotics therefore represents a logical approach to FBDs. Although systemic antimicrobials have been mostly used in the past, the availability of poorly absorbed antibiotics like rifaximin, being safe and effective, has represented a step forward in the treatment of this challenging clinical condition.

Introduction

Gas-related symptoms are a very frequent complaint in functional gastrointestinal disorders. In patients with irritable bowel syndrome (IBS), bloating may be the predominant symptom or it may occur as part of the symptom complex: up to 80–90% of these patients suffer from bloating [1] and they consider this symptom to be one of the most bothersome [2]. A recent survey in the general

US population [3] showed that around 16% of individuals experienced abdominal bloating in the month prior to the interview, and other studies [4, 5] suggest that this symptom may represent the second most common complaint in functional bowel disorders (FBDs), the first being abdominal pain.

The pathophysiology underlying gas-related symptoms is certainly multifactorial and not yet completely understood. Bloating is frequently present in conditions characterized by an obstruction of luminal flow and the restoration of a normal transit is followed by symptom relief [6, 7]; the production of excess intestinal gas has been proposed as another important mechanism [8] and, similarly, the reduction of gas production improves bloating and flatulence severity [8, 9]. However, the adoption of these therapeutic strategies in clinical practice does not always allow a satisfactory control of symptoms and alternative approaches have therefore been suggested. Probiotic modulation of intestinal flora, although promising [10], was shown not to be always effective [11–14]. On the contrary, pharmacological stimulation of intestinal peristaltic activity proved to be capable of improving both abdominal bloating and flatulence via an increased elimination of intraluminal gas [15].

The use of antibiotics in the treatment of FBDs has received growing attention. The presence of overlapping symptoms in FBDs and small intestinal bacterial overgrowth (SIBO) led to investigate the possibility of an overlapping pathophysiology in these two conditions [16]. Since the correct diagnosis of SIBO by using an indirect approach such as the lactulose-glucose hydrogen breath test is still a matter of debate and important symptoms of FBDs may have explanations other than SIBO, the results of antibiotic treatment of these two different clinical conditions will be analyzed separately.

Functional Bowel Disorders

According to Rome II criteria, the presence of bloating and symptoms related to intestinal gas is frequently encountered in clinical practice, particularly in IBS and functional abdominal bloating [17]. Levitt et al. [18] analyzed the relationship between abdominal bloating and intestinal gas by supplementing healthy volunteers' diet with fermentable (lactulose) or non-fermentable (methylcellulose) carbohydrates or placebo for a 1-week period. As far as passage of flatus is concerned, lactulose supplementation increased its frequency, while no difference was seen after methylcellulose and placebo (fig. 1a). On the contrary, both lactulose and methylcellulose caused an increase in abdominal bloating scores (fig. 1b). This finding could be explained on the basis of the increased fecal bulk by methylcellulose and on the enhanced gas production by lactulose. Both mechanisms are able to induce a stimulation of bowel wall

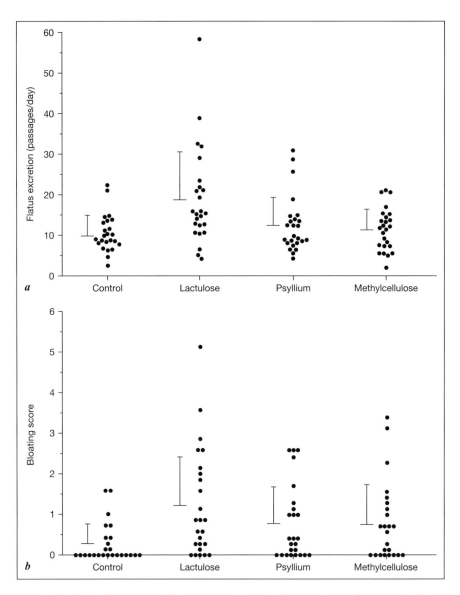

Fig. 1. Daily frequency of flatus passage (***a***) and daily score (sum of noon and bedtime scores) for abdominal bloating (***b***) for all 25 subjects in the control period (1 week) and in the weeks during which the diet was supplemented with lactulose, psyllium, or methylcellulose (from Levitt et al. [18]).

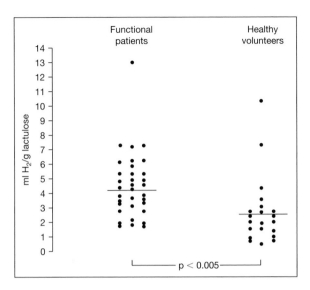

Fig. 2. Breath H_2 excretion (expressed in ml H_2 per gram of disaccharides ingested during the 6 h of testing after lactulose administration in 34 functional patients and 21 healthy volunteers (from Di Stefano et al. [8]).

mechanoceptors due to increased intraluminal pressure and subsequent enhancement of wall tension in the involved gastrointestinal tract [19]. Consequently, flatulence certainly represents a gas-related symptom, but abdominal bloating is not always related to an increased gas production. These observations are of course extremely important for the selection of patients who could benefit from antibiotic therapy.

After oral administration, carbohydrates are fermented by enteric bacterial flora to give water, short chain fatty acids and several gases, namely carbon dioxide (CO_2), hydrogen (H_2), methane (CH_4), hydrogen sulfide (SH_2) and methanethiol (CH_3SH) [20, 21]. These gases are absorbed through the colonic wall, carried to the lungs via the blood and excreted with expired air, allowing their measurement in the breath. This represents the basis for the hydrogen breath test, a simple method to detect carbohydrate malabsorption.

In a group of functional bloaters and in a group of healthy volunteers, the non-absorbable sugar lactulose was administered and breath hydrogen excretion monitored for a 6-hour period [8]. Functional patients showed a mean hydrogen excretion significantly higher than that of healthy volunteers, suggesting an increased gas production at intestinal level (fig. 2). However, a wide overlap between patients and healthy volunteers was observed, thus implying that intestinal gas production is not the only factor determining symptom

Table 1. Perception and discomfort thresholds to rectal distension after administration of lactulose or a control iso-osmotic electrolyte solution in healthy volunteers and patients with functional bloating (from Di Stefano et al. [22])

Subjects	Lactulose solution			Electrolyte solution		
	basal	post-infusion	significance	basal	post-infusion	significance
Thresholds for perception						
Healthy volunteers	4 ± 3	2 ± 1	NS	11 ± 9	9 ± 7	NS
Functional patients	6 ± 4	2 ± 2	$p < 0.05$	7 ± 4	3.5 ± 2	$p < 0.05$
Thresholds for discomfort						
Healthy volunteers	28 ± 17	24 ± 14	NS	25 ± 14	24 ± 5	NS
Functional patients	16 ± 8	9.5 ± 6	$p < 0.05$	17 ± 11	16.5 ± 6	NS

generation. As a consequence, inhibition of the fermentation process after antibiotic therapy may not always be fully effective.

Whether alterations of visceral sensitivity do exist in patients with functional bloating is presently unknown. Sensitivity thresholds to rectal distension were evaluated in a group of IBS patients with relevant bloating [22]. A basal series of distensions at rectal level was performed by a balloon connected to a barostat. Lactulose was then given per os and hydrogen excretion was monitored in expired air to detect the increase of hydrogen breath excretion indicating the beginning of colonic fermentation. At this point in time, a second evaluation of sensitivity thresholds was performed to test whether colonic fermentation may induce visceral hypersensitivity. On a separate day, the test was repeated with the administration of a non-fermentable, non-absorbable electrolyte solution to serve as a control. A small amount of barium was added to this solution and the timing of the second series of distensions was selected on the basis of an X-ray monitoring. In healthy volunteers neither lactulose nor the control solution induced any modification of sensitivity thresholds. On the contrary, only in the patient group was a reduction of perception and discomfort thresholds evident after lactulose but not after the control solution (table 1). This finding is consistent with the idea that a subgroup of patients may have a heightened visceral sensation (induced or unmasked by colonic fermentation), which allows even low amounts of fermentation products to trigger the symptoms. Accordingly, in this subgroup the reduction of colonic fermentation with antibiotics may hardly affect symptom severity and a complete suppression of enteric flora could be needed to obtain symptom relief.

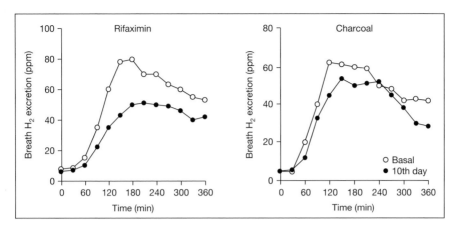

Fig. 3. Average breath H_2 concentration – time curves of patients treated with rifaximin or activated charcoal in basal conditions and 10 days after the end of 1 week of therapy (from Di Stefano et al. [8]).

A double-blind, randomized trial [8] comparing the effect of rifaximin and activated charcoal in patients with FBDs showed that, after 7 days of therapy, rifaximin (800 mg daily) induced a hydrogen breath excretion significantly lower than that observed after charcoal administration (fig. 3); rifaximin, but not charcoal, significantly improved flatulence and the overall severity of symptoms (table 2), and also reduced abdominal girth, but no effect was seen on bloating and pain; the variation of breath hydrogen excretion correlated significantly with the variation of flatulence, confirming the close relationship between breath hydrogen excretion and gas production [8].

Patients with FBDs often display several comorbidities, of which lactose intolerance is one of the most common [23, 24]. Whether the high rate of comorbidity reflects true malabsorption (i.e. lactase enzyme deficiency) or if symptoms result from fermentation of lactose in the small intestine (due to SIBO) and subsequent increase of gaseous by-products, continues to be investigated. In any case, it is worth mentioning that a recent open trial [25] showed that in patients with lactose intolerance a short course (10 days) of rifaximin (400 mg twice daily) was able to significantly reduce abdominal pain, distension and bloating.

All the above findings do suggest that – in the absence of hypersensitivity to colonic fermentation – treating increased gas production with antibiotics could represent a rational approach. Further studies in specific subgroups of patients are needed to evaluate the efficacy of this therapeutic option.

Table 2. Effect of rifaximin (800 mg daily for 7 days) or activated charcoal on symptoms severity in patients with FBDs (from Di Stefano et al. [8])

	Patients	Symptom score		
		before therapy	10th day after end of therapy	p value*
Bloating				
Rifaximin	16	17.1 ± 9.7	11.3 ± 12.3	NS
Charcoal	13	10.9 ± 9.2	13.5 ± 9.0	NS
Abdominal pain				
Rifaximin	12	10.5 ± 7.4	5.2 ± 8.6	NS
Charcoal	12	7.4 ± 6.8	6.0 ± 7.7	NS
Flatus passage				
Rifaximin	17	21.2 ± 21.3	9.2 ± 13.6	<0.05
Charcoal	11	19.8 ± 19.9	19.8 ± 22.4	NS
Abdominal girth				
Rifaximin	18	79.2 ± 8.7	77.0 ± 7.5	<0.02
Charcoal	16	82.8 ± 13.4	82.5 ± 13.7	NS
Overall severity				
Rifaximin	17	5.9 ± 2.1	3.2 ± 3.3	<0.02
Charcoal	13	5.4 ± 2.6	5.3 ± 2.3	NS

Mean ± SD values. NS =Not significant.
*Wilcoxon test with Bonferroni-type correction for multiple comparisons.

Small Bowel Bacterial Overgrowth

SIBO is a condition defined by the presence of pathological amounts or types of bacteria at the level of the small bowel, responsible for a malabsorption syndrome, clinically evident with a spectrum of symptoms such as diarrhea, flatulence, abdominal pain, bloating, and, in more severe cases, anemia, weight and bone loss [26, 27]. Bacterial overgrowth is associated with the presence of several predisposing conditions: conditions causing stasis, gastric resections with reduced efficacy of 'gastric filter' as well as intestinal resection with altered efficacy of the ileo-cecal valve [26, 27]. Although characterized by a very different pathophysiology, all these conditions are responsible for allowing bacteria to pass into or develop in the small bowel. A predisposing condition is crucial for SIBO to occur. Indeed, its prevalence in patients with one of these conditions is extremely high and larger than that seen in patients without [28].

A thoughtful review of Lin [16] has put forward the hypothesis that SIBO could represent a framework to understand IBS. The possibility that SIBO may explain bloating is suggested by the greater total hydrogen excretion after lactulose ingestion, the correlation between the pattern of bowel movement and the type of excreted gas, the prevalence of abnormal lactulose breath test in 84% of IBS patients, and the large improvement (up to 75%) of IBS symptoms after eradication of SIBO. Altered gastrointestinal motility and sensation, changed activity of the central nervous system, and increased sympathetic drive and immune activation may be interpreted as consequences of the host response to SIBO [16]. To further support abnormal enteric flora as the contributing cause of IBS, two recent studies have shown that metronidazole [29] and neomycin [30] are both able to cause a significant symptomatic improvement in this condition.

The original study [31] suggesting a high prevalence of SIBO in IBS patients was criticized because of the low accuracy of the lactulose breath test, which was used to define bacterial overgrowth. And indeed, glucose has now become the preferred substrate for hydrogen breath testing. However, the glucose breath test also presents some drawbacks, the most important being the negative interference on its accuracy by an accelerated gastrointestinal transit, which becomes responsible for glucose malabsorption, glucose fermentation at colonic level and consequent false-positive results [32]. Several preliminary reports aimed at clarifying the potential association between SIBO and IBS were presented during the 2005 Digestive Disease Week Meeting in Chicago. Lupascu et al. [33] assessed the prevalence of SIBO by glucose breath testing in IBS patients *versus* healthy controls. The study involved patients with IBS as defined by Rome II criteria; an appropriately matched group without IBS served as the control population. The investigators found a significantly increased ($p < 0.05$) proportion of patients with SIBO among patients in the IBS group: 20 of 65 (30.7%) compared with 4 of 102 (3.9%) controls. McCallum et al. [34] presented additional evidence on the association of SIBO with IBS. They evaluated only IBS patients with diarrhea using the glucose breath test and a prevalence rate of SIBO of 38.5% was found. However, in this work a 75-gram dose of glucose was administered and such a high carbohydrate load may be responsible for false-positive results, also taking into account that the enrolled subset of diarrhea patients was likely to have accelerated intestinal transit. For the breath-test analysis, 74.5% of patients were positive only by H_2 analysis, and 23.6% were positive only by the CH_4 analysis. The investigators suggested that both the H_2 and CH_4 analysis should be performed to optimize the interpretation of these breath tests in this population of patients. It was previously suggested [35], but not yet confirmed, that an improved accuracy of breath test for diagnosis of carbohydrate malabsorption may be achieved by taking into account not only hydrogen but also methane measurements, while absolute values of breath methane excretion by its own proved to be inadequate for diagnostic purposes [36, 37]. Fasting breath CH_4 excretion indeed shows a continuous fluctuation reflecting either variations in production or release from fecal material into the lumen. This latter phenomenon is more likely since methanogenic flora is primarily located in the semisolid fecal component of the left colon [38, 39] and bubbles of CH_4, trapped in the colon, may be intermittently released with the induction of fecal stirring [40].

It is worth mentioning that in IBS patients the prevalence of SIBO diagnosed according to the gold standard for this condition (i.e. culture of small bowel aspirate) is much lower than that reported by using indirect methods. In this connection, Simrén et al. [41] performed culture of small bowel aspirate in 33 IBS patients, diagnosed according to Rome II criteria and refractory to standard medical therapy, and found that only 3 (9%) patients showed >100,000 bacteria/ml of small bowel aspirate. In any event, a prevalence of 10% could be considered a reasonable figure. Given the high prevalence of IBS in the general population, this proportion of patients represents a relevant number of subjects, which makes the search for SIBO cost-effective.

Provided SIBO is diagnosed in IBS patients, the therapeutic strategy should be aimed first of all at removing the predisposing condition. Since this is not always possible, antibiotic administration represents – together with adequate nutritional support – the main strategy, albeit there is no agreement regarding the most effective drug and regimen. Moreover, there are no available studies dealing with composition of contaminating flora in IBS, so that no specific species or strains could be considered responsible for this abnormality. Up to now the contaminating flora has believed to be polymicrobic in nature and, therefore, the use of wide-spectrum antibiotics considered mandatory [26, 27]. Several antibiotics have shown to be effective (table 3) (for a review, see Di Stefano and Corazza [42]). Despite the fact that anaerobes are the bacteria responsible for the most important metabolic consequences of SIBO, tetracyclines (whose efficacy against those bacteria is quite low) have long been regarded as the drugs of choice [43–45]. Their action on anaerobes is probably indirect, i.e. mediated by their effect on aerobes. Indeed tetracyclines do increase oxygen availability, making the environment unfavorable for anaerobes. While metronidazole – being very active on anaerobes [45] – is still used, cephalosporins, lincomycin and chloramphenicol have been abandoned [44–46]. Quinolones and amoxicillin-clavulanic acid combination have also recently been employed thanks to their good tolerability [47].

Rifaximin, a poorly absorbed rifamycin derivative, is effective against aerobes and anaerobes, both Gram-positive and Gram-negative [48, 49]. In a double-blind, randomized trial [9] the effects of this antibiotic and of tetracycline were compared in a group of patients with SIBO. Rifaximin proved to be not only more effective than tetracycline on symptom severity (table 4) and

Table 3. Antimicrobial regimens used in the treatment of small intestine bacterial overgrowth

Drug	Dose	n	Predisposing conditions	Responders
Tetracycline				
Kahn et al., 1966 [43]	250 mg q.i.d.	4	Scleroderma	75%
Goldstein et al., 1961 [44]	250 mg q.i.d.	1	Billroth II	+
Gorbach and Tabaqchali, 1969 [51]	250 mg q.i.d.	1	Ileocolonic anastomosis in Crohn's disease	−
Bjorneklett et al., 1983 [45]	NA	3	Small bowel diverticulosis	100%
Di Stefano et al., 2000 [9]	333 mg t.i.d.	11	Gastrointestinal surgery, intestinal stasis	27%
Chloramphenicol				
Goldstein et al., 1961 [44]	500 mg q.i.d.	1	Billroth II	+
Lincomycin				
Bjorneklett et al., 1983 [45]	NA	1	Radiation fibrosis	−
Gorbach and Tabaqchali, 1969 [51]	500 mg t.i.d.	2	Small bowel diverticulosis	50%
Ampicillin				
Goldstein et al., 1970 [52]	250 mg q.i.d.	1	Diabetic autonomic neuropathy	+
Metronidazole				
Bjorneklett et al., 1983 [45]	NA	6	Radiation fibrosis, small bowel diverticulosis	83%
Cotrimoxazole				
Elsborg, 1977 [53]	400 mg b.i.d	1	Small bowel diverticulosis	+
Norfloxacin				
Attar et al., 1999 [54]	400 mg b.i.d.	10	Gastrointestinal surgery or intestinal stasis	30%
Amoxicillin-clavulanic acid				
Attar et al., 1999 [54]	500 mg t.i.d.	10	Gastrointestinal surgery or intestinal stasis	50%
Rifaximin				
Trespi and Ferrieri, 1999 [55]	400 mg t.i.d.	8	Chronic pancreatitis and Billroth II	100%
Di Stefano et al., 2000 [9]	400 mg t.i.d.	10	Gastrointestinal surgery or intestinal stasis	70%

NA = Not applicable; + = positive effect of therapy; − = no effect of therapy.

hydrogen breath excretion after glucose oral administration, but also better tolerated. Not all patients however showed an improvement of breath excretion and clinical symptoms and a lower effect of the drug was evident in those previously submitted to Billroth II operation [9], most likely because of a low bioavailability of the drug at the afferent loop. Indeed, in a study specifically performed in this subgroup of patients [50], both rifaximin and metronidazole induced an improvement of breath H_2 excretion but the statistical significance

Table 4. Effect of rifaximin (1,200 mg daily) or chlortetracycline (1,000 mg daily) for 7 days on symptom severity in patients with SIBO (from Di Stefano et al. [9])

	Symptom score		p value*
	before therapy	after therapy	
Diarrhea			
Rifaximin	1.9 ± 0.3	1.0 ± 0.5	0.05
Chlortetracycline	2.0 ± 0.2	1.8 ± 0.4	NS
Borborigmi			
Rifaximin	1.7 ± 0.3	0.9 ± 0.4	0.05
Chlortetracycline	1.8 ± 0.3	1.5 ± 0.4	NS
Lassitude			
Rifaximin	1.8 ± 0.3	1.1 ± 0.3	<0.03
Chlortetracycline	1.6 ± 0.2	1.3 ± 0.4	NS
Anorexia			
Rifaximin	1.0 ± 0.0	1.0 ± 0.0	NS
Chlortetracycline	1.8 ± 0.3	1.9 ± 0.3	NS
Abdominal pain			
Rifaximin	0.7 ± 0.2	0.7 ± 0.1	NS
Chlortetracycline	0.7 ± 0.1	0.7 ± 0.2	NS
Bloating			
Rifaximin	1.7 ± 0.3	1.6 ± 0.4	NS
Chlortetracycline	1.6 ± 0.3	1.6 ± 0.4	NS
Mean cumulative score			
Rifaximin	6.3 ± 1.2	5.2 ± 0.5	<0.01
Chlortetracycline	6.6 ± 1.3	6.4 ± 1.2	NS

Mean $\pm$ SD values. NS = Not significant.
*Wilcoxon test with Bonferroni-type correction for multiple comparisons.

was achieved only with metronidazole, a systemic antimicrobial. The same held true for symptom severity [50].

Conclusions

Therapy of both FBDs and SIBO can and must be considerably improved. A rigid protocol with one single therapeutic regimen for all patients is certainly questionable. Rather, a more flexible approach, tailored to the predisposing condition, represents the best approach. Obviously, the availability of better tolerated drugs, such as rifaximin, has represented a step forward in the treatment of this challenging clinical condition. In particular, this poorly absorbed antibiotic achieves good symptom relief and reduces H_2 breath excretion in patients with FBDs and increased gas production. Patients with hypersensitivity to colonic fermentation may show less benefit from *standard* antibiotic therapy but may take advantage from a profound suppression of enteric flora.

References

1 Dotevall G, Svedlund J, Sjodin I: Symptoms in irritable bowel syndrome. Scand J Gastroenterol Suppl 1982;79:16–19.

2 Lembo T, Naliboff B, Munakata J, Fullerton S, Saba L, Tung S, Schmulson M, Mayer EA: Symptom and visceral perception in patients with pain-predominant irritable bowel syndrome. Am J Gastroenterol 1999;94:1320–1326.

3 Sandler RS, Stewart WF, Liberman JN, Ricci JA, Zorich NL: Abdominal pain, bloating, and diarrhea in the United States: prevalence and impact. Dig Dis Sci 2000;45:1166–1171.

4 Manning AP, Thompson WG, Heaton KW, Morris AF: Towards positive diagnosis of the irritable bowel. Br Med J 1978;ii:653–654.

5 Maxton DG, Morris JA, Whorwell PJ: Ranking of symptoms by patients with irritable bowel syndrome. Br Med J 1989;299:1138.

6 Cameron IC, Stoddard JE, Treacy PJ, Patterson J, Stoddard CJ: Long-term symptomatic follow-up after Lind fundoplication. Br J Surg 2000;87:362–373.

7 Laine S, Rantala A, Gullichsen R, Ovaska J: laparoscopic vs. conventional Nissen fundoplication. A prospective randomized study. Surg Endosc 1997;11:441–444.

8 Di Stefano M, Strocchi A, Malservisi S, Vene-to G, Ferrieri A, Corazza GR: Non-absorbable antibiotics for managing intestinal gas production and gas-related symptoms. Aliment Pharmacol Ther 2000;14:1001–1008.

9 Di Stefano M, Malservisi S, Veneto G, Ferrieri A, Corazza GR: Rifaximin versus chlortetracycline in the short-term treatment of small intestine bacterial overgrowth. Aliment Pharmacol Ther 2000;14:551–556.

10 Gorbach SL: Probiotics and gastrointestinal health. Am J Gastroenterol 2000;95:S1–S4.

11 Koebnick C, Wagner I, Leitzmann P, Stern U, Zunft HJ: Probiotic beverage containing *Lactobacillus casei* Shirota improves gastrointestinal symptoms in patients with chronic constipation. Can J Gastroenterol 2003;17:655–659.

12 Kim HJ, Camilleri M, McKinzie S, Lempke MB, Burton DD, Thomforde GM, Zinsmeister AR: A randomized controlled trial of a probiotic, VSL#3, on gut transit and symptoms in diarrhoea-predominant irritable bowel syndrome. Aliment Pharmacol Ther 2003;17:895–904.

13 O'Sullivan MA, O'Morain CA: Bacterial supplementation in the irritable bowel syndrome. A randomised double-blind placebo-controlled crossover study. Dig Liver Dis 2000;32:294–301.

14 Nobaek S, Johansson ML, Molin G, Ahrne S, Jeppsson B: Alteration of intestinal microflora is associated with reduction in abdominal bloating and pain in patients with irritable bowel syndrome. Am J Gastroenterol 2000;95:1231–1238.

15 Caldarella MP, Serra J, Azpiroz F, Malagelada JR: Prokinetic effects in patients with intestinal gas retention. Gastroenterology 2002;122:1748–1755.

16 Lin HC: Small intestinal bacterial overgrowth: a framework for understanding irritable bowel syndrome. JAMA 2004;292:852–858.

17 Thompson WG, Longstreth GF, Drossman DA, Heaton KW, Irvine EJ, Muller-Lissner SA: Functional bowel disorders and functional abdominal pain. Gut 1999;45(suppl 2):43–47.

18 Levitt MD, Furne J, Olsson S: The relation of passage of gas and abdominal bloating to colonic gas production. Ann Intern Med 1996;124:422–424.

19 Distrutti E, Azpiroz F, Soldevilla A, Malagelada JR: Gastric wall tension determines perception of gastric distension. Gastroenterology 1999;116:1035–1042.

20 Levitt MD, Donaldson RM: Use of respiratory hydrogen (H_2) excretion to detect carbohydrate malabsorption. J Lab Clin Med 1970;75:937–945.

21 Strocchi A, Ellis C, Levitt MD: Reproducibility of measurements of trace gas concentrations in expired air. Gastroenterology 1991;101:175–179.

22 Di Stefano M, Miceli E, Missanelli A, Mazzocchi S, Corazza GR: Hypersensitivity to colonic gas in the pathophysiology of symptoms in functional patients. Gastroenterology 2004;126 (suppl 2):A378.

23 Frissora CL, Koch KL: Symptom overlap and comorbidity of irritable bowel syndrome with other conditions. Curr Gastroenterol Rep 2005;7:264–271.

24 Vernia P, Ricciardi MR, Frandina C, Bilotta T, Frieri G: Lactose malabsorption and irritable bowel syndrome. Effect of a long-term lactose-free diet. Ital J Gastroenterol 1995;27:117–121.

25 Cappello G, Marzio L: Rifaximin in patients with lactose intolerance. Dig Liver Dis 2005; 37:316–319.

26 King CE, Toskes PP: Small intestine bacterial overgrowth. Gastroenterology 1979;76:1035–1055.

27 Banwell JG, Kistler LA, Giannella RA, Weber FL, Lieber A, Powell DE: Small intestinal bacterial overgrowth syndrome. Gastroenterology 1981;80:834–845.

28 Corazza GR, Menozzi MG, Strocchi A, Rasciti L, Vaira D, Lecchini R, Avanzini P, Chezzi C, Gasbarrini G: The diagnosis of small bowel bacterial overgrowth. Gastroenterology 1990;98: 302–309.

29 Nayak AK, Karnad DR, Abraham P, Mistry FP: Metronidazole relieves symptoms in irritable bowel syndrome: the confusion with socalled 'chronic amebiasis'. Indian J Gastroenterol 1997;16:137–139.

30 Pimentel M, Chow EJ, Lin HC: Normalization of lactulose breath testing correlates with symptom improvement in irritable bowel syndrome. A double-blind, randomized, placebo-controlled study. Am J Gastroenterol 2003;98:412–419.

31 Pimentel M, Chow EJ, Lin HC: Eradication of small intestinal bacterial overgrowth reduces symptoms of irritable bowel syndrome. Am J Gastroenterol 2000;95:3503–3506.

32 Sellin JH, Hart R: Glucose malabsorption associated with rapid intestinal transit. Am J Gastroenterol 1992;87:584–589.

33 Lupascu A, Gabrielli M, Lauritano C, Scarpellini E, Santoliquido A, Cammarota G, Flore R, Tondi P, Pola P, Gasbarrini G, Gasbarrini A: Hydrogen glucose breath test to detect small intestinal bacterial overgrowth: a prevalence case-control study in irritable bowel syndrome. Aliment Pharmacol Ther 2005;22:1157–1160.

34 McCallum R, Schultz C, Sostarich S: Evaluating the role of small intestinal bacterial overgrowth in diarrhea predominant irritable bowel syndrome patients using the glucose breath test. Gastroenterology 2005;128(suppl 2):A460.

35 Rumessen JJ, Nordgaard-Andersen I, Gudmand-Hoyer E: Carbohydrate malabsorption: quantification by methane and hydrogen breath tests. Scand J Gastroenterol 1994;29:826–832.

36 Myo-Khin, Bolin TD, Khin-Mar-Oo, Tin-Oo, Kyaw-Hla S, Thein-Myint T: Ineffectiveness of breath methane excretion as a diagnostic test for lactose malabsorption. J Pediatr Gastroenterol Nutr 1999;28:474–479.

37 Corazza GR, Benati G, Strocchi A, Malservisi S, Gasbarrini G: The possible role of breath methane measurement in detecting carbohydrate malabsorption. J Lab Clin Med 1994;124:695–700.

38 Bond JH Jr, Engel RR, Levitt MD: Factors influencing pulmonary methane excretion in man. An indirect method of studying the in situ metabolism of the methane-producing colonic bacteria. J Exp Med 1971;133:572–588.

39 Flourie B, Etanchaud F, Florent C, Pellier P, Bouhnik Y, Rambaud JC: Comparative study of hydrogen and methane production in the human colon using caecal and faecal homogenates. Gut 1990;31:684–685.

40 Levitt MD, Duane WC: Floating stools – flatus versus fat. N Engl J Med 1972;286:973–975.

41 Simrén M, Ringstrom G, Agerforz P, Bjornsson ES, Abrahamsson H, Stotzer PO: Small intestinal bacterial overgrowth is not of major importance in the irritable bowel syndrome. Gastroenterology 2003;124(suppl 1):A163.

42 Di Stefano M, Corazza GR: Treatment of small intestine bacterial overgrowth and related symptoms by rifaximin. Chemotherapy 2005;51(suppl 1):103–109.

43   Kahn IJ, Jeffries GH, Sleisenger MH: Malabsorption in intestinal scleroderma: correction by antibiotics. N Engl J Med 1966;274:1339–1344.
44   Goldstein F, Wirts CW, Kramer S: The relationship of afferent loop stasis and bacterial flora to the production of postgastrectomy steatorrhea. Gastroenterology 1961;40:47–54.
45   Bjorneklett A, Fausa O, Midtvedt T: Bacterial overgrowth in jejunal and ileal disease. Scand J Gastroenterol 1983;18:289–298.
46   Joiner KA, Gorbach SL: Antimicrobial therapy of digestive diseases. Clin Gastroenterol 1979;8:3–35.
47   Bouhnik Y, Alain S, Attar A, Flourie B, Raskine L, Sanson-Le Pors MJ, Rambaud JC: Bacterial population contaminating the upper gut in patients with small intestinal bacterial overgrowth syndrome. Am J Gastroenterol 1999;94:1327–1331.
48   Scarpignato C, Pelosini I: Rifaximin, a poorly absorbed antibiotic: pharmacology and clinical potential. Chemotherapy 2005;51(suppl 1):36–66.
49   Jiang ZD, DuPont HL: Rifaximin: in vitro and in vivo antibacterial activity – a review. Chemotherapy 2005;51(suppl 1):67–72.
50   Di Stefano M, Miceli E, Missanelli A, Mazzocchi S, Corazza GR: Absorbable vs. non-absorbable antibiotics in the treatment of small intestine bacterial overgrowth in patients with blind loop syndrome. Aliment Pharmacol Ther 2005;21:985–992.
51   Gorbach SL, Tabaqchali S: Bacteria, bile and the small bowel. Gut 1969;10:963–972.
52   Goldstein F, Wirts CW, Kowlessar OD: Diabetic diarrhea and steatorrhea. Ann Intern Med 1970;72:215–218.
53   Elsborg L: Malabsorption in small intestinal diverticulosis treated with a low dosage sulphonamide-trimethoprim. Dan Med Bull 1977;24:33–35.
54   Attar A, Flourie B, Rambaud JC, Franchisseur C, Ruszniewski P, Bouhnik Y: Antibiotic efficacy in small intestinal bacterial overgrowth related chronic diarrhea: a crossover, randomized trial. Gastroenterology 1999;117:794–797.
55   Trespi E, Ferrieri A: Intestinal bacterial overgrowth during chronic pancreatitis. Curr Med Res Opin 1999;15:47–52.

Note Added in Proof

While this paper was being submitted, Lauritano et al. [1] did publish a dose-finding study to evaluate the effectiveness of rifaximin in patients with SIBO (based on positivity of glucose breath test). As expected, a dose-dependent eradication rate was observed, with the maximum effect (i.e. 60%) seen at 1,200 mg daily. Prolonging the duration of treatment (from 7 to 10 days) appears to increase the success of therapy [2].

The results of a double-blind, randomized, placebo-controlled study [3] on the rifaximin efficacy in patients with IBS were presented at the recent meeting of the *American College of Gastroenterology* in Honolulu (Hawaii, USA). Antibiotic treatment (1,200 mg daily for 10 days) resulted in a $37.7 \pm 5.8\%$ overall symptom improvement, a figure significantly ($p < 0.05$) higher than that observed with placebo (i.e. $23.4 \pm 4.3\%$). Amongst the patients with diarrhea, rifaximin benefit was seen in 49% of them. These findings overlapping those obtained with neomycin [4] suggest that the use of poorly absorbed antimicrobials is effective and should be preferred to the system ic ones, which can themselves lead to the development of abdominal symptoms, including those of the IBS, as well as other functional symptoms [5]. Whether the use of antibiotics should be followed by a course of probiotics to reconstitute intestinal flora, an approach often adopted in clinical practice, has never been formally assessed.

References

1   Lauritano EC, Gabrielli M, Lupascu A, San-toliquido A, Nucera G, Scarpellini E, Vincenti F, Cammarota G, Flore R, Pola P, Gasbarrini G, Gasbarrini A: Rifaximin dose-finding study for the treatment of small intestinal bacterial overgrowth. Aliment Pharmacol Ther 2005;22:31–35.
2   Di Stefano M, Malservisi S, Veneto G, Ferrieri A, Corazza GR: Rifaximin versus chlortetracycline in the short-term treatment of small intestine bacterial overgrowth. Aliment Pharmacol Ther 2000;14:551–556.
3   Pimentel M, Spark S, Kong Y, Wade R, Kane AV: Rifaximin, a non-absorbable antibiotic, improves symptoms of irritable bowel syndrome: a double-blind randomized controlled study. Am J Gastroenterol 2005;100(suppl):S324.
4   Pimentel M, Chow EJ, Lin HC: Normalization of lactulose breath testing correlates with symptom improvement in irritable bowel syndrome. A double-blind, randomized, placebo-controlled study. Am J Gastroenterol 2003;98:412–419.
5   Barbara G, Stanghellini V, Brandi G, Cremon C, Di Nardo G, De Giorgio R, Corinaldesi R: Interactions between commensal bacteria and gut sensorimotor function in health and disease. Am J Gastroenterol 2005;100:2560–2568.

Gino Roberto Corazza, MD
First Department of Internal Medicine, University of Pavia
IRCCS 'S. Matteo' Hospital, Viale Golgi 19
IT–27100 Pavia (Italy)
Tel. +39 0382 502 973
Fax +39 0382 502 618
E-Mail gr.corazza@smatteo.pv.it

This chapter should be cited as follows:

Corazza GR, Di Stefano M, Scarpignato C: Treatment of Functional Bowel Disorders: Is There Room for Antibiotics? Digestion 2006;73(suppl 1):38–46.

Scarpignato C, Lanas Á (eds): Bacterial Flora in Digestive Disease.
Focus on Rifaximin.

....

Colonic Diverticular Disease: Pathophysiology and Clinical Picture

Adolfo Parra-Blanco

Department of Gastroenterology, Hospital Universitario de Canarias,
Santa Cruz de Tenerife, Spain

Abstract

Colonic diverticulosis is the most frequent structural abnormality of the large bowel, although it was a rarity before the 20th century. Lifestyle changes in westernized societies with reduced fiber diet are supposed to be the main cause for its high prevalence nowadays. In African countries, where staple diet is rich in fiber, diverticulosis remains very infrequent. Prevalence increases with ageing too. A fiber-deficient diet and subsequent reduction in bowel content volume would lead to increased intraluminal pressures and colonic segmentation, thus promoting diverticula formation. Animal and human studies have shown increased intracolonic pressures in patients with diverticulosis. Alterations in colonic muscle properties, collagen metabolism and in the interactions of the extracellular matrix components may play a role in remodelling the gut wall in diverticular disease. At least one fourth of patients with diverticulosis will develop symptoms, sometimes overlapping with irritable bowel syndrome, but 10–25% will suffer diverticulitis and 3–5% diverticular bleeding. Conservative medical management is usually sufficient in the first episode of diverticulitis, but surgical treatment is generally advocated in recurrences. Diverticular bleeding is a major cause of lower digestive haemorrhage, but generally self-limited. With the application of therapeutic endoscopic and angiographic methods, emergency surgery can often be avoided.

Introduction

Colonic diverticulosis is a common disorder in the western world, which refers to acquired herniation of the colonic wall through low resistance sites in areas of vascular passage, producing small outpouchings of the mucosa frequently located in the sigmoid colon. Prevalence of diverticular disease has increased steadily during the 20th century, probably in relation to dietary changes in western societies [1]. During the last decades, different pathophysiological aspects of colonic diverticulosis have been studied, from the epidemiological to the basic research level. The results from those studies have provided a rationale for the currently accepted management of diverticular disease.

Epidemiology

In their seminal report, Painter and Burkitt [1] reviewed the initial descriptions of diverticulosis in the 18th and 19th centuries. Although diverticular disease was almost unknown of the 19th century, by 1920, basic understanding of the disease had been established, and it had become clear that prevalence was increasing [2]. Painter et al. [3] proposed that diets deficient in fiber would elevate intraluminal pressure, leading to segmentation of the colon and finally resulting in diverticulosis. Such diets, associated with developed societies, would be responsible for the striking geographical differences in prevalence of diverticulosis.

It is not possible to define accurately the true prevalence of diverticulosis, as most individuals are asymptomatic. Prevalence of diverticular disease increases with age. Autopsy studies in western countries indicate that over 30% of adults, and over 50% of individuals older than 40 have colonic diverticulosis [4]. The incidence of diverticulosis has risen dramatically during the last century. In 1930 the prevalence among the North American population estimated from barium enema studies was 5–8%, whereas a recent colonoscopy study found extensive distal diverticulosis in 23% of subjects with a mean age of 58.6 years [1, 5]. No overall sex differences have been clearly established although admissions for diverticulitis are more frequent in men in age groups <65 years, whereas in older patients female gender is more frequent [6].

Geographical differences have been recognized both in disease prevalence and in anatomic distribution of diverticula. Although prevalence can reach 50% in older age groups in western societies, it is less than 2% in rural Africa [6]. The prevalence rate in Singapore, a developed Eastern country, as estimated by barium enema, is comparable to that in western countries [7]. Japanese studies provide valuable information about the mechanisms involved in diverticular disease. As this country has changed its traditional diet for a more western-type diet, the prevalence of diverticulosis had increased steadily. One differential aspect between diverticular disease in the West and Asia is the predominant right location in the latter. Miura et al. [8] observed right colon location in 83% of patients, whereas only 17% had lesions located exclusively in the left colon. An autopsy study in Japanese Hawaiians showed high prevalence rates of diverticulosis, which were predominantly located in the right colon [9]. It seems that the adoption of western lifestyles in Asian countries results in a higher prevalence of diverticulosis, which are however located mainly in the right colon. Accordingly, it is thought that both right-sided diverticulosis in Asian countries and left-sided diverticula in western countries are associated with low fiber intake [10]. Therefore – although the cause for diverticular disease may be acquired – racial and congenital factors may control the site of development.

Pathophysiology

The pathophysiology of colonic diverticular disease has not yet been completely understood, but it is believed to involve multifactorial events. The main factors considered to play a role in the development of diverticular disease are dietary factors, colonic motility and structural changes affecting the colonic wall. The pathogenesis of acute diverticulitis and diverticular bleeding will also be briefly reviewed.

Diet
In 1971, Painter and Burkitt [1] hypothesized that colonic diverticulosis is a deficiency disease of western civilization, related to a removal of vegetable fiber from the diet, and therefore preventable in the same way as scurvy. They postulated a relation with the development of diverticulosis through a mechanism of colonic segmentation, which would be responsible for mucosal herniation by generating high intrasegmental pressures. This hypothesis suggests that high-fiber diets result in large volume of faeces and wide colon diameter, with less effective segmentation, decreased intracolonic pressure and reduced risk for developing diverticula. Gear et al. [11] found colonic diverticulosis by barium enema in 12% of vegetarians compared to 33% of non-vegetarians, with a significantly higher fiber intake in the former. This dietary hypothesis has been supported by some studies, but not by all [12–14]. Moreover, animal studies have shown an increased risk for developing diverticulosis in rats fed with a fiber-deficient diet compared to a high-fiber diet (42 *vs.* 0%, respectively) [15]. In another study, maternal high-fiber diet was associated with a decreased risk for diverticulosis in the offsprings [16]. Higher concentrations of short chain fatty acids were found in high-fiber fed rats, although no clear connection with collagen cross-linking could be established.

One report which evaluated a prospective cohort of over 47,000 health professionals found that total dietary fiber intake was inversely associated with the risk of diverticular disease, with a relative risk of 0.58 for men in the highest quintile of dietary fiber [17]. In another study on the same cohort, the insoluble component of fiber was significantly associated with a decreased risk of diverticular disease, and this inverse association was especially strong for cellulose [18].

Table 1. Intraluminal colonic pressure in patients with diverticular disease

	Resting	Post-prandial	Provocative	Symptoms
Painter et al., 1964 [3]	Normal	–	High	–
Arfwidsson, 1964 [21]	High	High	High	–
Parks and Connell, 1969 [27]	High	High	–	–
Attisha and Smith, 1969 [20]	Normal	High	High	–
Sugihara et al., 1983 [23]	High	–	High	Both
Trotman and Misiewicz, 1988 [28]	High	High	–	Symptomatic
Cortesini and Pantalone, 1991 [25]	High	High	–	Differentiates upon symptoms
Christopher et al., 2000 [22]	High	High	–	Asymptomatic

A negative correlation between dietary fiber intake and the incidence of colonic diverticulosis has been observed also for right-sided diverticulosis in Japan [10].

Colonic Motility

Colonic motility features in diverticular disease have been studied and differences in intracolonic pressure have been searched for between normal subjects and those with diverticulosis (table 1). Painter et al. [3, 19] used manometry and simultaneous cineradiography to show that the contraction of the circular muscle produced colonic segmentation with bladder formation. The coincidence of segmentation (obstructing contraction rings) and contraction of the bladder itself resulted in localized high pressure, which then led to diverticula formation. They found a greater increase in intraluminal pressure after injection of provocative agents (morphine or prostigmine) in patients with diverticulosis compared to healthy patients, but no differences were noted in the resting pressure [19]. Other investigators found excessive response to prostigmine but no basal differences with controls, or raised resting and food-provoked intracolonic pressure, and a greater increase after prostigmine injection [20, 21]. Christopher et al. [22] reported in abstract form abnormally strong pressure waves in the diverticular segment compared to adjacent segments or the normal colon, especially after meals and waking up. One Japanese study showed high resting and prostigmine-stimulated intraluminal pressures in right-sided diverticular disease [23].

Although some confusion arises from the results of the available studies, it is generally believed that there is an increased phasic activity that could be related to symptoms rather than to the existence of diverticula [24, 25]. Methodological shortcomings, such as recordings from short segments, for short periods, previous colonic cleansing and others, can account for discrepant results when studying colonic manometry, not only in patients with diverticulosis [24, 26].

Shafik et al. [29] investigated electromyographic activity of the sigmoid and descending colon, and intracolonic pressure, including patients with early or advanced diverticular disease and healthy volunteers. Three patterns of electrical activity were found in patients with diverticulosis: tachyrhythmic (early disease), bradyrhythmic and silent (advanced disease). The authors hypothesize that this abnormal activity may result from an alteration in the colonic pacemaker, and that persistent increased pressure in advanced diverticulosis despite decreased motor activity would be connected to sigmoid colon narrowing due to fibrosis.

Huizinga et al. [30] investigated electric activity from circular and longitudinal muscle tissue from 12 patients who had undergone surgery for diverticular disease. They found changes in electrical activity, with predominance of slow-wave activity and lack of periodic bursts normally associated with propulsive activity. This would favour segmental contractions causing localized high pressures, thus supporting Painter and Burkitt's hypothesis [1].

Increased cholinergic activity has been shown in smooth muscle in diverticular disease (in vitro studies) and it is believed to be related to a dominance of cholinergic nerves [31]. In the same study, nitric oxide appeared to mediate the muscle relaxation reaction in the normal colon and to a lesser extent in the diverticula bearing colon. However, the results from an immunohistochemistry and pharmacological study suggested that in diverticular disease increased cholinergic activity might be related to denervation hypersensitivity, with decreased cholinergic innervation and compensatory upregulation of smooth muscle M_3 receptors [32].

Structural Changes in the Colonic Wall

Both circular and longitudinal muscle in colonic diverticulosis show abnormalities on gross pathological examination. The taeniae coli are enlarged and shortened, a fact often attributed to contraction secondary to elastin deposition, which can be double than in normal subjects [33]. Shortening of the taenia coli produces abnormalities in the circular layer, with resulting shortening and thickening, luminal narrowing, and typical concertina-like appearance. Weakness of the colonic wall could account for the increased prevalence of diverticular disease in western countries compared to African individuals. An autopsy study compared the mechanical properties of colon specimens from the UK (16% with diverticulosis) and Uganda (none of which had diverticula) [34]. The tensile strength was reduced with increasing age in both populations, and the left colon had lower tensile strength and was narrower than the right colon. Specimens from the African population were stronger and wider.

The submucosal layer is composed mainly by collagen fibrils, and plays the most important part in maintaining the integrity and properties of the colonic wall. The viscoelastic properties of elastin and collagen give the colonic wall its stability, strength and maintenance of the shape [15, 16, 34, 35]. Collagen has inter- and intramolecular cross-links that stabilize and give strength to the tissue where it is located, but excessive cross-linking of collagen is believed to lead to rigidity and loss of tensile strength [36]. An autopsy study by Wess et al. [36] showed that – although the total amount of collagen was not elevated in diverticular colon compared to controls – differences in collagen nature with increased cross-linking were noted with increasing age and in diverticular colon, which might cause the rigidity and inflexibility of the colonic wall. Two animal studies from the same group also suggested that fiber content in diet might determine the nature of collagen, and the development of diverticular disease [15, 16]. Bode et al. [37] observed and increased synthesis of type III collagen in diverticulosis, although its significance remains to be elucidated.

Matrix metalloproteinases (MMPs) are a family of zinc-containing endopeptidases capable of degrading extracellular matrix, and are regulated by tissue inhibitors of MMPs (TIMPs). They are involved in normal physiological processes such as morphogenesis, wound healing and tissue remodelling, but they have also been implicated in pathological conditions like rheumatoid arthritis, inflammatory bowel disease, tumour invasion and metastasis [38]. Mimura et al. [39] observed increased collagen content in the mucosal and submucosal layer in both complicated and uncomplicated diverticulosis, and increased expression of TIMP-1 and TIMP-2 in the proper muscle layer in complicated diverticulosis compared to normal subjects. Increased collagen I expression and a decrease in the expression of the collagenase MMP-1 was found in colonic tissue in patients with diverticulitis by immunohistochemistry [40]. Collagen metabolism and interactions of the extracellular matrix components may play a role in remodelling the gut wall in diverticular disease. The mechanisms involved in the formation of diverticula are summarized in figure 1.

Pathogenesis of Diverticulitis

Diverticula may contain particles of faecal matter (fig. 2). Although it was believed that the obstruction of the diverticula by those faecaliths would increase intraluminal pressure and cause perforation, currently it is accepted that it is the abrasion of the mucosa that results in inflammation [41]. Inflammation can be initially low grade and chronic, with associated hyperplasia of lymphoid tissue, and eventually progress to active inflammation in the mucosa (figs. 3 and 4). A small microperforation may occur within the diverticulum forming an abscess, which may remain localized or lead to phlegmon in the surrounding pericolic and mesenteric fat, or involving adjacent organs producing fistula or obstruction,

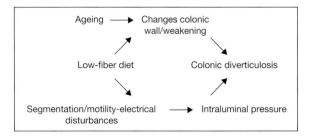

Fig. 1. Pathophysiology of diverticula formation (modified from Mimura et al. [35]).

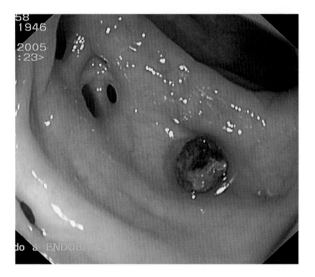

Fig. 2. Diverticula in the sigmoid colon; one of them shows faecal impaction.

or even freely perforate. Rupture of an abscess rather than rupture of an inflamed diverticulum per se is believed to be the most common cause of acute peritonitis [41].

Colonic inflammation in patients with diverticulosis can occur not only in the diverticulum itself, but segmental active sigmoid colitis mimicking Crohn's disease has been reported [41–44]. The cause for Crohn's disease-like changes may be multifactorial, including mucosal redundancy and prolapse with ischaemic phenomena, peridiverticular inflammation, increased exposure to intraluminal antigens and toxins, and bacterial flora changes related to stasis [41, 43]. Nevertheless, this entity is infrequently observed; in one study it was present in 1.3% of the colons resected for diverticulitis [44].

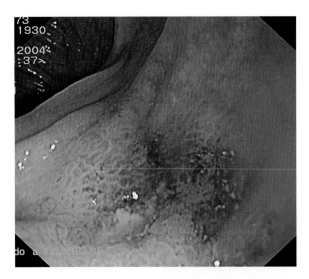

Fig. 3. Endoscopic findings in acute diverticulitis: mucosal erythema and discharge of purulent material.

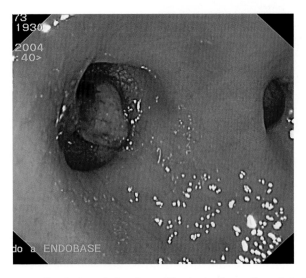

Fig. 4. Granulation tissue (histologically confirmed) inside a diverticulum, indicating post-inflammatory state.

Small intestinal bacterial overgrowth has been shown in acute uncomplicated diverticulitis, which could be secondary at least in part to colonic bacterial overgrowth; it might play a role in the development of symptoms in those patients [45]. The sequence of events leading to acute diverticulitis is summarized in figure 5.

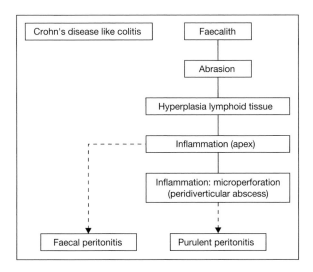

Fig. 5. Pathophysiology of diverticulitis [adapted from 41].

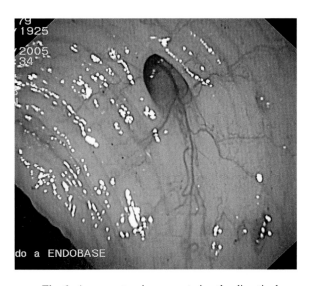

Fig. 6. A *vas rectum* is seen entering the diverticulum.

Pathogenesis of Diverticular Bleeding

As diverticula herniate, the *vasa recta* penetrating through the circular muscle layer are displaced to the dome of the diverticulum where they are exposed to injury in the luminal aspect (fig. 6). Meyers et al. [46] performed a pathological study of colons resected for bleeding, in which the bleeding site had been

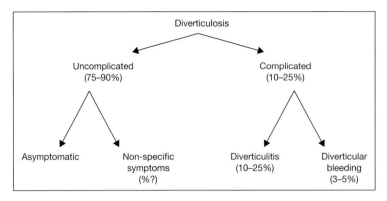

Fig. 7. Possible clinical status in patients with colonic diverticulosis.

identified. In all cases the cause was rupture of the vasa recta with ulceration of the overlying mucosa, which had occurred in 75% of cases at the dome, and in the remaining cases at the margin near the neck. The vasa recta showed structural abnormalities both at and near the site of rupture, such as eccentric fibromuscular intimal thickening and thinning of the media layer. However, acute or chronic diverticulitis was not present. In more than 50% of diverticular bleeding cases requiring surgery, the lesion is right-sided [46, 47]. This could be due to the wider necks and domes of right-sided diverticula, with vasa recta exposed to injury over a greater length [43]. Non-steroidal anti-inflammatory drugs may be an important risk factor for diverticular bleeding [47, 48].

Clinical Picture

The spectrum of the clinical picture of diverticulosis is summarized in figure 7.

Uncomplicated Diverticulosis
Colonic diverticulosis is a highly prevalent condition in western societies, but 75–80% of patients with anatomical diverticulosis will never develop symptoms [49–51]. Asymptomatic patients are diagnosed during examinations carried out for another reason, or with increasing frequency during colonoscopy for colorectal cancer screening [6]. Although such individuals do not require any further diagnostic evaluation, it is reasonable to recommend a high-fiber diet [51]. A significant inverse association has been observed between insoluble fiber intake and the risk of developing symptomatic diverticulosis [18].

A proportion of patients with diverticulosis report recurrent colicky abdominal pain, and/or changed bowel habits without any findings consistent with diverticulitis, which has been called uncomplicated symptomatic diverticulosis. Bouts of abdominal pain in these patients may be related to abnormal colon motility. In a controlled study, episodes of cramping abdominal pain were coincident with a regular colonic contractile pattern, as assessed by 24-hour colonic manometry [52].

Considering the high prevalence of irritable bowel syndrome (IBS) (5–25%) and diverticulosis (10–66%), both conditions may coexist frequently [51, 53]. One study showed heightened visceral perception of rectosigmoid perception (and not only in the area with diverticula), not due to altered compliance of the bowel wall [54]. This situation of hyperperception resembles IBS. In a community-based survey, Simpson et al. [55] studied 261 patients with diverticulosis diagnosed by barium enema, and observed that 14% met the Rome I criteria for IBS, 36% had recurrent short-lived pain, and 19% had episodes of prolonged pain lasting for 1 day or longer, which in more than 60% required emergency medical attention. In greater than half of the patients with prolonged pain, there was also short-lived pain as part of their usual bowel habit. The authors concluded that recurrent short-lived pain (similar to that seen in IBS) often occurs in patients who have experienced prolonged pain attributable to diverticulitis. However, the presence of colonic diverticula does not seem to change the natural history of IBS [53]. The connection and/or differences between uncomplicated symptomatic diverticulosis and IBS should be further clarified in future studies.

A high-fiber diet is recommended for patients with symptomatic uncomplicated diverticulosis [51]. Although there is theoretically no rationale for the use of antibiotics in this group of patients, two Italian randomized trials comparing daily fiber supplementation alone or with cyclic administration of oral rifaximin for 12 months showed that significantly more patients in the rifaximin group were free of symptoms, and in one of the studies the incidence of complications (mainly diverticulitis) was also reduced [56, 57]. Although the mechanism for such improvement is unknown, the authors postulate that it could be related to a reduction in gas production and in bacterial overgrowth.

Diverticulitis

Between 10 and 25% of the patients with known diverticular disease suffer diverticulitis [58]. A grading system was developed by Hinchey et al. [59], including four stages: stage I confined pericolic abscess, stage II distant abscess, stage III generalized purulent peritonitis by rupture of a pericolic or pelvic abscess, and stage IV faecal peritonitis with free perforation of a diverticulum. Left lower quadrant pain is almost universal in sigmoid diverticulitis except for immunocompromised patients, whereas right-sided diverticula present symptoms suggestive of acute appendicitis with right-quadrant pain. Constipation takes place in 43–60% of the cases by entrapment of small bowel loops in the inflammatory process, in case of peritoneal irritation, or in the presence of colonic stenosis [41]. Fever is common in patients suffering from diverticulitis, but hypotension and shock are rare and generally found in more severe cases. Perforation into an adjacent organ can lead to the formation of fistulae. In one study from the Cleveland Clinic, 65, 25 and 6% of all internal fistulas were colovesical, colovaginal and coloenteric, respectively [60]. After recurrent episodes of diverticulitis, strictures may develop, presenting usually with insidious symptoms but sometimes as an obstruction. Surgery is the treatment of choice, and endoscopic management may be attempted only for selected cases unfit for surgery [61]. Klein et al. [62] reported three cases with extraintestinal manifestations typical of inflammatory bowel disease (arthritis and pyoderma gangrenosum) unresponsive to medical treatment, which resolved after surgical resection for diverticulitis.

About 75% of cases correspond to 'non-complicated' diverticulitis (stage I), which usually respond to conservative treatment. In the remaining cases surgery is advocated.

In 25–30% of the cases, symptoms of diverticulitis will recur after a first episode. Therefore, elective resection is generally recommended after two well-documented episodes of diverticulitis [51, 63–65]. Immunocompromised patients have a higher risk of complicated disease and surgery might be indicated after one single attack [64]. In younger patients (<40 years) the first attack is usually more severe, requiring surgery more frequently, and the risk for recurrence after initial response to conservative treatment is also increased [66, 67]. Resection after the first episode of diverticulitis can be considered in young patients, although evidence from controlled studies is lacking and the natural history of diverticulitis in young patients is not clearly defined [51, 63, 65].

Diverticular Bleeding

Significant bleeding occurs in 3–5% of patients with diverticulosis and accounts for approximately 40% of lower haemorrhage episodes [68–70]. Rectal bleeding should not be attributed to diverticula until other sources of bleeding have been ruled out (especially vascular lesions and neoplasms). Diverticular bleeding remains the major cause for acute lower bleeding in most series, followed by angiodysplasia, although these results may vary depending on the criteria employed to define the bleeding episode [70]. Bleeding ceases spontaneously in 75–80% of the patients, out of whom 25–35% will present rebleeding [69, 70]. The diagnosis of definite diverticular bleeding requires the recognition of bleeding stigmata [71] (figs. 8, 9). Most case series report

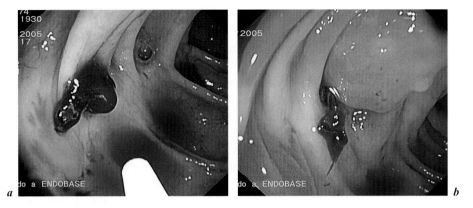

Fig. 8. Adherent clot attached to diverticulum in a patient with acute lower gastro-intestinal bleeding before (*a*) and after (*b*) 1:10,000 epinephrine injection.

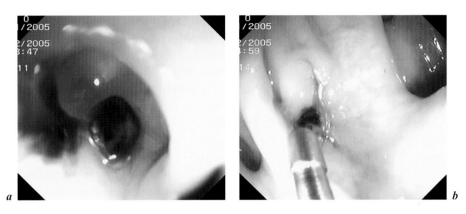

Fig. 9. *a* Red protuberance at the bottom of a diverticulum. *b* One Hemoclip is applied after injection of 1:10,000 epinephrine solution.

successful endoscopic haemostasis in patients with stigmata of bleeding [70–72]. In one study by Jensen et al. [71], 22% of patients with lower haemorrhage had diverticula with bleeding stigmata. Bleeding recurred in 53% of patients treated medically, one-third of which required emergency surgery. However, no early or delayed recurrence (after a median follow-up of 2 years) took place in the patients who underwent endoscopic haemostatic treatment with epinephrine injection and/or bipolar coagulation, a statistically significant difference. However in another study, 38% of the patients experienced recurrent bleeding after endoscopic haemostasis [73]. Endoscopic treatment may modify the natural history of diverticular bleeding by preventing recurrences, but its role has to be further clarified in larger studies with longer follow-up periods. In the hands of an expert interventional radiologist, superselective microcoil embolization achieved successful haemostasis in 81% of cases of acute lower haemorrhage, most of which corresponded to diverticular bleeding [74]. In cases of persisting or recurrent bleeding despite colonoscopic and/or angiographic treatment, all reasonable efforts are justified in order to localize the bleeding lesion preoperatively, as the outcome of blind colectomy in the situation of massive bleeding is dismal. In a case review study made on patients who underwent emergency total colectomies for unknown bleeding sites, 57% developed peritonitis and 29% died [75].

Conclusions and Perspectives for the Future

Diverticular disease of the colon covers a wide clinical spectrum: from an incidental finding to symptomatic uncomplicated disease to diverticulitis. A quarter of patients with diverticulitis will develop potentially life-threatening complications including perforation, fistulae, obstruction or stricture. In Western countries, diverticular disease predominantly affects the left colon, its prevalence increases with age and its causation has been linked to a low dietary fiber intake. Right-sided diverticular disease is more commonly seen in Asian populations and affects younger patients. Pathogenesis of the disease remains unclear. However, it is the result of complex interactions between colonic structure, intestinal motility, diet and genetic factors.

Why symptoms develop is still unclear. Results of recent experimental studies on IBS suggest that low-grade inflammation of colonic mucosa, induced by changes in bacterial microflora, could affect the enteric nervous system, which is crucial for normal gut function, thus favoring symptom development. This hypothesis could be extrapolated also for diverticular disease, since bacterial overgrowth is present, at least in a considerable proportion of patients [76].

Diverticular disease of the colon is a significant cause of morbidity and mortality in the Western world and its frequency has increased throughout the whole of the 20th century. As our elderly population continues to grow, a concomitant rise can be anticipated in the number of patients with diverticular disease, who will absorb an increasing portion of our gastroenterological and surgical workload.

Diagnosis is primarily by barium enema and colonoscopy, but more sophisticated imaging procedures such as high-resolution ultrasound [77] and computed tomography [78] are increasingly being used to assess and treat complications such as abscess or fistula, or to provide alternative diagnoses if diverticulosis is not confirmed.

Acknowledgements

Adolfo Parra-Blanco is supported in part by a grant from the Instituto de Salud Carlos III (C03/02) and by a grant from Fundación Canaria de Investigación (P21/02), Canary Islands, Spain.

References

1   Painter NS, Burkitt D: Diverticular disease of the colon: a deficiency disease of western civilization. Br Med J 1971;ii:450–454.
2   Schoetz DJ: Diverticular disease of the colon: a century-old problem. Dis Colon Rectum 1999;42:703–709.
3   Painter NS, Truelove SC, Ardran GM, Tuckey M: Segmentation and the localization of intraluminal pressures in the human colon, with special reference to the pathogenesis of colonic diverticula. Gastroenterology 1965;49:169–177.
4   Hugues LE: Post-mortem survey of diverticular disease in the colon. I. Diverticulosis and diverticulitis. Gut 1969;10:336–344.
5   Kieff BJ, Eckert GJ, Imperiale TF: Is diverticulosis associated with colorectal neoplasia? A cross-sectional colonoscopic study. Am J Gastroenterol 2004;10:2007–2011.
6   Jun S, Stollman N: Epidemiology of diverticular disease. Best Pract Res Clin Gastroenterol 2002; 16:529–542.
7   Chia JG, Wilde CC, Ngoi SS, Goh PM, Ong CL: Trends of diverticular disease of the large bowel in a newly developed country. Dis Colon Rectum 1991;34:498–501.
8   Miura S, Kodaira S, Shatari T, Nishioka M, Hosoda Y, Hisa K: Recent trends in diverticulosis of the right colon in Japan: retrospective review in a regional hospital. Dis Colon Rectum 2000;43: 1383–1389.
9   Stemmermann GN, Yatani R: Diverticulosis and polyps of the large intestine: a necropsy study of Hawaii Japanese. Cancer 1973;31:1260–1270.
10 Nakaji S, Danjo K, Munakata A, Sugawara K, MacAuley D, Kernohan G, Baxter D: Comparison of etiology of right-sided diverticula in Japan with that of left-sided diverticula in the West. Int J Colorectal Dis 2002;17:365–373.
11 Gear JSS, Fursdon P, Nolan DJ, Ware A, Mann JI, Brodribb AJM: Symptomless diverticular disease and intake of dietary fibre. Lancet 1979;i:511–514.
12 Taylor I, Duthue HL: Bran tablets and diverticular disease. Br Med J 1976;i:988–990.
13 Brodribb AJM: Treatment of symptomatic diverticular disease with a high-fibre diet. Lancet 1977;i:664–666.
14 Ornstein MH, Littlewood ER, McLean Baird I, Fowler J, North WRS, Cox AG: Are fibre supplements really necessary in diverticular disease in the colon? A controlled clinical trial. Br Med J 1981;282:1353–1356.
15 Wess L, Eastwood MA, Edwards CA, Busuttil CA, Miller A: Collagen alteration in an animal model of colonic diverticulosis. Gut 1996;38:701–706.
16 Wess L, Eastwood M, Busuttil A, Edwards C, Miller A: An association between maternal diet and colonic diverticulosis in an animal model. Gut 1996;39:423–427.
17 Aldoori WH, Giovanucci EL, Rimm EB, Wing AL, Trichopoulos DV, Willet WC: A prospective study of diet and the risk of symptomatic diverticular disease in men. Am J Clin Nutr 1994;60: 757–764.

18   Aldoori WH, Giovanuci EL, Rockett HR, Sampson L, Rimm EB, Willett WC: A prospective study of dietary fibre types and symptomatic diverticular disease in men. J Nutr 1998;128:714–719.

19   Painter NS, Truelove SC: The intraluminal pressure patterns in diverticulosis of the colon. Gut 1964;5:365–369.

20   Attisha RP, Smith AN: Pressure activity of the colon and rectum in diverticular disease before and after sigmoid myotomy. Br J Surg 1969;56:891–894.

21   Arfwidsson S: Pathogenesis of multiple diverticula of the sigmoid colon in diverticular disease. Acta Chir Scand 1964;342(suppl):1–68.

22   Christopher K, Sadeghi P, Rao S: Investigation of the pathophysiology of diverticular disease. Gastroenterology 2000;118:A833.

23   Sugihara K, Muto T, Morioka Y: Motility study in right sided diverticular disease of the colon. Gut 1983;24:1130–1134.

24   Simpson J, Scholefield JH, Spiller RC: Pathogenesis of colonic diverticula. Br J Surg 2002; 89:546–554.

25   Cortesini C, Pantalone D: Usefulness of colonic motility studies in identifying patients at risk for complicated diverticular disease. Dis Colon Rectum 1991;34:339–342.

26   Rao SS, Sadeghi P, Beaty J, Kavlock R, Ackerson K: Ambulatory 24-hour colonic manometry in healthy humans. Am J Physiol 2001;280:G629–G639.

27   Parks T, Connell A: Motility studies in diverticular disease of the colon. Gut 1969;10:538–542.

28   Trotman IF, Misiewicz JJ: Sigmoid motility in diverticular disease and the irritable bowel syndrome. Gut 1988;29:218–222.

29   Shafik A, Ahmed I, Shafik AA, El Sibai O: Diverticular disease: electrophysiologic study and a new concept of pathogenesis. World J Surg 2004;28:411–415.

30   Huizinga JD, Waterfall WE, Stern HS: Abnormal response to cholinergic stimulation in the circular muscle layer of the human colon in diverticular disease. Scand J Gastroenterol 1999;34: 683–688.

31   Tomita R, Fujisaki S, Tanjoh K, Fukuzawa M: Role of nitric oxide in the left-sided colon of patients with diverticular disease. Hepatogastroenterology 2000;33:692–696.

32   Golder M, Burleigh DE, Belai A, Ghali L, Ashby D, Lunniss P, Navsaria HA, Williams NS: Smooth muscle cholinergic denervation hypersensitivity in diverticular disease. Lancet 2003; 361:1945–1951.

33   Whiteway J, Morson BC: Elastosis in diverticular disease of the sigmoid colon. Gut 1985; 26:258–266.

34   Watters D, Smith A, Eastwood MA, Anderson KC, Elton RA, Mugerwa JW: Mechanical properties of the colon: comparison of the features of the African and European colon in vitro. Gut 1985;26:384–392.

35   Mimura T, Emanuel A, Kamm M: Pathophysiology of diverticular disease. Best Pract Res Clin Gastroenterol 2002;16:563–576.

36   Wess L, Eastwood MA, Wee TJ, Busuttil CA, Miller A: Cross-linking of collagen is increased in colonic diverticulosis. Gut 1995;37:91–94.

37   Bode MK, Karttunen TJ, Mäkelä J, Risteli L, Risteli J: Type I and III collagens in human colon cancer and diverticulosis. Scand J Gastroenterol 2000;35:747–752.

38   Medina C, Santana A, Quintero E, Radomski MW, Guarner F: Matrix metalloproteinases in diseases of the gastrointestinal tract (in Spanish). Gastroenterol Hepatol 2004;27:491–497.

39   Mimura T, Bateman AC, Lee EL, Johnson PA, McDonnald PJ, Talbot IC, Kamm MA, MacDonnald TT, Pender SLF: Up-regulation of collagen and tissue inhibitors of matrix metalloproteinase in colonic diverticular disease. Dis Colon Rectum 2004;47:371–379.

40   Stumpf M, Cao W, Klinge U, Klosterhalfen B, Kasperk R, Schumpelick V: Increased distribution of collagen III and reduced expression of matrix metalloproteinase-1 in patients with diverticular disease. Int J Colorectal Dis 2001;16:271–275.

41   Ludeman L, Warren BF, Shepherd N: The pathology of diverticular disease. Best Pract Res Clin Gastroenterol 2002;16:543–562.

42   Goldstein NS, Leon-Armin C, Mani A: Crohn's colitis-like changes in sigmoid diverticulitis specimens is usually an idiosyncratic inflammatory response to the diverticulosis rather than Crohn's colitis. Am J Surg Pathol 2000;24:668–675.

43   Peppercorn MA: The overlap of inflammatory bowel disease and diverticular disease. J Clin Gastroenterol 2004;38:S8–S10.
44   Makapugay LM, Dean PJ: Diverticular disease-associated chronic colitis. Am J Surg Pathol 1996;20:94–102.
45   Tursi A, Brandimarte G, Giorgetti GM, Elisei W: Assessment of small intestinal bacterial overgrowth in uncomplicated acute diverticulitis of the colon. World J Gastroenterol 2005;11: 2773–2776.
46   Meyers MA, Alonso DR, Gray GF, Baer JW: Pathogenesis of bleeding colonic diverticulosis. Gastroenterology 1976;71:577–583.
47   Foutch G: Diverticular bleeding: Are non-steroidal anti-inflammatory drugs risk factors of hemorrhage and can colonoscopy predict outcome for patients? Am J Gastroenterol 1995; 90:1780–1784.
48   Lanas A, Sekar MC, Hirschowitz BI: Objective evidence of aspirin use in both ulcer and non-ulcer upper and lower gastrointestinal bleeding. Gastroenterology 1992;103:862–869.
49   Almy TP, Howell DA: Diverticular disease of the colon. N Engl J Med 1980;302:324–331.
50   Stollman N, Raskin J: Diverticular disease of the colon. Lancet 2004;363:631–639.
51   Stollman NH, Raskin JB: Diagnosis and management of diverticular disease of the colon in adults. Ad Hoc Practice Parameters Committee of the American College of Gastroenterology. Am J Gastroenterol 1999;94:3110–3121.
52   Bassotti G, Battaglia E, De Roberto G, Morelli A, Tonini M, Villanacci V: Alterations in colonic motility and relationship to pain in colonic diverticulosis. Clin Gastroenterol Hepatol 2005;3:248–253.
53   Otte JJ, Larsen L, Andersen JR: Irritable bowel syndrome and symptomatic diverticular disease – different diseases? Am J Gastroenterol 1986;81:529–531.
54   Clemens CHM, Samsom M, Roelofs J, van Berge Henegouwen GP, Smout AJPM: Colorectal visceral perception in diverticular disease. Gut 2004;53:717–722.
55   Simpson J, Neal KR, Scholefield JH, Spiller RC: Patterns of pain in diverticular disease and the influence of acute diverticulitis. Eur J Gastroenterol Hepatol 2003;15:1005–1010.
56   Latella G, Pimpo MT, Sottili S, Zippi M, Viscido A, Chiaramonte M, Frieri G: Rifaximin improves symptoms of acquired uncomplicated diverticular disease of the colon. Int J Colorectal Dis 2003;18:55–62.
57   Papi C, Ciaco A, Koch M, Capurso L: Efficacy of rifaximin in the treatment of symptomatic diverticular disease of the colon. A multicentre double-blind placebo-controlled trial. Aliment Pharmacol Ther 1995;9:33–39.
58   Parks TG: Natural history of diverticular disease of the colon. A review of 521 cases. Br Med J 1969;iv:639–645.
59   Hinchey EJ, Schaal PH, Richards MB: Treatment of perforated diverticular disease of the colon. Adv Surg 1978;12:85–109.
60   Woods RJ, Lavery IC, Fazio VW, Jagelman DG, Weakley FL: Internal fistulas in diverticular disease. Dis Colon Rectum 1988;31:591–596.
61   Halligan S, Saunders B: Imaging diverticular disease. Best Pract Res Clin Gastroenterol 2002;16:595–610.
62   Klein S, Mayer L, Present DH, Youner KD, Cerulli MA, Sachar DB: Extraintestinal manifestations in patients with diverticulitis. Ann Intern Med 1988;108:700–702.
63   Roberts P, Abel M, Rosen L, Cirocco W, Fleshman J, Leff E, Levien D, Pritchard T, Wexner S, Hicks T, Kennedy H, Oliver G, Reznick R, Robeertson W, Ross T, Rothenberger D, Senatore P, Surrell J, Wong D: Practice parameters for sigmoid diverticulitis. The Standards Task Force American Society of Colon and Rectal Surgeons. Dis Colon Rectum 1995;38:125–132.
64   Schoetz DJ: Uncomplicated diverticulitis: indications for surgery and surgical management. Surg Clin N Am 1993;73:965–974.
65   Aydin HN, Remzi FH: Diverticulitis: when and how to operate? Dig Liver Dis 2004;36:435–445.
66   Spivak H, Weinrauch S, Harvey J, Surick B, Ferstenberg H, Friedman I: Acute diverticulitis in the young. Dis Colon Rectum 1997;40:570–574.
67   Ambrosetti P, Robert JH, Witzig JA, Mirescu D, Mathey P, Borst F, Rohner A: Acute left colonic diverticulitis: a prospective analysis of 226 consecutive cases. Surgery 1994;115:546–550.

68 Lingenfelser T, Ell C: Lower intestinal bleeding. Best Pract Res Clin Gastroenterol 2001;15: 135–153.
69 McGuire HH, Haynes BW: Massive hemorrhage from diverticulosis of the colon. Guidelines for therapy based on bleeding patterns observed in fifty cases. Ann Surg 1972;175: 847–853.
70 Elta G: Urgent colonoscopy for acute lower gastrointestinal bleeding. Gastrointest Endosc 2004;59:402–408.
71 Jensen DM, Machicado GA, Jutabha R, Kovacs TO: Urgent colonoscopy for the diagnosis and treatment of severe diverticular hemorrhage. N Engl J Med 2000;342:78–82.
72 Foutch PG, Zimmermann K: Diverticular bleeding and the pigmented protuberance (sentinel clot): clinical implications, histopathological correlation, and results of endoscopic intervention. Am J Gastroenterol 1996;91:2589–2593.
73 Bloomfeld RS, Rockey DC, Shetzline MA: Endoscopic therapy of acute diverticular hemorrhage. Am J Gastroenterol 2001;96:2367–2372.
74 Funaki B, Kostelic JK, Lorenz J, Van Ha T, Yip DL, Rosenblum JD, Leef JA, Straus C, Zaleski GX: Superselective microcoil embolization of colonic haemorrhage. Am J Roentgenol 2001;177: 829–836.
75 McGuire HH: Bleeding colonic diverticula. A reappraisal of natural history and management. Ann Surg 1994;220:653–656.
76 Colecchia A, Sandri L, Capodicasa S, Vestito A, Mazzella G, Staniscia T, Roda E, Festi D: Diverticular disease of the colon: new perspectives in symptom development and treatment. World J Gastroenterol 2003;9:1385–1389.
77 Vijayaraghavan SB: High-resolution sonographic spectrum of diverticulosis, diverticulitis, and their complications. J Ultrasound Med 2006;25:75–85.
78 Lawrimore T, Rhea JT: Computed tomography evaluation of diverticulitis. J Intensive Care Med 2004;19:194–204.

Adolfo Parra-Blanco, MD, PhD
Department of Gastroenterology, Hospital Universitario de Canarias
Ofra s/n, La Laguna
ES–38320 Santa Cruz de Tenerife (Spain)
Tel. +34 922 678 039, Fax +34 922 678 554, E-Mail parrablanco@hotmail.com

This chapter should be cited as follows:

Parra-Blanco A: Colonic Diverticular Disease: Pathophysiology and Clinical Picture. Digestion 2006;73(suppl 1):47–57.

Scarpignato C, Lanas Á (eds): Bacterial Flora in Digestive Disease.
Focus on Rifaximin.

······················

Management of Colonic Diverticular Disease

Giuseppe Frieri[a], Maria Teresa Pimpo[a], Carmelo Scarpignato[b]

[a]Gastroenterology Unit, School of Medicine and Dentistry, University of L'Aquila,
L'Aquila, [b]Laboratory of Clinical Pharmacology, Department of Anatomy,
Pharmacology and Forensic Sciences, University of Parma, Parma, Italy

Abstract

Diverticular disease of the colon is a complex syndrome that includes several clinical conditions, each needing different therapeutic strategies. In patients with asymptomatic diverticulosis, only a fiber-rich diet can be recommended in an attempt to reduce intraluminal pressure and slow down the worsening of the disease. Fiber supplementation is also indicated in symptomatic diverticulosis in order to get symptom relief and prevent acute diverticulitis. In this regard, the best results have been obtained by combination of soluble fiber, like glucomannan, and poorly absorbed antibiotics, like rifaximin, given 7–10 days every month. For uncomplicated diverticulitis the standard therapy is liquid diet and oral antimicrobials, usually ciprofloxacin and metronidazole. Hospitalization, bowel rest, and intravenous antibacterial agents are mandatory for complicated diverticulitis. Haemorrhage is usually a self-limited event but may require endoscopic or surgical treatment. Once in remission, continuous fiber intake and intermittent course of rifaximin may improve symptoms and reduce diverticulitis recurrence. These preventive strategies will likely improve patients' quality of life and reduce management costs. A surgical approach in diverticular disease is needed in 15–30% of cases and consists of removing the intestinal segment affected by diverticula. It is indicated in diffuse peritonitis, abscesses, fistulas, stenosis and after the second to fourth attack of uncomplicated diverticulitis. Young people and immunocompromised patients are more likely to be operated.

The presence of diverticula in the sigmoid colon, even in absence of symptoms, represents the result of long-lasting increased intraluminal pressure. In fact, pathophysiological studies have demonstrated that a higher than normal colonic luminal pressure, together with a longer intestinal transit time and a smaller stool volume, predisposes first to diverticular herniation and then to diverticular inflammation and complication [1–3].

Asymptomatic Diverticular Disease

In patients with asymptomatic diverticulosis, a treatment aimed to reduce intraluminal pressure and colonic transit time could theoretically be useful in order to prevent worsening of the disease and, consequently, reduce the risk of complications. In this regard, the most frequent recommendation to these patients is to adopt a diet rich in fiber (vegetables and fruits) whose intake accelerates the transit of colonic contents and reduces intraluminal pressure. In fact, population studies have shown that individuals eating a refined western diet low in fiber (and rich in fat), have colonic transit times of approximately 80 h, and mean stool weights of about 110 g/day, whilst the rural Ugandans, eating very high-fiber diets, have a significantly shorter transit times (about 34 h), and stool weights >450 g/day [4–6].

In patients with asymptomatic diverticulosis, the greatest benefits in preventing the diverticular inflammation are seen in those individuals consuming an average of 32 g/day of total fiber as demonstrated in a prospective study following 51,529 US males over a 6-year period [7]. A significant inverse association between insoluble dietary fiber intake (especially fruit and vegetable) and the risk of subsequent development of symptomatic diverticular disease (relative risk = 0.63, 95% CI 0.44–0.91) does exist. It should be noted that gas production from fiber metabolism may limit acceptance. This is particularly true for bran [8] and other insoluble fibers. On the contrary, soluble fibers (psyllium, ispaghula, calcium polycarbophil, glucomannan) appear to be better tolerated and accepted [9].

Symptomatic Diverticular Disease

Patients can present with non-specific abdominal complaints, e.g. lower abdominal pain, usually left-sided, and subsequently be shown to have diverticulosis coli; a causal relation is sometimes difficult to establish. Such patients do not usually manifest signs of inflammation, such as fever or increased white blood cell count, which could indicate diverticulitis. Pain is generally exacerbated by eating and diminished with defecation or flatus, which suggests colonic wall tension due to raised intraluminal pressure [10]. Patients might also report other symptoms such as bloating or alteration in bowel habit, which overlap those seen in irritable bowel syndrome [11].

The aim of treatment is of course to reduce the frequency and severity of diverticular-related symptoms and prevent the complications. Fibers, antispasmodics and poorly absorbed antimicrobials are generally used in this clinical setting.

Fibers

Several uncontrolled studies have suggested a good effect of a fiber-rich diet in patients with intestinal symptoms and diverticulosis. The first randomized, double-blind, placebo-controlled trial of a high-fiber diet in patients with symptomatic diverticular disease has shown – after 3 months of fiber intake – a statistically significant decrease in bowel symptoms in all the 18 patients studied [12]. However, these favourable results have not been confirmed in a large controlled study where patients were treated with wheat bran (24 g/day) for up to 4 months [13].

Although epidemiological data and pathogenic mechanisms strongly suggest that some symptom relief can be expected in patients with uncomplicated disease on a high-fiber diet, results from clinical trials have so far been conflicting. In any case, historically, food containing large pieces of fiber (such as nuts, corn, seeds) has been excluded from such diets due to the fear that they might become entrapped in diverticula; however, controlled studies that support this belief are lacking. Furthermore, there are no data to support a role for any specific 'elimination' diet in this disorder.

Antispasmodics

The documented hypermotility of the colon in diverticular disease suggests that anticholinergic and antispasmodic agents may improve symptoms by inducing muscle relaxation. However, randomized controlled trials failed to clearly document the efficacy of these agents [14]. Intravenous glucagon has been reported in one study to offer short-term relief of pain [15], most likely thanks to its muscle-relaxing activity.

Poorly Absorbed Antimicrobials

Some observations suggest a possible role of gut microflora in determining symptoms related to diverticular disease. Indeed, bacterial metabolism is the major source of intestinal gas such as H_2, CO_2 and CH_4 via carbohydrate fermentation [16]. Excessive production of bowel gas can play a role in determining abdominal symptoms such as bloating, pain and discomfort [17]. Antimicrobial drugs have been shown to reduce colonic H_2 production [18,19] and gas-related symptoms [20, 21]. In addition, antimicrobial therapy causes a rise in mean stool weight in subjects on a constant fiber intake, most likely because of a reduced fiber degradation consequent to the decline in bacterial population [22]. Both these findings represent a rationale for antibiotic use in diverticular disease. The reduction in gas production and the increase of faecal mass both reduce the intraluminal pressure thus improving symptoms and decreasing the enlargement and stretching of diverticula as well as the generation of new diverticula [14]. Nevertheless, the use of antibiotics in uncomplicated diverticular disease without signs of inflammation is still debated. In a pilot multicentre open trial, 217 patients with symptomatic uncomplicated diverticular disease were treated with glucomannan (a soluble fiber) 2 g/day or with glucomannan plus rifaximin (a poorly absorbed antibiotic with a wide spectrum of antibacterial activity [24]) 400 mg twice a day for 7 days each month [25] (table 1). Clinical evaluation was performed at admission and at 2-month intervals for 12 months. At the end of the study period, 58% of patients treated with rifaximin and glucomannan were symptom-free compared to 24% of patients treated with glucomannan only (p < 0.001). Similar results were obtained in a large prospective open trial including 968 outpatients with symptomatic diverticular disease (table 1) [26]. Patients were randomly assigned to receive fiber supplementation (glucomannan 4 g/day) or fiber supplementation plus rifaximin (400 mg twice a day for 7 days every month) for 12 months. At the end of the study, 56.5% of patients in the rifaximin group were symptom-free compared to 29.2% of patients in the fiber supplementation group (p < 0.001) (fig. 1). These results have also been confirmed by a multicentre double-blind placebo-controlled trial conducted on 168 patients with symptomatic uncomplicated diverticular disease (table 1) [27]. In this study the patients were randomly assigned to receive fiber supplementation (glucomannan 2 g/day) plus rifaximin (400 mg twice a day for 7 days every month for 12 months), or fiber supplementation plus placebo. Patients treated with rifaximin showed a significantly greater reduction in the symptom score compared to patients treated with placebo with an expected therapeutic gain of approximately 30% compared to fiber supplementation alone after 1 year of treatment.

Further support to rifaximin use in diverticular disease comes from a recent study [28] showing that rifaximin achieved a good symptomatic response also without supplementation of dietary fiber. Patients were only advised to follow a high-fiber diet. In the same study, rifaximin was compared with mesalazine, an anti-inflammatory compound widely used in the treatment of inflammatory bowel disease, which showed comparable efficacy. As expected, addition of mesalazine to rifaximin did exert a synergistic effect [29], most likely because the two drugs target different pathophysiological abnormalities (namely enteric bacteria and mucosal inflammation). It is however worth mentioning that rifamycins display a *topical* anti-inflammatory activity [24], which could – in addition to the antimicrobial one – be useful in this clinical condition.

Uncomplicated Diverticulitis

Need for admission is the initial decision to be made in uncomplicated diverticulitis, which is based on patient's presentation, their ability to tolerate

Table 1. Studies addressing rifaximin in the treatment of symptomatic diverticular disease

Study	Patients	Study design	Treatment	Study period, months	Asymptomatic patients, %	RD, % (95% CI)	Complications, %	RD, % (95% CI)
Papi et al. 1992 [25]	217	Open	Glucomannan 2 g	12	24	34.3	2.7	−1.8
			Glucomannan 2 g + rifaximin[1]		58	(22.0–46.5)	0.9	(−5.3 to 1.7)
Latella et al. 2003 [26]	968	Open	Glucomannan 4 g	12	29	27.0	3.3	−1.8
			Glucomannan 4 g + rifaximin[1]		56	(20.9–33.1)	1.3	(−3.8 to 0.1)
Papi et al.	168	Double-blind	Glucomannan 2 g + placebo	12	39	29.7	2.3	0
			Glucomannan 2 g + rifaximin[1]	12	69	(15.3–44.1)	2.3	(−4.6 to 4.6)

RD = Rate difference.
[1]Rifaximin 400 mg b.i.d. for 7 days each month for 12 months.

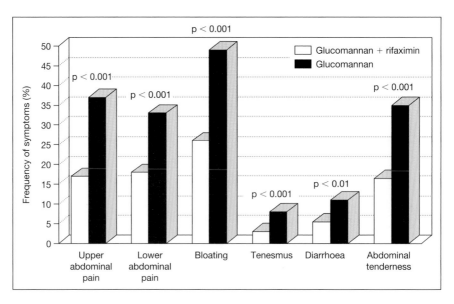

Fig. 1. Frequency of symptoms of colonic diverticulosis after 12 months of treatment with rifaximin plus glucomannan compared to glucomannan alone (from Latella et al. [26]).

oral intake, severity of illness, comorbid disease, and adequate outpatient support. Outpatients should be treated with a clear liquid diet and broad-spectrum oral antimicrobials with activity against anaerobes and Gram-negative rods (in particular, *Escherichia coli* and *Bacteroides fragilis*) [30].

Symptomatic improvement should generally be evident within 2–3 days, at which time diet can be slowly advanced. Antibiotic treatment should also be continued for 7–10 days. Patients needing admission should have clear liquids or nothing by mouth and intravenous fluids. Intravenous antimicrobials should also be started [30]. Improvement of symptoms is to be expected within 2–4 days, at which point diet can be resumed. If improvement continues, patients may be discharged to complete a 7- to 10-day oral antibiotic course at home. Failure of conservative medical treatment warrants a diligent search for complications, consideration of alternative diagnoses, and surgical consultation. Most patients admitted with acute diverticulitis will respond to conservative treatment, but 15–30% will need surgery during that time [31–33].

As far as antimicrobials are concerned, in absence of clinical trials, recommendations are suggested by clinical experience. Ampicillin, gentamycin, metronidazole, piperacillin, clindamycin and tazobactam are the most used antibiotics.

Combination regimens such as anaerobic coverage with metronidazole or clindamycin and Gram-negative coverage with an aminoglycoside (e.g. gentamycin, tobramycin), monobactam (e.g. aztreonam, tazobactam), or third-generation cephalosporins (e.g. ceftazidime, cefotaxime, ceftriaxone) are also suggested [30, 34]. However, a single intravenous antibiotic active against aerobes and anaerobes shows similar efficacy of antibiotic combination therapy in resolving acute diverticulitis [35, 36]. The second-generation cephalosporins are frequently used followed by ampicillin/sulbactam [37]. Many physicians prefer to use a combination of ciprofloxacin and metronidazole as indicated in the treatment of the uncomplicated diverticular disease, but using the intravenous route of administration [34, 38, 39].

Probiotic use has recently been attempted in acute diverticulitis. Probiotics are live microbial food ingredients acting on the enteric flora with a favourable effect on health [40]. Their use in uncomplicated diverticulitis has the same rationale of the antibiotic therapy and is strongly suggested by the efficacy of probiotics in mild forms of inflammatory bowel disease, in post-infectious diarrhea, in irritable bowel syndrome and in preventing antibiotic-related gastrointestinal adverse effects [41, 42]. The action of probiotics includes production of antimicrobial substances, competitive metabolic interactions with pro-inflammatory organisms, and inhibition of adherence and translocations of pathogens. They may also influence mucosal defence at the levels of immune and epithelial function, such as the decreasing of tumour necrosis factor-α, interleukin-1α and interferon-γ. Lactobacilli, bifidobacteria and other non-pathogenic bacterial strains, including certain *E. coli* and enterococci, as well as some yeasts such as *Saccharomyces boulardii*, have been used. A pilot study has been performed on 15 patients using the non-pathogenic *E. coli* strain Nissle (2.5×10^{10} viable bacteria/capsule, one capsule on days 1–4, and then two capsules after day 5) added to an antimicrobial (dichlorchinolinol) and an absorbent (active coal tablets) for acute uncomplicated diverticulitis. The study showed that the remission period in patients treated with combined therapy was longer in comparison to that observed in with patients treated without probiotic [43].

Complicated Diverticulitis

Complicated diverticulitis usually results from worsening of the infection. If this is the case, large perforations develop with consequent abscesses, peritonitis and fistulas. Obstruction may suddenly develop during an episode of diverticulitis or be a late complication. Haemorrhage however represents a non-infective complication.

Abscess

When an abscess is suspected, diagnostic imaging should be sought. Staging of patients by CT scan may allow selecting the patients most likely to respond to conservative therapy. Small pericolic abscesses (stage I) can often be treated conservatively with antimicrobials and bowel rest [44]. Their good prognosis may be attributed to a persistent fistula between the abscess and the colon, permitting spontaneous internal drainage. When surgery is necessary, a single-stage *en bloc* resection and subsequent anastomosis can generally be performed. For patients with distant abscesses (stage II) or unresolved pericolic abscesses, a CT-guided percutaneous drainage is indicated [32].

Drainage of abdominal abscesses has assumed a prominent complementary role to surgery [45]. The immediate advantage of percutaneous catheter drainage is rapid control of sepsis and patient stabilization, without the risk of general anaesthesia. More generally, it will often eliminate the need for a two-stage procedure with colostomy, instead allowing for temporary palliative drainage and subsequent single-stage resection in 3–4 weeks. Two retrospective series have reported success rates of 74 and 80% in stabilizing patients and safely allowing for subsequent single-stage procedures [46, 47]. An initial surgical procedure is required in the 20–25% of patients in whom the abscess is multiloculated, anatomically inaccessible for drainage, or not responding to drainage. A single-stage procedure is preferable, although not always possible [48]. Laparoscopic resections have also been described for treatment of abscesses [49], although this technique is not yet widely applied.

Pyogenic liver abscesses may also occur as a complication of colonic diverticulitis [50–52]. Antibacterial agents, percutaneous drainage, and surgery each have a role in their management.

Peritonitis

When an abscess opens into abdominal cavity, a purulent peritonitis will develop (stage III). A faecal peritonitis (stage IV) may be the consequence of larger perforations. In both cases, surgery and intensive care are mandatory due to the high mortality of these two conditions (6 and 35% respectively) [53–55].

Fistulas

When a diverticular phlegmon or abscess extends or ruptures into an adjacent organ, fistulas may occur. Treatment is surgical resection with fistula closure. Spontaneous colo-cutaneous fistulas are very rare and usually follow a prior surgical repair [48, 54].

Obstruction

Acute obstruction during an episode of acute diverticulitis is usually self-limiting and responds well to conservative therapy. Colonic ileus or pseudo-obstruction are more infrequent conditions that usually improve with effective medical therapy. If obstruction does not resolve rapidly, surgical intervention is mandatory. Also, recurrent attacks of diverticulitis, which may be subclinical, can initiate progressive fibrosis and stricturing of the colonic wall in the absence of ongoing inflammation. In this case a surgical option should be considered before an obstruction ensues [48, 54].

Haemorrhage

The bleeding from diverticula is not associated with underlying acute inflammation. The presumed cause of this complication is an erosion of a submucosal blood vessel by impacted stool at the neck of a diverticulum. Severe haemorrhage has been reported to occur in 3–5% of all patients with diverticulosis [56, 57].

The management of bleeding diverticula requires a coordinated approach by gastroenterologists, radiologists, and surgeons. For the majority of patients, diverticular bleeding is self-limited. Subsequent colonoscopy should generally be performed to potentially elucidate the bleeding source, but more importantly to exclude neoplasia. Angiography and colonoscopy may be therapeutically useful in patients with ongoing bleeding, and surgery required in those in whom these approaches are unsuccessful.

The role of endoscopic therapy in acute diverticular bleeding is being refined. A case report in 1985 first described cessation of haemorrhage from an actively bleeding diverticulum by local irrigation with 1:1,000 epinephrine [58]. Later reports have demonstrated the haemostatic abilities of the heater probe, bicap probe, injection therapies, and fibrin sealant in patients with bleeding diverticula [59–63]. Recently, an endoscopic description of diverticular 'stigmata' thought to have prognostic values, similar to those associated with peptic ulcers, in patients with acute lower gastrointestinal bleeding 'unequivocally' due to diverticula, has been reported [64, 65]. Cumulative results from nine studies of endoscopically treated diverticular bleeding reveal a 95% homeostasis rate with no procedure-related morbidity [66]. Although this intervention is promising, more controlled data are required before endoscopic therapy becomes a standard approach in this setting.

Surgery in acute lower gastrointestinal bleeding is usually reserved when medical, endoscopic, or angiographic therapies fail. Segmental resection is most commonly performed if the bleeding site is definitively known from a therapeutically unsuccessful angiographic or endoscopic procedure. The rebleeding rate compiled from seven series was 6% in 167 patients who underwent segmental resections [67]. In patients with persistent bleeding, and no angiographic or endoscopic identification of a definite bleeding site, a subtotal colectomy may be required.

Surgery: When and How

Surgery consists of resection of the intestinal segment affected by diverticula, followed by end-to-end anastomosis. It is necessary in 15–30% of cases of acute diverticulitis and is often elective [67].

Emergency Surgery

Urgent surgery is rarely required for diverticular disease and mainly includes free perforation with severe peritonitis or no otherwise stopped haemorrhage. In patients <40 years, urgent surgery is required in 50–75% of cases, and in patients <50 years in 25–80%. In case of purulent or faecal peritonitis, mortality ranges from 6 to 35% [31, 68, 69].

Elective Surgery

The decision to perform an elective surgery should take into account that after the first attack, only 20–30% of patients (7–62%) have a second episode of diverticulitis but, after this recurrence, the probability of a third attack is greater than 50%. After each recurrent episode the patient is less likely to respond to medical therapy (70% chance of response to medical therapy after the first attack vs. 6% chance after the third). Furthermore, the complications of diverticulitis may be severe and mortality of surgery high [31, 70, 71]. For these reasons most authors suggest surgery after the second to fourth episode of diverticulitis, in accordance with the patient's general conditions and severity of episodes [32, 33].

Younger patients who initially respond to conservative medical measures have a significantly higher risk of recurrences or complications than older patients and a lower response rate to medical treatment [72–76]. Therefore, surgical resection may be reasonably considered after one well-documented episode of uncomplicated diverticulitis in the younger patient. A similar approach should be followed for immunocompromised patients.

Surgical Procedure

Although diverticula may be present throughout the colon, it is not necessary to remove all colon containing diverticula since the proximal margin of resection is determined by the abnormally thickened colonic wall. The distal margin of resection should involve the rectum to reduce the risk of postoperative recurrence. Up to 10% of patients will have symptomatic recurrent diverticulitis after surgical resection. Re-operation may be required in about 3% of patients and is often technically more difficult because of inflammation and adhesions [32, 77, 78]. In a series of 501 patients from the Mayo Clinic who had resection and re-anastomosis for diverticular disease, a higher recurrence rate

Table 2. Patients discharged from hospital, re-admitted to hospital, and those who underwent surgery (from Porta et al. [84])

Patient groups	Antibiotics	No antibiotics	Total
Discharged[1]	350	155	505
Newly admitted[2]	22 (6.3%)*	19 (12.3%)	41 (8.1%)
Operations[3]	3 (13.6%)**	10 (52.6%)	13 (32%)

[1]Patients discharged from hospital with or without antibiotic prescription after recovery from a complication of diverticular disease (occlusion, perforation, fistula or bleeding).

[2]Percentage of those patients, taking or not taking antibiotics, who were re-admitted to hospital because of a further complication.

[3]Number and percentage of the re-admitted patients, taking or not taking antibiotics, who needed to undergo surgical operation.

*$\chi^2 = 4.37$; p = 0.037.

**Fischer's exact test (two-sided), p = 0.017.

was found when the sigmoid colon was used for the distal resection margin as compared to the rectum. This suggests that the entire distal colon should routinely be removed during resections for diverticular disease with a rectal (rather than sigmoid) anastomosis [32, 79–83].

Prevention of Diverticulitis Recurrence

Since each repeated episode of diverticulitis responds less to medical therapy and is more susceptible of complications, great attention has been paid to attain preventive strategies [31, 68]. The combination of soluble dietary fiber and the poorly absorbed antibiotic, rifaximin, seems to be effective in this respect. Indeed, in two out of three clinical trials performed with such a therapeutic regimen the occurrence of complications was reduced by more than 50% (table 1). Although the only double-blind study [27] available did not show a benefit, most likely because of a small sample size, such combination can be safely recommended in diverticular disease since it achieves a symptomatic benefit in the vast majority of patients. This approach is further supported from retrospective data [84] showing that treatment with poorly absorbed antibiotics, including rifaximin, not only halves the relative risk of hospital re-admission for complications, but also reduces by 73% the risk of re-operation (table 2). Like for symptomatic relief, the addition of mesalazine to rifaximin almost completely prevented the recurrence of diverticulitis, whose rate in patients treated with both drugs fell to only 2.7% [29]. Similarly, starting probiotic administration after a course of rifaximin – if done cyclically – is effective in controlling symptoms and reducing the number of episodes of acute diverticulitis [85].

Conclusions

Asymptomatic diverticular disease does not require any treatment. However, when inflammation of one or more diverticula occurs, diverticulitis and the potential complications need to be carefully addressed. Once in remission, continuous fiber intake and intermittent course of poorly absorbed antibiotics, like rifaximin [86], may improve symptoms and reduce diverticulitis recurrence. These preventive strategies will likely improve patients' quality of life and reduce management costs [87].

References

1   Trotman IF, Misiewicz JJ: Sigmoid motility in diverticular disease and the irritable bowel syndrome. Gut 1988;29:218–222.
2   Sugihara K, Muto T, Morioka Y: Motility study in right-sided diverticular disease of the colon. Gut 1983;24:1130–1134.
3   Painter NS, Truelove SC, Ardran GM: Segmentation and localization of intraluminal pressures in the human colon, with special reference to the pathogenesis of colonic diverticula. Gastroenterology 1965;49:169–177.
4   Painter NS, Burkitt DP: Diverticular disease of the colon: a deficiency disease of western civilization. Br Med J 1971;ii:450–454.
5   Burkitt DP, Walker ARP, Painter NS: Effect of dietary fibre on stools and transit times, and its role in the causation of disease. Lancet 1972;ii:1408–1411.
6   Baird IM, Walters RL, Davies PS, Hill MJ, Drasar BS, Southgate DA: The effects of two dietary fiber supplementation on gastrointestinal transit, stool weight and frequency, bacterial flora and fecal bile acids in normal subjects. Metabolism 1977;26:117–128.
7   Aldoori WH, Giovannucci EL, Rockett HR, Sampson L, Rimm EB, Willett WC: A prospective study of dietary fiber types and symptomatic diverticular disease in men. J Nutr 1998;128: 714–719.
8   Francis CY, Whorwell P: Bran and irritable bowel syndrome: time for reappraisal. Lancet 1994;344:39–40.
9   Bijkerk CJ, Muris JW, Knottnerus JA, Hoes AW, de Wit NJ: Systematic review: the role of different types of fibre in the treatment of irritable bowel syndrome. Aliment Pharmacol Ther 2004; 19:245–251.
10   Stollman N, Raskin JB: Diverticular disease of the colon. Lancet 2004;363:631–639.
11   Parra-Blanco A: Colonic diverticular disease: pathophysiology and clinical picture. Digestion 2006;73(suppl 1):41–50.
12   Brodribb AJM: Treatment of symptomatic diverticular disease with a high fibre diet. Lancet 1977;i:664–665.
13   Ornstein MH, Littlewood ER, Baird IM, Fowler J, North WR, Cox AG: Are fiber supplements really necessary in diverticular disease of the colon? A controlled clinical trial. Br Med J 1981; 282: 1353–1356.

14   Stollman NH, Raskin B: Diagnosis and management of diverticular disease of the colon in adults. Am J Gastroenterol 1999;94:3110–3121.
15   Daniel O, Basup K, Al-Samarrae HM: Use of glucagon in the treatment of acute diverticulitis. Br Med J 1974;iii:720–722.
16   Levitt MD, Bond JH: Volume, composition and source of intestinal gas. Gastroenterology 1970;59: 921–929.
17   Strocchi A, Levitt MD: Intestinal gas; in Sleisenger MH, Fordtran JS (eds): Gastrointestinal Disease: Pathophysiology, Diagnosis, Management, ed 5. Philadelphia, Saunders, 1993, pp 1035–1042.
18   Bjorneklett A, Midvedt T: Influence of three antimicrobial agents – penicillin, metronidazole and doxycyclin – on the intestinal microflora of healthy humans. Scand J Gastroenterol 1981;16:473–480.
19   Rao SS, Edwards CA, Austen CJ, Bruce C, Read NW: Impaired colonic fermentation of carbohy-drate after ampicillin. Gastroenterology 1988;94:928–932.
20   Di Stefano M, Strocchi A, Malservisi S, Veneto G, Ferrieri A, Corazza GR: Non-absorbable antibiotics for managing intestinal gas production and gas-related symptoms. Aliment Pharmacol Ther 2000;14:1001–1008.
21   Corazza GR, Di Stefano M, Scarpignato C: Treatment of functional bowel disorders: is there room for antibiotics? Digestion 2006;73(suppl 1):33–40.
22   Kurpad AV, Shetty PS: Effects of antimicrobial therapy on fecal bulking. Gut 1986;27:55–58.
23   Papi C, Koch M, Capurso L: Management of diverticular disease: is there room for rifaximin? Chemotherapy 2005;51(suppl 1):110–114.
24   Scarpignato C, Pelosini I: Experimental and clinical pharmacology of rifaximin, a gastrointestinal selective antibiotic. Digestion 2006;73(suppl 1):13–27.
25   Papi C, Ciaco A, Koch M, Capurso L, Camarri E, Ferrieri A, Guardascione F, Miglio F, Minoli G, Terruzzi V, Parodi MC, Riegler G, Russo A: Efficacy of rifaximin of symptoms of uncomplicated diverticular disease of the colon. A pilot multicenter open trial. Ital J Gastroelterol 1992;24: 452–456.
26   Latella G, Pimpo MT, Sottili S, Zippi M, Viscido A, Chiaramonte M, Fieri G: Rifaximin improves symptoms of acquired uncomplicated diverticular disease of the colon. Int J Colorectal Dis 2003;18:55–62.
27   Papi C, Ciaco A, Koch M, Capurso L, Diverticular Disease Study Group: Efficacy of rifaximin in the treatment of symptomatic diverticular disease of the colon. A multicentre double-blind placebo-controlled trial Aliment. Pharmacol Ther 1995;9:33–39.
28   Di Mario F, Aragona G, Leandro G, Comparato G, Fanigliulo L, Cavallaro LG, Cavestro GM, Iori V, Maino M, Moussa AM, Gnocchi A, Mazzocchi G, Franze A: Efficacy of mesalazine in the treat-ment of symptomatic diverticular disease. Dig Dis Sci 2005;50:581–586.
29   Tursi A, Brandimarte G, Daffinà R: Long-term treatment with mesalazine and rifaximin versus rifaximin alone for the patients with recurrent attacks of acute diverticulitis of the colon. Digest Liver Dis 2002;34:510–515.
30   Chow A: Appendicitis and diverticulitis; in Hoeprich PD, Jordan MC, Ronald AL (eds): Infectious Disease: A Treatise of Infectious Processes. Philadelphia, Lippincott, 1994, pp 878–881.
31   Roberts PL, Veidenheimer MC: Current management of diverticulitis. Adv Surg 1994;27: 189–208.
32   Standards Task Force of the American Society of Colon and Rectal Surgeons: Practice parameters for sigmoid diverticulitis: supporting documentation. Dis Colon Rectum 1995;38:126–132.
33   Parks TG: Natural history of diverticular disease of the colon: a review of 521 cases. BMJ 1969;iv:639–642.
34   Ferzoco LB, Raptopoulos V, Silen W: Acute diverticulitis. N Engl J Med 1998;338:1521–1526.
35   Kellum JM, Sugerman HJ, Coppa GF, Way LR, Fine R, Herz B, Speck EL, Jackson D, Duma RJ: Randomized prospective comparison of cefoxitin and gentamycin-clindamycin in the treatment of acute colon diverticulitis. Clin Ther 1992;14:376–384.
36   Drusano GL, Warren JW, Saah AJ, Caplan ES, Tenney JH, Hansen S, Granados J, Standiford HC, Miller EH Jr: A prospective randomized controlled trial of cefoxitin versus clindamycin-aminoglycoside in mixed anaerobic-aerobic infections. Surg Gynecol Obstet 1982;154:715–720.
37   Schechter S, Mulvey J, Eisenstat TE: Management of uncomplicated acute diverticulitis: results of a survey. Dis Colon Rectum 1999;42:470–476.

38   Berman LG, Burdick D, Heitzman ER, Prior JT: A critical reappraisal of sigmoid peridiverticulitis. Surg Gynecol Obstet 1968;127:481–491.

39   Williams RA, Davis IP: Diverticular disease of the colon; in Haubrich WS, Schaffner F (eds): Bockus Gastroenterology, ed 5. Philadelphia, Saunders, 1995, pp 1637–1656.

40   Sanders ME: Probiotics. Food Technol 1999;53:67–77.

41   Gionchetti P, Amadini C, Rizzello F, Venturi A, Palmonari V, Morselli C, Romagnoli R, Campieri M: Probiotics – role in inflammatory bowel disease. Digest Liver Dis 2002;34(suppl 2):S58–S62.

42   Isolauri E: Probiotics for infectious diarrhoea. Gut 2003;52:436–437.

43   Fric P, Zavoral M: The effect of non-pathogenic *Escherichia coli* in symptomatic uncomplicated diverticular disease of the colon. Eur J Gastroenterol Hepatol 2003;15:313–315.

44   Ambrosetti P, Robert J, Witzig JA, Ambrosetti P, Robert J, Witzig JA, Mirescu D, de I Gautard R, Borst F, Rohner A: Incidence, outcome, and proposed management of isolated abscesses complicating acute left-sided colonic diverticulitis: a prospective study of 140 patients. Dis Colon Rectum 1992;35:1072–1076.

45   Gerzof SG, Robbins AH, Johnson WC, Birkett DH, Nabseth DC: Percutaneous catheter drainage of abdominal abscesses. N Engl J Med 1981;305:653–657.

46   Schechter S, Eisenstat TE, Oliver GC, Rubin RJ, Salvati EP: Computed tomographic scan-guided drainage of intra-abdominal abscesses. Dis Colon Rectum 1994;37:984–988.

47   Stabile BE, Puccio E, vanSonnenberg E, Neff CC: Preoperative percutaneous drainage of diverticular abscesses. Am J Surg 1990;159:99–105.

48   Wedell J, Banzhaf G, Chaoui R, Fischer R, Reichmann J: Surgical management of complicated colonic diverticulitis. Br J Surg 1997;84:380–383.

49   Franklin ME, Dorman JP, Jacobs M, Plasencia G: Is laparoscopic surgery applicable to complicated colonic diverticular disease? Surg Endosc 1997;11:1021–1025.

50   Yoshida M, Mitsuo M, Kutsumi H, Fujita T, Soga T, Nishimura K, Kawabata K, Kadotani Y, Kinoshita Y, Chiba T, Kuroiwa N, Fujimoto S: A successfully treated case of multiple liver abscesses accompanied by portal venous gas. Am J Gastroenterol 1996;91:2423–2425.

51   Nosher JL, Guidici M, Needell GS, Brolin RE: Elective one-stage abdominal operations after percutaneous catheter drainage of pyogenic liver abscess. Am Surg 1993;59:658–663.

52   Read DR, Hambrick E: Hepatic abscesses in diverticulitis. South Med J 1980;73:881–883.

53   Hinchey EF, Schaal PG, Richards GK: Treatment of perforated diverticular disease of the colon. Adv Surg 1978;12:85–109.

54   Tudor RG, Keighley MR: The options in surgical treatment of diverticular disease. Surg Annu 1987;19:135–149.

55   Krukowski ZH, Matheson NA: Emergency surgery for diverticular disease complicated by generalized and faecal peritonitis: a review. Br J Surg 1984;71:921–927.

56   Reinus JF, Brandt LJ: Vascular ectasias and diverticulosis: common causes of lower intestinal bleeding. Gastroenterol Clin North Am 1994;23:1–20.

57   McGuire HH, Haynes BW: Massive hemorrhage from diverticulosis of the colon: guidelines for therapy based on bleeding patterns observed in 50 cases. Ann Surg 1972;175:847–855.

58   Mauldin JL: Therapeutic use of colonoscopy in active diverticular bleeding. Gastrointest Endosc 1985;31:290–291.

59   Johnston J, Sones J: Endoscopic heater probe coagulation of the bleeding colonic diverticulum. Gastrointest Endosc 1986;32:A160.

60   Savides TJ, Jensen DM: Colonoscopic hemostasis for recurrent diverticular hemorrhage associated with a visible vessel: a report of three cases. Gastrointest Endosc 1994;40:70–73.

61   Bertoni G, Conigliaro R, Ricci E, Mortilla MG, Bedogni G, Fornaciari G: Endoscopic injection hemostasis of colonic diverticular bleeding: a case report. Endoscopy 1990;22:154–155.

62   Kim YI, Marcon NE: Injection therapy for colonic diverticular bleeding: a case study. J Clin Gastroenterol 1993;17:46–48.

63   Andress HJ, Mewes A, Lange V: Endoscopic hemostasis of a bleeding diverticulum of the sigma (sic) with fibrin sealant. Endoscopy 1993;25:193.

64   Foutch PG: Diverticular bleeding: are nonsteroidal anti-inflammatory drugs risk factors for hemorrhage and can colonoscopy predict outcome for patients? Am J Gastroenterol 1995;90: 1779–1784.

65   Foutch PG: Diverticular bleeding and the pigmented protuberance (sentinel clot): clinical implications, histopathological correlation, and results of endoscopic intervention. Am J Gastroenterol 1996;91:2589–2593.
66   Foutch PG: Utility of endoscopic hemoclipping for colonic diverticular bleeding (response to Dr. Hokama). Am J Gastroenterol 1997;92:543–545.
67   Browder W, Cerise EJ, Litwin MS: Impact of emergency angiography in massive lower gastrointestinal bleeding. Ann Surg 1986;204:530–536.
68   Sleisenger & Fordtran's Gastrointestinal and Liver Disease: Pathophysiology, Diagnosis, Management. Philadelphia, Saunders, 2002, pp 2100–2112.
69   Elliot TB, Yego S, Irvin TT: Five-year audit of the acute complications of diverticular disease. Br J Surg1997;84:535–539.
70   Almy TP, Howell DA: Diverticular disease of the colon. N Engl J Med 1980;302:324–331.
71   Munson KD, Hensien MA, Jacob LN, et al: Diverticulitis. A comprehensive follow-up. Dis Colon Rectum 1996;39:318–322.
72   Chodak GW, Rangel DM, Passaro E Jr: Colonic diverticulitis in patients under age 40: need for earlier diagnosis. Am J Surg 1981;141:699–702.
73   Eusebio EB, Eisenberg MM: Natural history of diverticular disease of the colon in young patients. Am J Surg 1973;125:308–311.
74   Freischlag J, Bennion RS, Thompson JE Jr: Complications of diverticular disease of the colon in young people. Dis Colon Rectum 1986;29:639–643.
75   Spivak H, Weinrauch S, Harvey JC, Surick B, Ferstenberg H, Friedman I: Acute colonic diverticulitis in the young. Dis Colon Rectum 1997;40:570–574.

Giuseppe Frieri, MD
Gastroenterology Unit
Department of Internal Medicine and Public Health
Piazzale Tommasi, Coppito, IT–67100, L'Aquila (Italy)
Tel. +39 0862 368 796/324, E-Mail g.frieri@libero.it

This chapter should be cited as follows:

Frieri G, Pimpo MT, Scarpignato C: Management of Colonic Diverticular Disease.
Digestion 2006;73(suppl 1):58–66.

Scarpignato C, Lanas Á (eds): Bacterial Flora in Digestive Disease.
Focus on Rifaximin.

....

Inflammatory Bowel Disease: Current Therapeutic Options

Eugeni Domènech

Department of Digestive Diseases, Hospital Universitari Germans Trias i Pujol,
Badalona, Spain

Abstract

Medical management of inflammatory bowel diseases (IBD) includes two treatment strategies: induction and maintenance of remission. 5-Aminosalycilates are mostly used for mild
active IBD and for maintenance treatment in ulcerative colitis (UC). Glucocorticoids remain,
despite their frequent (and occasionally severe) side effects, as the mainstay for induction of
remission in moderate to severe active IBD, both UC and Crohn's disease (CD). Cyclosporine
and infliximab have emerged as the main, rapid-acting, alternatives in steroid-refractory UC and
CD, respectively. Thiopurines (azathioprine and 6-mercaptopurine) are the most efficient and
used immunomodulators in IBD; steroid refractoriness, steroid dependency, and long-term
maintenance of remission for both UC and CD are their main indications. Methotrexate and
infliximab may be used in the same clinical settings as thiopurines in CD, but not in UC; however, these drugs are a second-line treatment because of safety profile and economic costs.

Introduction

Inflammatory bowel diseases (IBD) are chronic, idiopathic, inflammatory
disorders that involve a longer or shorter segment of the small intestine and/or
the colon. Natural history of IBD is characterized by repeated periods during
which the patients are symptomatic because of a severe inflammatory process
of the intestinal mucosa or even the bowel wall (flare-ups), followed by periods
with 'quiescent disease'. As a consequence, therapeutic strategies in IBD must
be directed to: (1) induce remission of acute flares, and (2) maintain long-term
disease remission.

Current pathogenic hypothesis of IBD holds that, in subjects with a genetic
susceptibility, exposure to certain environmental factors (much of them still

Table 1. Main factors influencing therapeutic decisions in active IBD

Ulcerative colitis
Disease activity (mild, moderate, severe)
Disease extent (distal vs. extensive)
Lack of response to other drugs in the same flare-up
Drug intolerance and/or contraindications
Time from diagnosis

Crohn's diseases
Pattern of disease behaviour (penetrating, stenosing, inflammatory)
Disease activity (mild, moderate, severe)
Disease location (ileal, colonic, ileocolonic)
Patient's age
Lack of response to other drugs in the same flare-up
Drug intolerance and/or contraindications

unknown) may trigger IBD development. In these circumstances (genetics and environment), a maintained immunological response to normal bacterial flora will occur in the gut, leading to the initiation and perpetuation of gut inflammatory lesions. By this point of view, several therapeutic approaches could be adopted in IBD. Unfortunately, we are still far from gene therapy in Crohn's disease (CD) and ulcerative colitis (UC). Tobacco is the only known environmental factor involved in IBD, and smoking habit withdrawal has become a cornerstone in the general management of CD. Bacterial modulation for the treatment of IBD will be discussed elsewhere. Thus, modulation of the inflammatory process itself has been the only therapeutic approach in IBD for many years, and it is still the most widely used therapeutic strategy.

Since the response to different drugs is not the same in CD and UC, and that surgery remains as a 'curative' treatment in those UC patients refractory to medical treatment, these entities are discussed separately in this therapeutic overview.

Ulcerative Colitis

Treatment of Acute Flare-Ups of UC

Several factors may influence therapeutic decisions in active UC, but disease activity and UC extension are the most important ones (table 1). The aminosalicylates (5-aminosalicylic acid derivatives or 5-ASA, also called mesalazine) remain the mainstays of therapy for mild to moderately active UC. A recent meta-analysis [1] has confirmed their efficacy over placebo in inducing remission (table 2). 5-ASA is usually well tolerated and adverse effects seem to be less

Table 2. Effectiveness of 5-ASA compounds in inducing clinical remission or improvement in active ulcerative colitis depending on dosage (from Sutherland and MacDonald [1])

Study	Treatment n/N	Control n/N	Peto odds ratio, 95 % CI	Weight (%)	Peto odds ratio 95% CI
Dose of 5-ASA: <2 g					
Hanauer, 1993	27/92	14/30		11.0	0.46 [0.19, 1.10]
Schroeder, 1987	8/11	15/19		2.8	0.71 [0.13, 4.02]
Sninsky, 1991	34/53	21/26		8.1	0.46 [0.17, 1.27]
Subtotal (95% CI)	156	75		21.9	0.49 [0.26, 0.90]
Total events: 69 (treatment), 50 (control)					
Test for heterogeneity $\chi^2 = 0.21$, d.f. = 2, p = 0.90, $I^2 = 0.0\%$					
Test for overall effect z = 2.28, p = 0.02					
Dose of 5-ASA: 2–2.9 g					
Feurle, 1989	25/52	29/53		14.3	0.77 [0.36, 1.65]
Hanauer, 1993	20/97	14/30		9.8	0.27 [0.11, 0.67]
Hetzel, 1986	9/15	13/15		3.3	0.27 [0.05, 1.31]
Robinson, 1988	29/50	34/48		12.3	0.58 [0.25, 1.31]
Sninsky, 1991	32/53	21/26		3.3	0.40 [0.15, 1.08]
Sutherland, 1990	37/45	18/22		4.8	1.03 [0.27, 3.85]
Subtotal (95% CI)	312	194		52.9	0.51 [0.34, 0.76]
Total events: 152 (treatment), 129 (control)					
Test for heterogeneity $\chi^2 = 5.01$, d.f. = 5, p = 0.41, $I^2 = 0.2\%$					
Test for overall effect z = 3.31, p = 0.009					
Dose of 5-ASA: ≥3 g					
Hanauer, 1993	19/95	13/30		8.6	0.21 [0.08, 0.55]
Schroeder, 1987	10/38	16/19		6.9	0.10 [0.03, 0.30]
Sutherland, 1990	26/47	18/22		7.6	0.32 [0.11, 0.92]
Zinberg, 1990	3/7	6/8		2.1	0.29 [0.04, 2.12]
Subtotal (95% CI)	187	79		25.2	0.20 [0.11, 0.35]
Total events: 54 (treatment), 53 (control)					
Test for heterogeneity $\chi^2 = 2.43$, d.f. = 3, p = 0.49, $I^2 = 0.0\%$					
Test for overall effect z = 5.50, p < 0.00001					
Total (95% CI)	655	348		100.0	0.40 [0.30, 0.53]
Total events: 275 (treatment), 232 (control)					
Test for heterogeneity $\chi^2 = 15.17$, d.f. = 12, p = 0.23, $I^2 = 20.9\%$					
Test for overall effect z = 6.23, p < 0.00001					

0.1 0.2 0.5 1 2 5 10

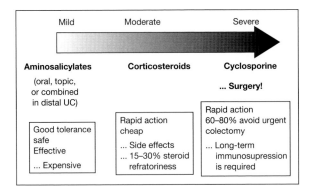

Fig. 1. Medical therapeutic approach in acute attacks of ulcerative colitis, depending on disease activity.

frequent with mesalazine (the main 5-ASA derivative) than with sulfasalazine (the first aminosalicylate molecule used for active UC treatment), because of the lack of the sulfamidic moiety of the latter. Main adverse effects of 5-ASA are acute pancreatitis (allergic), gastrointestinal symptoms (abdominal pain, diarrhea, nausea), and headache (dose-related) [2]. Although new formulations of 5-ASA derivatives have been developed in the last two decades, it seems that there are no relevant differences in terms of clinical efficacy and safety profile, and only marginal benefits for distal forms of UC could be observed with the more recent developed molecules [3]. In distal UC, mild to moderate flare-ups can also be successfully managed with topical treatment; in this sense, topical 5-ASA (enemas, foam, suppositories) is more effective than topical steroids, and it must be the drug of choice in this setting [4]. Whether 5-ASA must be administered orally, topically or in combination, to better treat distal UC is still a subject of controversy, because the results of the few randomized clinical trials (RCTs) addressing this question are not conclusive.

Systemic corticosteroids are the treatment of choice in those patients not responding to 5-ASA or those with a severe attack of UC (fig. 1). Since the initial trial of Truelove and Jewell [5], corticosteroids remain the cornerstone of the treatment of acute moderate to severe UC. Corticosteroids are rapid acting (lack of response in UC is defined after 3–7 days of intravenous steroid treatment), and cheap. However, only 60–70% of UC patients treated with systemic glucocorticoids achieve remission [6]. Although steroid refractoriness may be related to colonic reactivation of latent CMV infection in one third of these patients [7], the underlying mechanisms of this phenomenon are still unknown.

In patients with initial clinical response to glucocorticoids, these are administered at least for 2–3 months. In this scenario, the development of side effects is the rule; the most frequent ones, although mild in severity, may be troublesome in such young patients (i.e. acne, obesity, fluid retention). Major side effects such as myopathy, osteoporosis, aseptic necrosis, psychosis, glaucoma, cataracts, hypertension, hyperglycaemia, or hyperlipaemia are not exceptional. Moreover, long-term toxicity is even higher and become unacceptable. It has to be pointed out that up to one third of patients become 'steroid-dependent', with disease relapse when steroids are withdrawn or doses reduced.

Until the last decade of the 20th century, urgent colectomy was the only alternative if systemic steroids were not able to induce disease remission. Lichtiger et al. [8] demonstrated the clinical efficacy of intravenous cyclosporine (CyA) in this setting, in the only RCT comparing CyA to placebo in patients with well-defined steroid-resistant UC. Since then, CyA has become another therapeutic step before surgical treatment is considered, avoiding urgent colectomy in 60–80% of patients. As glucocorticoids, intravenous CyA is rapid acting and its use is often associated with side effects such as arterial hypertension, nephrotoxicity, tremor, seizures, or hyperglycaemia, specially when used for long periods. In addition, in those patients achieving remission with CyA for a steroid-refractory UC attack, immunosuppressant maintenance treatment with thiopurines is advised. In recent years, CyA in monotherapy has also become an efficient alternative to systemic steroids in severe attacks of UC [9]. This approach is particularly attractive in patients with previous intolerance or contraindication to glucocorticoids (i.e. psychosis, glaucoma, uncontrolled hyperglycaemia, severe osteoporosis). Recently, excellent results have been obtained with infliximab (a chimeric anti-TNF-α antibody) in steroid-refractory active UC [10], showing that this approach is also effective.

Unfortunately, the therapeutic armamentarium in UC is not as extensive as in CD, and patients not responding to 5-ASA, steroids, and CyA must be colectomized. Promising results have been achieved with some drugs or therapeutic devices such as tacrolimus [11], or granulocyte apheresis [12], but still large RCTs are needed to establish their role in UC treatment. Biologic agents, mainly infliximab, that have started a therapeutic revolution in the management of CD, have not been adequately evaluated in UC, and the results of large RCTs are eagerly waited.

Maintenance Treatment of UC

Once disease remission has been medically induced, most patients require maintenance treatment because of the natural trend of the disease to relapse. It is not clearly known which patients benefit from maintenance treatment, and how long maintenance treatment must be kept. However, recent data suggest that the more the disease remains inactive, the less is the risk of dysplasia or carcinoma of the colon. Moreover, 5-ASA itself could have a chemoprotective effect against carcinogenesis as has been suggested by some recent studies [13, 14]; it is not known which is the main antineoplastic or chemopreventive action of 5-ASA in IBD, although several mechanisms have been proposed [15]. From this point of view, all patients should follow maintenance treatment indefinitely. 5-ASA is the most used drug for maintenance treatment in UC, because of its proven efficacy and safety profile (table 3) [16]. Although renal toxicity after long-term use of 5-ASA compounds was initially described, clinical practice and a small number of clinical studies suggest that this adverse event is uncommon, and that renal impairment could be related to the disease itself more than to 5-ASA therapy [17, 18]. The economic cost of long-term 5-ASA treatment is high. In fact, mesalazine is, apart from biologic agents, the most expensive drug of those used in IBD treatment. Although sulfasalazine is cheaper and equivalent in efficacy to mesalazine, its safety profile is worse, and its use is not advised in young men because of drug-induced oligospermia.

The only alternative to 5-ASA in the maintenance treatment of UC are thiopurines [azathioprine (AZA) and 6-mercaptopurine (6-MP)]. Although clinical efficacy in UC has only been recently evaluated in clinical trials [19], AZA/6-MP are the most widely used immunomodulators in clinical practice for UC treatment. Thiopurines are cheaper than new 5-ASA derivatives; nevertheless, up to 10–20% of patients must discontinue thiopurines because of side effects [20]. The safety profile is hampered by early allergic untoward reactions (acute pancreatitis, flu-like syndrome, gastrointestinal intolerance), and dose-dependent adverse effects (mainly myelotoxicity and hepatotoxicity). The latter may occur anytime during treatment; in turn, periodic haematological and liver function tests must be performed while on thiopurines. The effect of AZA/6-MP on dysplasia development remains still unknown. Because of this AZA/6-MP are considered the second-line maintenance treatment in UC, after 5-ASA. Accepted indications for thiopurines in these patients are 5-ASA intolerance or contraindication, steroid dependency, or maintenance of CyA-induced remission. Age, time from diagnosis of UC, and disease extent (risk of dysplasia) are important factors to be taken into account when long-term treatment with thiopurines may be indicated, because colectomy still remains the only 'curative' therapy in UC.

Crohn's Disease

CD is much more heterogeneous in clinical manifestations and anatomical location than UC. Thus, in addition to those factors previously mentioned in

Table 3. Effectiveness of 5-ASA compounds in maintaining clinical or endoscopic remission in ulcerative colitis depending on dosage (from Sutherland et al. [16])

Study	Treatment n/N	Control n/N	Peto odds ratio 95% CI	Weight %	Peto odds ratio 95% CI
Dose of 5-ASA:<1g					
Hanauer, 1996	50/90	31/43		13.6	0.50 [0.24, 1.05]
Subtotal (95% CI)	90	43		13.6	0.50 [0.24, 1.05]
Total events: 50 (treatment),					
31 (control)					
Test for heterogeneity:					
not applicable					
Test for overall effect z = 1.82, p = 0.07					
Dose of 5-ASA: 1–1.9 g					
Hanauer, 1996	49/87	31/44		13.7	0.55 [0.26, 1.16]
Hawkey, 1997	40/99	66/111		25.6	0.47 [0.27, 0.80]
Sandberg, 1986	12/52	22/49		11.1	0.38 [0.17, 0.86]
Subtotal (95% CI)	238	204		50.4	0.47 [0.32, 0.69]
Total events: 101 (treatment), 119 (control)					
Test for heterogeneity χ² = 0.45, d.f. = 2,					
p = 0.80, I² = 0.0%					
Test for overall effect z = 3.86, p = 0.0001					
Dose 5-ASA: ≥ 2g					
Miner, 1995	44/103	68/102		24.9	0.38 [0.22, 0.66]
Wright, 1993	31/49	36/52		11.1	0.77 [0.34, 1.75]
Subtotal (95% CI)	152	154		36.0	0.47 [0.30, 0.75]
Total events: 75 (treatment), 104 (control)					
Test for heterogeneity χ² = 1.91,					
d.f. = 1, p = 0.17, I² = 47.7%					
Test for overall effect z = 3.21, p = 0.001					
Total (95% CI)	480	401		100.0	0.47 [0.36, 0.62]
Total events: 226 (treatment), 254 (control)					
Test for heterogeneity χ² = 2.39, d.f. = 5,					
p = 0.79, I² = 0.0%					
Test for overall effect z = 5.33, p < 0.00001					

0.1 0.2 0.5 1 2 5 10

UC, disease behaviour and location are the most important factors to be kept in mind when a therapeutic approach has to be tailored in CD patients (table 1). Recently, a new classification of CD defined three different patterns of disease behaviour [21]. Stenosing CD is characterized by fibrostenosing lesions of the intestine, with proximal gut dilation, and limited inflammatory component; this

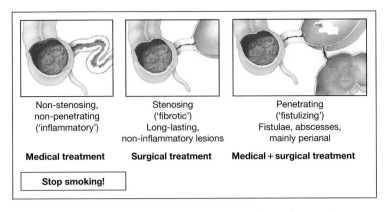

Non-stenosing, non-penetrating ('inflammatory')	Stenosing ('fibrotic') Long-lasting, non-inflammatory lesions	Penetrating ('fistulizing') Fistulae, abscesses, mainly perianal
Medical treatment	**Surgical treatment**	**Medical + surgical treatment**
Stop smoking!		

Fig. 2. Therapeutic options in Crohn's disease depending on disease pattern.

situation must be almost always treated surgically. Fistulizing CD courses with the development of intra-abdominal fistulae and/or abscesses; although most of those patients may be initially treated medically, in some instances a surgical approach is the best option. Although included as a variant of the fistulizing pattern, perianal disease (and the less frequent spontaneous enterocutaneous fistulae to abdominal wall) must be always actively treated, and a combined medical/surgical approach is often necessary. Finally, those patients not meeting criteria for stenosing or fistulizing CD are defined as 'non-stenosing, non-fistulizing'; this is the most purely 'inflammatory' pattern of the disease, its therapeutic approach is always medical, and surgery is only considered in refractory cases. There is only one therapeutic measure that must be advised in all CD patients whatever the disease pattern might be: stop smoking. Smokers have a worse disease evolution, with higher requirements of surgical resections and immuno-modulator treatments, and a higher risk of disease recurrence after surgical-induced remission (fig. 2) [22].

Treatment of Active 'Inflammatory' CD

Although glucocorticoids are still the gold standard treatment for active 'inflammatory' CD, several alternatives are available in mild to moderately active CD (fig. 3). Enteral nutrition, administered orally or tube-feeding, is an excellent alternative in some instances. Despite its efficacy in inducing remission is lower than that of corticosteroids, the lack of serious side effects and its beneficial effects on nutritional status make enteral nutrition the treatment of choice in paediatric patients and in adults with concomitant malnutrition [23]. The mechanism of action of nutritional therapy is not exactly known, although

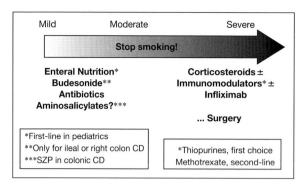

| Mild | Moderate | Severe |

Stop smoking!

Enteral Nutrition*
Budesonide**
Antibiotics
Aminosalicylates?***

Corticosteroids ±
Immunomodulators* ±
Infliximab

... Surgery

*First-line in pediatrics
**Only for ileal or right colon CD
***SZP in colonic CD

*Thiopurines, first choice
Methotrexate, second-line

Fig. 3. Medical therapeutic approach in 'inflammatory' active Crohn's disease.

modulation of inflammatory process (by means of administration of anti-inflammatory cytokine precursors such as fatty acids), and regulation of the intestinal bacterial ecosystem (prebiotic effect) could be involved. Budesonide was the first synthetic steroid developed to have the same efficacy than conventional glucocorticoids with a better safety profile, in IBD; this drug is associated with significantly fewer side effects and less suppression of the hypothalamic-pituitary-adrenal axis, but also with a lower efficacy in inducing remission. Moreover, it only acts topically on the intestinal segment where drug is released, limiting its use to CD of the terminal ileum and right colon [24]. There is no placebo-controlled evidence for the efficacy of 5-ASA derivatives in active CD. Although commonly used in clinical practice, sulfasalazine (for colonic CD) and mesalazine seem to have only a marginal benefit over placebo in mild active disease [25].

The efficacy of conventional corticosteroids in CD is similar to that previously described in UC, with a proportion of patients being refractory to full doses of steroids, and some of the initial responders developing steroid dependency [6, 26]. In these circumstances, thiopurines (AZA/6-MP), methotrexate (MTX), and infliximab (IFX) have been demonstrated to be clinically effective. Thiopurines have been used in IBD since the early 1980s, and they have become the most widely used immunomodulator agents. Their clinical efficacy has been evaluated in a recent meta-analysis (table 4) [27], and their supposed potential carcinogenic and teratogenic effects have not been confirmed. One of the drawbacks for the use of thiopurines is the latency period prior to achieving their therapeutic effects. Since these drugs have a mean latency period of 3 to 6 months (although there is a wide variation among individuals), their use for inducing remission treatment in acute IBD would be unreasonable. Therefore, since the use of AZA/6-MP has always to be envisaged in a long-term setting,

Table 4. Effectiveness of thiopurines in inducing remission in active Crohn's disease depending on the time under therapy (from Sandborn et al. [27])

Study	Treatment n/N	Control n/N	Peto odds ratio 95% CI	Weight %	Peto odds ratio 95% CI
Trials ≥ 17 weeks					
Ewe, 1993	16/21	8/21		11.2	4.57 [1.36, 15.27]
Klein, 1974	6/13	6/13		7.1	1.00 [0.22, 4.54]
Oren, 1997	13/32	12/26		15.2	0.80 [0.28, 2.26]
Present, 1980	26/36	5/36		19.0	10.45 [4.14, 26.38]
Summers, 1979	21/59	20/77		30.1	1.57 [0.75, 3.29]
Willoughby, 1971	6/6	1/6		3.4	23.17 [2.57, 208.60]
Subtotal (95% CI)	167	179		86.1	2.61 [1.69, 4.03]
Total events: 88 (treatment), 52 (control)					
Test for heterogeneity χ² = 21.58, d.f. = 5, p = 0.0006, I² = 76.8%					
Test for overall effect z = 4.32, p = 0.00002					
Trials < 17 weeks					
Candy, 1995	25/33	20/30		13.9	1.55 [0.52, 4.59]
Rhodes, 1971	0/9	0/7		0.0	Not estimable
Subtotal (95% CI)	42	37		13.9	1.55 [0.52, 4.59]
Total events: 25 (treatment), 20 (control)					
Test for heterogeneity: not applicable					
Test for overall effect z = 0.79, p = 0.4					
Total (95% CI)	209	216		100.0	2.43 [1.62, 3.64]
Total events: 113 (treatment), 72 (control)					
Test for heterogeneity χ² = 22.34, d.f. = 6, p = 0.001, I² = 73.1%					
Test for overall effect z = 4.30, p = 0.00002					

0.1 0.2 0.5 1 2 5 10

the treatment should start while inducing response in acute IBD with other methods (steroids, antibiotics, IFX, etc.).

MTX is a second-line immunomodulator for active CD. In fact, its efficacy has only been demonstrated when administered intramuscularly in a unique RCT [28]. Similarly to thiopurines, MTX has a slow onset of action, but beneficial effects may become evident in 1–3 months. One of the major concerns when using MTX in long-term situations in chronic diseases is its potential hepatotoxicity; severe liver damage seems to be less frequent than initially expected, but the risk may increase in those patients with concomitant risk factors for hepatotoxicity (chronic alcohol consumption, obesity, hypergly-caemia, chronic viral hepatitis).

IFX is the only biological agent approved for clinical use in IBD. Its efficacy in CD has been shown in large clinical trials [29–31], and it has been widely used in the last 5 years in Europe and North America. One of the main characteristics of IFX is its rapid onset of action; however, this is an expensive therapy with associated side effects such as an increased risk of serious infections (tuberculosis, listeriosis, aspergillosis). In addition, the chimeric nature of the drug seems to be the explanation of the development of antibodies to IFX, that are responsible of acute reactions to drug infusion, tachyphylaxis, or loss of initial response to IFX. For these reasons, in Europe the use of IFX has only been approved in active CD refractory to conventional therapy (including steroids and immunomodulators) [32]. In America, IFX is not limited to refractory CD, but some American authors agree to restrict the use of this agent only in this subgroup of patients [33].

An important number of new biological agents and new therapeutic approaches are being evaluated. Some of them, such as natalizumab, adalimumab, thalidomide, or even bone marrow transplantation, have shown promising results in pilot studies.

Treatment of Active Fistulizing CD

The fistulizing pattern of CD entails two major clinical conditions. First, the occurrence of intra-abdominal or perianal abscesses. In these cases, control of sepsis must be the first aim of treatment, and antibiotherapy together with surgical or US-guided drainage are mandatory. The second problem is the development of fistulae; entero-enteric fistulae do not require specific treatment unless malabsorption due to intestinal bypass is present. Organ-enteric fistulae are treated surgically almost always. The more frequent fistulae are located in the perianal region; although not life-threatening, they impair significantly the quality of life and represent a very disabling problem associated with CD. There is little evidence for medical treatment in perianal disease. Antibiotics, thiopurines, and IFX are the most used drugs in fistulizing CD; however, only IFX has been adequately evaluated in placebo-controlled trials [34, 35]. AZA/6-MP seem to have a beneficial effect, only demonstrated in a recent meta-analysis [27], and antibiotics are thought to have a transient, partial effect on fistulae drainage [36, 37]. Nevertheless, the most optimistic results achieve long-term fistulae closure (disease remission) in less than one half of those patients treated with thiopurines and/or IFX. In view of these poor response rates, most authors agree in prolonging the treatment (immunomodulators, IFX, or both) indefinitely if a complete response is obtained [32].

Table 5. Effect of 5-ASA compounds on Crohn's disease maintenance of remission compared to placebo in RCTs (from Akobeng and Gardener [39])

Study	Treatment n/N	Control n/N	Odds ratio (random) 95% CI	Weight %	Odds ratio (random) 95% CI
12 months					
Anonymous, 1990	17/93	29/100		16.9	0.55 [0.28, 1.08]
Arber, 1995	6/22	15/27		8.4	0.30 [0.09, 1.00]
Mahmud, 2001	55/112	59/134		21.4	1.23 [0.74, 2.03]
Prantera, 1992	19/54	32/56		14.9	0.41 [0.19, 0.88]
Sutherland, 1997	30/94	47/107		19.4	0.60 [0.34, 1.07]
Thomson, 1995	33/86	38/102		19.0	1.05 [0.58, 1.89]
Subtotal (95% CI)	461	526		100.0	0.68 [0.45, 1.02]

Total events: 160 (treatment), 220 (control)
Test for heterogeneity
$\chi^2 = 10.94$, d.f. = 5,
$p = 0.05$, $I^2 = 54.3\%$
Test for overall effect z = 1.85,
p = 0.06

24 months					
Gendre, 1993	31/57	36/62		100.0	0.86 [0.42, 1.78]
Subtotal (95% CI)	57	62		100.0	0.86 [0.42, 1.78]

Total events: 31 (treatment), 36 (control)
Test for heterogeneity: not applicable
Test for overall effect z = 0.40, p = 0.7

```
      0.01  0.1    1    10   100
        Favours      Favours
       treatment      control
```

Only another drug, tacrolimus, has been evaluated in the treatment of fistulizing CD, with even worse results, although more RCTs comparing this drug to IFX are advisable [38].

Maintenance Treatment of CD

Because of the relapsing nature of CD and the impossibility to surgically 'cure' the disease, it seems reasonable that almost all patients have to follow maintenance treatment in order to avoid disease relapses and/or associated complications. In contrast to UC, 5-ASA derivatives have not been clearly demonstrated to be beneficial in this setting (table 5) [39]; however, in clinical practice it is not uncommon to prescribe aminosalicylates in those patients with less 'aggressive' CD, because of the inconclusive results of even several meta-analysis [40]. As I mentioned above, thiopurines are the most used immuno-modulators in IBD, especially in CD; steroid refractoriness, steroid dependency, fistulizing CD, and even prevention of CD recurrence (after surgically induced remission) are widely accepted indications to start AZA/6-MP. In most of these settings, AZA/6-MP have demonstrated their clinical efficacy [41]. The possibility of early use of AZA in new onset disease is an attractive approach, especially in youngsters, adolescents and children [42]. In the last two groups, disease may take an aggressive type of evolution and a profound deleterious effect on growth and sexual development, which can be worsened by the use of repeated steroid treatments. The combination of enteral nutrition, and AZA/6-MP in this case, may be of use, since both can induce and maintain disease remission and prevent growth and sexual development arrest.

Intramuscular MTX (at lower doses than in active CD) has been shown to successfully maintain disease remission induced by steroids and MTX [43], but the scarce available data on long-term efficacy make this treatment only an alternative therapy in patients intolerant or refractory to thiopurines.

IFX has been shown to be superior to placebo in maintaining remission induced by the same drug, in both inflammatory and fistulizing CD [30, 31, 35]. However, immunomodulator concomitant therapy (AZA/6-MP, MTX) is advised in order to prevent associated immunogenicity to IFX administration [32]. As mentioned previously, this long-term strategy is restricted for most authors to immunomodulator-refractory CD because of the economic costs and safety profile.

Conclusions and Perspectives for the Future

Although recent advances in the knowledge of the pathogenesis of IBD have allowed new therapeutical approaches like biological agents (i.e. IFX), we are still far from a fully effective treatment. Current medical therapy in IBD is still based on the administration of aminosalicylates, steroids, and immunomodulators like thiopurines or MTX. Immediate perspectives might be targeted to evaluate combined medical strategies (including new biological agents and immunomodulators), in order to fight the inflammatory process at different levels. Basic research is essential to understand the initial events that trigger the development of the inflammatory process, in which intestinal flora and genetically determined gut immunological tolerance seem to be the cornerstones.

References

1 Sutherland L, MacDonald JK: Oral 5-amino-salicylic acid for induction of remission in ulcerative colitis. Cochrane Database Syst Rev 2003;(3):CD000543.

2 Baker DE, Kane S: The short- and long-term safety of 5-aminosalicylate products in the treatment of ulcerative colitis. Rev Gastroenterol Disord 2004;4:86–91.

3 Klotz U: Colonic targeting of aminosalicylates for the treatment of ulcerative colitis. Dig Liver Dis 2005;37:381–388.

4 Cohen RD, Woseth DM, Thisted RA, Hanauer SB: A meta-analysis and overview of the literature on treatment options for left-sided ulcerative colitis and ulcerative proctitis. Am J Gastroenterol 2000;95:1263–1276.

5 Truelove SC, Jewell DP: Intensive intravenous regimen for severe attacks of ulcerative colitis. Lancet 1974;i:1067–1070.

6 Faubion WA Jr, Loftus EV Jr, Harmsen WS, Zinsmeister AR, Sandborn WJ: The natural history of corticosteroid therapy for inflammatory bowel disease: a population-based study. Gastroenterology 2001;121:255–260.

7 Cottone M, Pietrosi G, Martorana G, Casà A, Pecoraro G, Oliva L, Rosselli M, Rizzo A, Pagliaro L: Prevalence of cytomegalovirus infection in severe refractory ulcerative and Crohn's colitis. Am J Gastroenterol 2001;96:773–775.

8 Lichtiger S, Present DH, Kornbluth A, Gelernt I, Bauer J, Galler G, Michelassi F, Hanauer S: Cyclosporine in severe ulcerative colitis refractory to steroid therapy. N Engl J Med 1994;330:1841–1845.

9 D'Haens G, Lemmens L, Geboes K, Vandeputte L, Van Acker F, Mortelmans L, Peeters M, Vermeire S, Penninckx F, Nevens F, Hiele M, Rutgeerts P: Intravenous cyclosporine versus intravenous corticosteroids as single therapy for severe attacks of ulcerative colitis. Gastroenterology 2001;120:1323–1329.

10 Järnerot G, Hertervig E, Friis-Liby I, Blom-quist L, Karlen P, Grännö CH, Vilien M, Strom M, Danielsson A, Verbaan H, Hellström PM, Magnuson A, Curman B: Infliximab as rescue therapy in severe to moderately severe ulcerative colitis: a randomised, placebo-controlled study. Gastroenterology 2005;128:1805–1811.

11 Fellermann K, Tanko Z, Herrlinger KR, Witthoeft T, Homann N, Bruening A, Ludwig D, Stange EF: Response of refractory colitis to intravenous or oral tacrolimus (FK506). In-flamm Bowel Dis 2002;8:317–324.

12 Domènech E, Hinojosa J, Esteve-Comas M, Gomollón F, Herrera JM, Bastida G, et al: Granulocyte apheresis in steroid-dependent inflammatory bowel disease: a prospective, open, pilot study. Aliment Pharmacol Ther 2004;20:1347–1352.

13 Eaden J: The data supporting a role for aminosalicylates in the chemoprevention of colorectal cancer in patients with inflammatory bowel disease. Aliment Pharmacol Ther 2003;18(suppl 2): 15–21.

14 Velayos FS, Terdiman JP, Walsh JM: Effect of 5-aminosalicylate use on colorectal cancer and dysplasia risk: a systematic review and meta-analysis of observational studies. Am J Gastroenterol 2005;100:1345–1353.

15 Allgayer H: Mechanisms of action of mesalazine in preventing colorectal carcinoma in inflammatory bowel disease. Aliment Pharmacol Ther 2003;18(suppl 2):10–14.

16 Sutherland L, Roth D, Beck P, May G, Makiyama K: Oral 5-aminosalicylic acid for maintenance of remission in ulcerative colitis. Cochrane Database Syst Rev 2002;(4):CD000544.

17 Corrigan G, Stevens PE: Review article: interstitial nephritis associated with the use of mesalazine in inflammatory bowel disease. Aliment Pharmacol Ther 2000;14:1–6.

18 Herrlinger KR, Noftz MK, Fellermann K, Schmidt K, Steinhoff J, Stange EF: Minimal renal dysfunction in inflammatory bowel disease is related to disease activity but not to 5-ASA use. Aliment Pharmacol Ther 2001;15:363–369.

19 López-Sanromán A, Bermejo F, Carrera E, García-Plaza A: Efficacy and safety of thiopurine immunomodulators (azathioprine and mercaptopurine) in steroid-dependent ulcerative colitis. Aliment Pharmacol Ther 2004;20:161–166.

20   Fraser AG, Orchard TR, Jewell DP: The efficacy of azathioprine for the treatment of inflammatory bowel disease: a 30-year review. Gut 2002;50:485–489.

21   Gasche C, Scholmerich J, Brynskov J, D'Haens G, Hanauer SB, Irvine EJ, Jewell DP, Rachmilewitz D, Sachar DB, Sandborn WJ, Sutherland LR: A simple classification of Crohn's disease: report of the working party for the World Congresses of Gastroenterology, Vienna 1998. Inflamm Bowel Dis 2000;5:8–15.

22   Cosnes J, Beaugerie L, Carbonnel F, Gendre JP: Smoking cessation and the course of Crohn's disease: an intervention study. Gastroenterology 2001;120:1093–1099.

23   Gassull MA: The role of nutrition in the treatment of inflammatory bowel disease. Aliment Pharmacol Ther 2004;20(suppl 4):79–83.

24   Rutgeerts P, Löfberg R, Malchow H, Lamers C, Olaison G, Jewell D, Danielsson A, Goebell H, Thomsen OO, Lorenz-Meyer H, Hodgson H, Persson T, Seidegard C: A comparison of budesonide to prednisolone for active Crohn's disease. N Engl J Med 1994;331:842–845.

25   Hanauer SB, Stromberg U: Oral Pentasa in the treatment of active Crohn's disease: a meta-analysis of double-blind, placebo-controlled trials. Clin Gastroenterol Hepatol 2004;2:379–388.

26   Munkholm P, Langholz E, Davidsen M, Binder V: Frequency of glucocorticoid resistance and dependency in Crohn's disease. Gut 1994;35:360–362.

27   Sandborn W, Sutherland L, Pearson D, May G, Modigliani R, Prantera C: Azathioprine or 6-mercaptopurine for inducing remission of Crohn's disease. Cochrane Database Syst Rev 2000;(2):CD000545.

28   Feagan BG, Rochon J, Fedorak RN, Irvine EJ, Wild G, Sutherland L, Steinhart AH, Greenberg GR, Gillies R, Hopkins M, Hanauer SB, McDonald JWD: Methotrexate for the treatment of Crohn's disease. The North American Crohn's Study Group of Investigators. N Engl J Med 1995;332:292–297.

29   Targan SR, Hanauer SB, van Deventer SJ, Mayer L, Present DH, Braakman T, DeWoody KL, Schaible TF, Rutgeerts PJ: A short-term study of chimeric monoclonal antibody cA2 to tumor necrosis factor-α for Crohn's disease. Crohn's Disease cA2 Study Group. N Engl J Med 1997;337:1029–1035.

30   Hanauer SB, Feagan BG, Lichtenstein GR, Mayer LLF, Schreiber S, Colombel JF, Rachmilewitz D, Wolf DC, Olson A, Bao W, Rutgeerts P: Maintenance infliximab for Crohn's disease: the ACCENT I randomised trial. Lancet 2002;359:1541–1549.

31   Rutgeerts P, Feagan BG, Lichtenstein GR, Mayer LF, Schreiber S, Colombel JF, Rachmilewitz D, Wolf DC, Olson A, Bao W, Hanauer SB: Comparison of scheduled and episodic treatment strategies of infliximab in Crohn's disease. Gastroenterology 2004;126:402–413.

32   Rutgeerts P, Van Assche G, Vermeire S: Optimizing anti-TNF treatment in inflammatory bowel disease. Gastroenterology 2004;126:1593–1610.

33   Egan LJ, Sandborn WJ: Advances in the treatment of Crohn's disease. Gastroenterology 2004;126:1574–1581.

34   Present DH, Rutgeerts P, Targan S, Hanauer SB, Mayer LL, van Hozegand RA, Podolsky DK, Sands BE, Braakman T, DeWoody KL, Schaible TF, Van Deventer SJH: Infliximab for the treatment of fistulas in patients with Crohn's disease. N Engl J Med 1999;340:1398–1405.

35   Sands BE, Anderson FH, Bernstein CN, Che WY, Feagan BG, Fedorak RN, Kamm MA, Korzenik JR, Lashner BA, Onken JE, Rachmilewitz D, Rutgeerts P, Wild G, Wolf DC, Marsters PA, Travers SB, Blank MA, Van Deventer SJ: Infliximab maintenance therapy for fistulizing Crohn's disease. N Engl J Med 2004;350:876–885.

36   Present DH: Crohn's fistula: current concepts in management. Gastroenterology 2003;124:1629–1635.

37   Rutgeerts P: Treatment of perianal fistulizing Crohn's disease. Aliment Pharmacol Ther 2004;20(suppl 4):106–110.

38   Sandborn WJ, Present DH, Isaacs KL, Wolf DC, Greenberg E, Hanauer SB, Feagan BG, Mayer L, Johnson T, Galanko J, Martin C, Sandler RS: Tacrolimus for the treatment of fistulas in patients with Crohn's disease: a randomised, placebo-controlled trial. Gastroenterology 2003;125:380–388.

39   Akobeng AK, Gardener E: Oral 5-amino-salicylic acid for maintenance of medically induced remission in Crohn's disease. The Cochrane Database of Systematic Reviews 2005, Issue 1. Art No CD003715.pub2. DOI: 10.1002/14651858.CD003715.pub2.

40   Lim WC, Hanauer SB: Controversies with aminosalicylates in inflammatory bowel disease. Rev Gastroenterol Disord 2004;4:104–117.

41   Pearson DC, May GR, Fick GH, Sutherland LR: Azathioprine and 6-mercaptopurine in Crohn's disease. A meta-analysis. Ann Intern Med 1995;122:132–142.

42   Markowitz J, Grancher K, Kohn N, Lesser M, Daum F: A multicenter trial of 6-mercaptopurine and prednisone in children with newly diagnosed Crohn's disease. Gastroenterology 2000;119: 895–902.

43   Feagan BG, Fedorak RN, Irvine EJ, Wild G, Sutherland L, Steinhart AH, Greenberg GR, Koval J, Wong CJ, Hopkins M, Hanauer SB, McDonald JWD: A comparison of methotrexate with placebo for the maintenance of remission in Crohn's disease. North American Crohn's Study Group of Investigators. N Engl J Med 2000;342:1627–1632.

Eugeni Domènech, MD
Department of Digestive Diseases
Hospital Universitari Germans Trias i Pujol
5ª planta, Ctra del Canyet, s/n
ES–08916 Badalona (Spain)
Tel. +34 93 497 8909, Fax +34 93 497 8951
E-Mail domenech@ns.hugtip.scs.es

This chapter should be cited as follows:

Domènech E: Inflammatory Bowel Disease: Current Therapeutic Options. Digestion 2006;73(suppl 1):67–76.

Scarpignato C, Lanas Á (eds): Bacterial Flora in Digestive Disease.
Focus on Rifaximin.

....

Antimicrobials in the Management of Inflammatory Bowel Disease

Paolo Gionchetti, Fernando Rizzello, Karen M. Lammers,
Claudia Morselli, Rosy Tambasco, Massimo Campieri

Department of Internal Medicine and Gastroenterology, University of Bologna,
Bologna, Italy

Abstract

Many experimental and clinical observations suggest a potential role for intestinal microflora in the pathogenesis of inflammatory bowel disease (IBD). Manipulation of the luminal content using antibiotics may therefore represent a potentially effective therapeutic option. However, the available studies do not support the use of antimicrobials in ulcerative colitis and larger studies are required. These drugs are however effective in treating septic complications of Crohn's disease (CD). The use of antibacterial agents as primary therapy for CD is more controversial, although this approach is frequently and successfully adopted in clinical practice. Despite the fact that properly controlled trials have been not carried out, antimicrobials are the mainstay of the treatment of pouchitis. Rifaximin is a poorly absorbed, broad-spectrum antibiotic that, thanks to its efficacy and long-term safety, could represent the preferred tool of manipulating enteric flora in patients with IBD. Preliminary data suggest that rifaximin may be beneficial in the treatment of active ulcerative colitis (and pouchitis), mild to moderate CD as well as prevention of post-operative recurrence of CD.

Introduction

The rationale for using antibiotics in inflammatory bowel disease (IBD) is based upon convincing evidence showing that intestinal bacteria are implicated in the pathogenesis of the disease [1]. Indeed, the distal ileum and the colon, which are the areas with the highest bacterial concentrations, represent the sites of inflammation in IBD. This loss of immune tolerance [2, 3] might be due to a lack of regulatory mediators or cells, or a breakdown in barrier function which allows the access of inflammatory bacterial products to the local immune

Table 1. Antibiotics m IBD: suggested mechanisms of action

Eradication of bacterial antigenic trigger
Elimination of bacterial overgrowth
Reduction of proinflammatory bacterial toxins
Potential immunosuppressive properties

system, thereby overwhelming normal regulation [2]. This sequence of events is supported by several studies reporting in patients with active IBD an important role for T cells in the proliferative response to intestinal flora [2], T-cell-mediated immune responses to different species of bacteria [3], and enhanced IgG levels against cytoplasmic bacterial proteins. Patients with Crohn's disease (CD) consistently improved after diversion of fecal stream, with immediate recurrence of inflammation after restoration of intestinal continuity or infusion of luminal content into the bypassed ileum [4, 5]. Furthermore, pouchitis does not occur prior to closure of the ileostomy.

An alteration of the enteric flora has been reported in patients with IBD, with an increased number of aggressive bacteria (such as *Bacteroides,* adherent/invasive *Escherichia coli,* and enterococci) and decreased number of protective lactobacilli and bifidobacteria [6].

The most compelling proof that intestinal bacteria play a role in IBD is derived from animal models. Despite great diversity in genetic defects and immunopathology, a consistent feature of many transgenic and knockout mutant murine models of colitis is that the presence of normal enteric flora is required for full expression of inflammation [7]. All of these observations suggest that IBD may be treated via manipulation of intestinal microflora [8]. As a consequence, increasing evidence supports a therapeutic role for antimicrobials in the management IBD. Suggested mechanisms of action for this class of drugs are shown in table 1.

Lessons from Animal Models

In several rodent models the use of broad-spectrum antibiotics can either prevent onset of and treat experimental colitis, whereas metronidazole and ciprofloxacin can only prevent experimental colitis but not reverse established disease [9–13]. Broad-spectrum antibiotics are effective in almost all models of acute and chronic colitis [13–16] but have only a transient efficacy in HLA-B27 transgenic rats [17]. Interestingly enough, ciprofloxacin and metronidazole had selective efficacy in different colonic regions in IL-10 knockout mice, suggesting that different bacteria may cause inflammation in different colonic segments [15]. These results are consistent with the idea that most clinical forms of IBD may respond to suppression of bacterial flora, provided a proper combination of broad-spectrum antimicrobials be used.

Studies in Patients with Ulcerative Colitis

Only few trials of antibacterial agents have been carried out in ulcerative colitis (UC) and results are controversial. Most clinicians have used antimicrobial agents as add-on medications in severe UC. Dickinson et al. [18] have carried out a double-blind controlled trial on the use of oral vancomycin as adjuvant therapy in acute exacerbations of idiopathic colitis. No significant difference was found between the two treatment groups with only a trend towards a reduction in the need for surgery in patients treated with the antibiotic [18]. Similarly, intravenous metronidazole, used in addition to steroids, did not improve the remission rate of patients with severe UC compared to placebo [19]. When oral tobramycin was added to steroids in patients with relapse of UC a significant (p < 0.003) benefit was obtained, the remission rate being 74 and 43% in the antibiotic and placebo groups, respectively [20]. In this study, patients on vancomycin displayed a trend towards a reduction in the need for operative intervention (i.e. colectomy), a finding not confirmed by subsequent investigations with other antimicrobials [18, 19, 21, 23] (fig. 1).

Ciprofloxacin has been tested in a randomized, placebo-controlled study; 70 patients with mild to moderate active UC were randomized to receive ciprofloxacin 250 mg b.i.d. or placebo for 14 days. At the end of the study, 70.5% of patients in the ciprofloxacin group vs. 72% in the placebo group achieved remission [22]. Similarly, a short course of intravenous ciprofloxacin was not effective as adjunctive treatment to corticosteroids in severe UC in a prospective, randomized, double-blind, placebo-controlled trial [23]. Nevertheless, a more recent randomized, placebo-controlled trial, in which ciprofloxacin was administered for 6 months to patients with active UC poorly responding to conventional therapy with steroids and mesalamine, did show a benefit. Indeed, at the end of the study, the treatment success rate was 79% in the ciprofloxacin-treated group and 66% in the placebo group (p < 0.002). It is worth mentioning that, based on endoscopic and histological findings, the antibiotic benefit, evident already at 3 months, disappeared 3 months later [24].

A first open, uncontrolled study [25], performed in 12 patients with active IBD refractory to standard treatment who all had positive stool culture, suggested that adding rifaximin (800 mg daily) could be beneficial. A further small but controlled investigation performed in our unit [26] evaluated the efficacy and

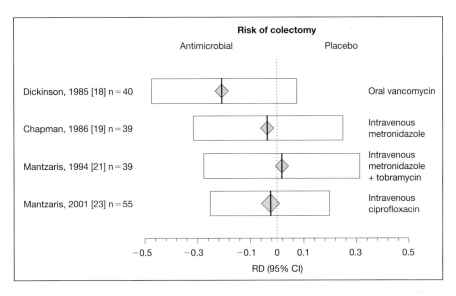

Fig. 1. Risk of colectomy following antimicrobial treatment in severe UC in comparison with placebo in four different studies.

systemic absorption of rifaximin in patients with moderately to severely active UC refractory to steroid treatment. Patients were eligible if they had no response to intravenous corticosteroid therapy (methylprednisolone 1 mg/kg/day) after 7–10 days. Twenty-eight patients were randomized to receive rifaximin 400 mg b.i.d. or placebo for 10 days as an add-on medication to standard steroid treatment. Clinical and endoscopic evaluations were performed before and after the treatment, and stool frequency, consistency and presence of blood were also recorded. Plasma and urine samples were collected before and after the treatment to determine the systemic absorption of rifaximin. Although there was no significant difference in overall clinical efficacy between the two treatments, only rifaximin determined a significant improvement of stool frequency, rectal bleeding and sigmoidoscopic score [26]. The cumulative excretion of rifaximin in 24-hour urine after 10 days was 64,617 ng, confirming the poor systemic absorption also in presence of colonic inflammation [26]. The efficacy of this rifamycin derivative as add-on medication in patients with mild to moderate UC was recently confirmed in another open-label study [27], where the clinical activity index decreased by 30% after 4 weeks of treatment.

In patients who experienced a clinical exacerbation of UC and who had a past history of serious adverse reactions to steroids, the antibiotic (400 mg b.i.d. for 4 weeks) was added to mesalazine (2.4 g daily) treatment [28]. In 7 out of

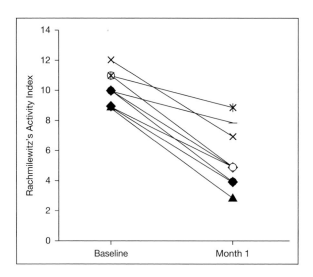

Fig. 2. Individual values of Rachmilewitz's Activity Index in patients with relapse of UC before (baseline) and after 1 month of treatment with rifaximin + mesalamine (from Guslandi et al. [27]).

10 patients (i.e. 70%) a clinical remission was achieved without corticoid use, thus showing that rifaximin displays a steroid-sparing effect (fig. 2).

Studies in Patients with Crohn's Disease

Antimicrobial Therapy

Broad-spectrum antibiotics are widely used to treat CD [29], but large, controlled trials have not been performed (table 2).

Metronidazole has been the mostly investigated agent. In 1978, Blichfeldt et al. [30] in a placebo-controlled, double-blind, cross-over trial did not find a difference between metronidazole and placebo-treated patients, but a positive trend in favor of metronidazole was observed when only the colon was involved. In the National Cooperative Swedish study, metronidazole was compared to sulfasalazine as primary treatment for CD; no significant difference was found between the two groups, but, interestingly, in the cross-over section of the study, the antimicrobial was effective in patients not responding to sulfasalazine [31]. Metronidazole was used as single therapy or associated to cotrimoxazole and compared to cotrimoxazole alone and placebo in patients with a symptomatic relapse of CD. At the end of the 4 weeks of treatment there was no

Table 2. Clinical studies with antimicrobials in active CD

Study	Patients	Weeks	Main outcome	Study design	Treatment schedules
Blichfeldt, 1978 [30]	28	8	Improvement (clinical/ lab score)	DB Crossover study	MZ (+ SASP/CS) Placebo (+SASP/CS)
Ursing, 1982 [31]	78	16	Change in CDAI and orosomucoid	DB Crossover study	MZ SASP
Ambrose, 1985 [32]	72	4	Improvement (clinical/lab score)	DB RCT	MZ CO, MZ/CO, placebo
Sutherland, 1991 [33]	99	16	Change in CDAI from baseline	DB RCT	MZ (10/20 mg/kg) Placebo
Prantera, 1996 [34]	41	12	Clinical remission (CDAI < 150)	DB RCT	MZ + Cipro Steroids
Colombel, 1999 [36]	40	6	Clinical remission (CDAI < 150)	DB RCT	Cipro 5-ASA
Arnold, 2002 [37]	47	24	Change in CDAI	NB RCT	Cipro (+ conc. drugs) Placebo (+ conc. drugs)
Steinhart 2002 [35]	134	8	Clinical remission (CDAI < 150)	DB RCT	MZ + Cipro (+ Bud 9 mg) Placebo (+ Bud 9 mg)

CDAI = Crohn's Disease Activity Index; DB = double blind; RCT = randomized clinical trial; NB = not blinded; MZ = metronidazole; SASP = sulfasalazine; CS = corticosteroids; CO = cortimoxazole; Cipro = ciprofloxacin; 5-ASA = 5-aminosalicylic acid; Bud = budesonide.

difference in response among the three groups [32]. In a Canadian randomized, placebo-controlled trial, Sutherland et al. [33] have shown that treatment with metronidazole for 16 weeks significantly decreased the Crohn's Disease Activity Index (CDAI), but no difference was found in the rates of remission compared with placebo; the benefit was dose-dependent, with 20 mg/kg being more effective than 10 mg/kg [33]. As in the case of the Swedish study, in the Canadian study metronidazole was effective for colonic and ileocolonic CD but not for ileitis. Metronidazole has important side effects that include nausea, anorexia, dysgeusia, dyspepsia, and peripheral neuropathy that limit its use in approximately 20% of patients. An antimicrobial combination was used in an Italian randomized controlled study in which metronidazole 250 mg four times daily plus ciprofloxacin 500 mg twice daily were compared to a standard steroid treatment for 12 weeks. No differences were reported in the rates of remission between treatments (46% with ciprofloxacin plus metronidazole vs. 63% with methylprednisolone) suggesting that this antimicrobial therapy could be an

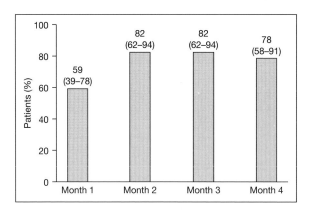

Fig. 3. Percentage of patients (95% CI) with at least a 70-point reduction in CDAI score during 4 months of treatment of active CD with rifaximin (n = 29) (from Shafran and Johnson [39]).

alternative to steroid treatment in acute phases of CD [34]. Combination of metronidazole and ciprofloxacin was associated to budesonide (9 mg/day) in active CD; no difference was observed compared to placebo, but surprisingly the overall response in the two groups was lower than that seen in previous studies with budesonide. Also in this study, antimicrobial treatment was more effective when the colon was involved [35].

Ciprofloxacin 1 g daily was compared to mesalamine 4 g daily in a controlled study dealing with mild-to-moderate active CD. After 6 weeks, both treatments were equally effective, the remission rate being 56 and 55% in patients receiving ciprofloxacin or mesalamine respectively [36]. In a small study [37], ciprofloxacin was shown to be effective in association to standard treatment in patients with resistant disease. In an open-label trial, Leiper et al. [38] reported an impressive positive response (64% patients improved or were in remission after 4 weeks) of clarithromycin in a group of 25 patients with active CD, many of whom were unresponsive to other treatments, including steroids and immunosuppressives.

Poorly absorbed antibiotics have been tested. Shafran and Johnson [39] reported recently an open-label study on the efficacy and safety of rifaximin (600 mg/day for 16 weeks) in the treatment of mildly to moderately active CD. At the end of the study, 59% of patients were in remission (as defined by CDAI, <150) with a significant reduction of the mean CDAI score compared to baseline (p < 0.0001) (fig. 3). Only one non-serious drug-related adverse event was reported, confirming the safety of the drug.

Manipulation of bacterial flora has been attempted in prevention of postoperative recurrence. Metronidazole at the dose of 20 mg/kg/day was compared to placebo in double-blind, controlled trial by Rutgeerts et al. [40]. Sixty patients were randomized to receive metronidazole or placebo for 12 weeks. At the end of the treatment, endoscopic relapse was evaluated by a specifically designed score. Metronidazole significantly decreased the incidence of severe endoscopic relapse (grade 3 or 4) in the neoterminal ileum 6 months after surgery and the clinical recurrence rates at 1 year, with a trend towards a protective effect after 3 years. More recently, ornidazole, another nitroimidazole compound, used continuously for 1 year was significantly more effective than placebo in the prevention of severe endoscopic recurrence in the neoterminal ileum both at 3 and 12 months [41].

Finally, Campieri et al. [42] performed a randomized trial to evaluate the efficacy in the prevention of postoperative recurrence of rifaximin 1.8 g daily for 3 months followed by a probiotic mixture (i.e. VSL#3) 6 g daily for 9 months vs. mesalazine 4 g daily for 12 months in 40 patients after curative resection for CD. After 3 months of treatment, patients on rifaximin had a significantly lower incidence of severe endoscopic recurrence compared to those on mesalazine, namely 2/20 (10%) vs. 8/20 (40%). This difference was maintained I after the end of the study using probiotics, namely 4/20 1 (20%) vs. 8/20 (40%). The results of this pilot study suggest therefore that the efficacy of the sequential combination of rifaximin and the highly concentrated probiotic preparation VSL#3 is effective in the prevention of severe endoscopic recurrence of CD after surgical resection [42].

Antimycobacterial Therapy

Several studies have tried to evaluate the efficacy of antimycobacterial drugs in patients with CD [43], pursuing the possibility that a strain of *Mycobacteria* might be an etiological agent in CD [44]. A meta-analysis of all randomized clinical trials [45] in which antimycobacterial therapy was compared to placebo concluded that antimycobacterial therapy is effective as a maintenance treatment only in patients who went on remission after a combined treatment with steroids and antimycobacterial agents (fig. 4). The incidence of adverse effects was, however, rather high and, since a small number of studies was included in the analysis, the conclusions should be interpreted with caution.

The same antimicrobials used to treat luminal CD have been reported to be beneficial in the treatment of perianal CD, but no controlled trials have been performed [46]. Metronidazole 20 mg/kg proved to achieve fistulae closure in 62–83% of patients [47, 48]. The combination of metronidazole and ciprofloxacin determined an improvement in 64% of patients and fistulae closure in 21% [49]. Unfortunately, fistulae tend to recur in most patients after stopping

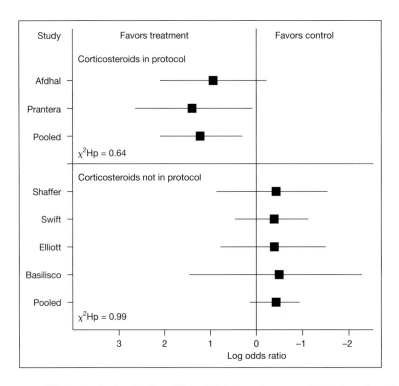

Fig. 4. Analysis of fully published trials based on use of antituberculous therapy with or without tapering course of corticosteroids (from Borgaonkar et al. [45]).

treatment. Although the results of these uncontrolled studies are not conclusive, metronidazole, ciprofloxacin or their combination are used by most clinicians as first-line treatment in patients with perianal disease, in combination with surgical abscess drainage.

Studies in Patients with Pouchitis

The awareness of the crucial importance that fecal stasis and the bacterial overgrowth may represent in the pathogenesis of acute pouchitis has led the clinicians to treat patients with antimicrobials, which – despite the lack of controlled trials – have become the mainstay of treatment. Usually, metronidazole represents the most common first therapeutic approach, and most patients with acute pouchitis respond quickly to administration of 1–1.5 g/day [50, 51]. A double-blind, randomized, placebo-controlled, cross-over trial was carried out by Madden et al. [52] to assess the efficacy of 400 mg three times a day of metronidazole per os in 13 patients (11 completed both arms of the study) with chronic, unremitting pouchitis. Patients were treated for 2 weeks and metronidazole was significantly more effective than placebo in reducing the stool frequency (73 vs. 9%), even without improvement of endoscopic appearance and histologic grade of activity. Some (55%) patients taking metronidazole experienced adverse effects including nausea, vomiting, abdominal discomfort, headache, skin rash and metallic taste.

Recently, Shen et al. [53] have compared the effectiveness and adverse effects of ciprofloxacin and metronidazole for treating acute pouchitis in a randomized clinical trial. Seven patients received ciprofloxacin 1 g/day and 9 patients metronidazole 20 mg/kg/day for a period of 2 weeks. The results of this study have shown that both ciprofloxacin and metronidazole are efficacious as treatment of acute pouchitis: they reduced the total Pouchitis Disease Activity Index (PDAI) scores and led to a significant improvement of symptoms and endoscopic and histologic scores. However, ciprofloxacin was significantly better leading to a greater degree of reduction in total PDAI score, to a greater improvement in symptoms and endoscopic scores; furthermore, ciprofloxacin was better tolerated than metronidazole. Indeed, 33% of the metronidazole-treated patients reported adverse effects, while none of the ciprofloxacin-treated patients did [54].

Medical treatment of patients with chronic refractory pouchitis is particularly difficult and disappointing [55]. A possible therapeutic alternative for chronic refractory pouchitis is the use of a combined antimicrobial treatment. In an open trial, 18 patients with active pouchitis not responding to the standard therapy (metronidazole or ciprofloxacin) for 4 weeks, were treated orally with rifaximin 2 g/day + ciprofloxacin 1 g/day for 15 days; symptoms assessment, endoscopic and histological evaluations were performed at screening and after 15 days according with PDAI. Sixteen out of 18 patients (88.8%) either improved (n = 10) or went into remission (n = 6); the median PDAI scores before and after therapy were 11 and 4, respectively ($p < 0.002$) [56]. A combination therapy with metronidazole (800 mg to 1 g/day) and ciprofloxacin (1 g/day) for 28 days was used in 44 patients with refractory pouchitis. Thirty-six patients (82%) went into remission; the median PDAI scores before and after therapy were 12 and 3, respectively ($p < 0.0001$). Patients' quality of life significantly improved with the treatment (median IBDQ increased from 96.5 to 175) [57].

A more recent study confirmed the efficacy of rifaximin-ciprofloxacin combination therapy in chronic active refractory pouchitis: after 2 weeks, 7 out of 8 patients either went into remission (n = 5) or improved (n = 2) and the median PDAI scores before and after therapy were 12 (range 9–18) and 0 (range 0–15), respectively ($p = 0.018$) (fig. 5) [58].

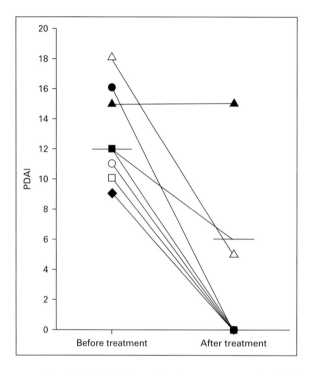

Fig. 5. PDAI before and after treatment with rifaximin-ciprofloxacin combination therapy ($p < 0.05$, Wilcoxon rank sum test; from Abdelrazeq et al. [58]).

Conclusions

There is strong evidence that enteric commensal bacteria are involved in the pathogenesis of IBD. As a consequence, suppression of intestinal flora should be beneficial in achieving and/or maintaining remission. However, the available literature does not support the use of antimicrobials in UC, and large studies with broad-spectrum antibacterial agents are required.

On the contrary, these drugs have an essential role in treating the septic complications of CD, including intra-abdominal and perianal abscesses and perianal fistulae. There is also evidence that ciprofloxacin, metronidazole or their combination are effective in Crohn's colitis and ileocolitis, but not in isolated ileal disease. The use of antibiotics as primary therapy in CD is poorly documented, and large, controlled trials are needed to define the optimal antibiotic regimens. On the contrary, the use of antimicrobials in pouchitis is largely justified on the basis of clinical results, despite the fact that proper controlled trials have not yet been conducted.

Rifaximin, a poorly absorbed antibiotic whose antibacterial spectrum includes several mycobacteria, has recently been studied in patients with UC (including pouchitis) and CD showing a good efficacy. Provided these preliminary results are confirmed in larger randomized trials, this antibiotic could represent – thanks to its efficacy and long-term safety – the preferred tool of manipulating enteric flora in patients with IBD. To better exploit rifaximin's potential in this clinical setting, a new high-dose (800 mg) formulation (i.e. sachets containing enteric-coated microgranules) has been developed, and clinical trials with this formulation are ongoing.

References

1 Sartor RB: Enteric microflora in IBD: pathogens or commensal? Inflamm Bowel Dis 1997;3: 230–235.
2 Duchmann R, Kaiser I, Hermann E, Mayet W, Ewe K, Meyer zum Buschenfelde KH: Tolerance exists towards resident intestinal flora but is broken in active inflammatory bowel disease. Clin Exp Immunol 1995;102:448–455.
3 Duchmann R, May E, Heike M, Knolle P, Neurath M, Meyer zum Buschenfelde KH: T-cell specificity and cross-reactivity towards enterobacteria, bacteroides, bifidobacterium and antigens from resident intestinal flora in humans. Gut 1999;44:812–818.
4 Rutgeerts P, Geboes K, Peeters M, Hiele M, Penninckx F, Aerts R, Kerremans R, Vantrappen G: Effect of faecal stream diversion on recurrence of Crohn's disease in the neoterminal ileum. Lancet 1991;338:771–774.
5 D'Haens GR, Goboes K, Peeters M, Penninckx F, Rutgeerts P: Early lesions of recurrent Crohn's disease caused by infusion of intestinal contents in excluded ileum. Gastroenterology 1998; 114:262–267.
6 Neut C, Bulois P, Desreumaux P, Membre JM, Lederman E, Gambiez L, Cortot A, Quandalle P, van Kruningen H, Colombel JF: Changes in bacterial flora of the neoterminal ileum after ileo-colonic resection for Crohn's : disease. Am J Gastroenterol 2002;97:939–946.
7 Sartor RB: Targeting enteric bacteria in treatment of inflammatory bowel diseases: why, how, and when? Curr Opin Gastroenterol 2003;19:358–365.
8 Sartor RB: Therapeutic manipulation of the enteric microflora in inflammatory bowel diseases: antibiotics, probiotics, and prebiotics. Gastroenterology 2004;126:1620–1633.
9 Rath HC, Schultz M, Freitag R, Dieleman LA, Li F, Linde HJ, Scholmerch J, Sartor RB: Different subsets of enteric bacteria induce and perpetuate experimental colitis in rats and mice. Infect Immun 2001;69:2277–2285.
10 Madsen KL, Doyle JS, Tavernini MM, Jewell LD, Rennie RP, Fedorak RN: Antibiotic therapy attenuates colitis in interleukin-10 gene-deficient mice. Gastroenterology 2000;118: 1094–1105.
11 Hoentjen F, Harmsen HJ, Braat H, Torrice CD, Mann BA, Sartor RB, Dieleman LA: Antibiotics with a selective aerobic or anaerobic spectrum have different therapeutic activities in various regions of the colon in interleukin-10 gene-deficient mice. Gut 2003;52:1721–1727.
12 Fiorucci S, Distrutti E, Mencarelli A, Barbanti M, Palazzini E, Morelli A: Inhibition of intestinal bacterial translocation with rifaximin modulates lamina propria monocytic cells reactivity and protects against inflammation in a rodent model of colitis. Digestion 2002;66:246–256.
13 Bamias G, Marini M, Moskaluk CA, Odashima M, Ross WG, Rivera-Nieves J, Cominelli F: Down-regulation of intestinal lymphocyte activation and Th1 cytokine production by antibiotic therapy in a murine model of Crohn's disease. J Immunol 2002;169:5308–5314.
14 Yamada T, Deitch E, Specian RD, Perry MA, Sartor RB, Grisham MB: Mechanisms of acute and chronic intestinal inflammation induced by indomethacin. Inflammation 1993;17:641–662.

15   Onderdonk AB, Hermos JA, Dzink JL, Bartlett JG: Protective effect of metronidazole in experimental ulcerative colitis. Gastroenterology 1978;74:521–526.

16   Videla S, Villaseca J, Guarner F, Salas A, Treserra F, Crespo E, Antolin M, Malagelada JR: Role of intestinal microflora in chronic inflammation and ulceration of the rat colon. Gut 1994;35: 1090–1097.

17   Dieleman LA, Goerres M, Arends A, Sprengers D, Torrice C, Hoentjen J, Grenther WB, Sartor RB: *Lactobacillus* GG prevents recurrence of colitis in HLA-B27 transgenic rats after antibiotic treatment. Gut 2003;52:370–376.

18   Dickinson RJ, O'Connor HJ, Pinder I, Hamilton I, Johnston D, Axon AT: Double-blind controlled trial of oral vancomycin as adjunctive treatment in acute exacerbations of idiopathic colitis. Gut 1985;26:1380–1384.

19   Chapman RW, Selby WS, Jewell DP: Controlled trial of intravenous metronidazole as adjunct to corticosteroids in severe ulcerative colitis. Gut 1986;27:1210–1212.

20   Burke DA, Axon ATR, Clayden SA, Dixon MF, Johnston D, Lacey RW: The efficacy of tobramycin in the treatment of ulcerative colitis. Aliment Pharmacol Ther 1990;4:123–129.

21   Mantzaris GJ, Hatzis A, Kontogiannis P, Triadaphyllou G: Intravenous tobramycin and metronidazole as an adjunct to corticosteroids in acute, severe ulcerative colitis. Am J Gastroenterol 1994;89:43–46.

22   Mantzaris GJ, Archavlis E, Christoforidis P, Kourtessas D, Amberiadis P, Florakis N, Petraki K, Spiliadi C, Triantafyllou G: A prospective randomised controlled trial of oral ciprofloxacin in acute ulcerative colitis. Am J Gastroenterol 1997;92:454–456.

23   Mantzaris GJ, Petraki K, Archavlis E, Amberiadis P, Kourtessas D, Christoforidis P, Triantafyllou G: A prospective randomised controlled trial of intravenous ciprofloxacin as an adjunct to corticosteroids in acute, severe ulcerative colitis. Scand J Gastroenterol 2001;36: 971–974.

24   Turunen UM, Farkkila MA, Hakala K, Seppala K, Sivonen A, Ogren M, Vuoristo M, Valtonen VV, Miettinen TA: Long-term treatment of ulcerative colitis with ciprofloxacin: a prospective, double-blind, placebo-controlled study. Gastroenterology 1998;115:1072–1078.

25   Pinto A, Borrutto G, Deall'Anna A, Turco L, Ferrieri A: An open, uncontrolled trial of oral rifaximin, a non-absorbable antibiotic, in inflammatory bowel disease refractory to conventional therapy. Eur J Clin Res 1997;9:217–224.

26   Lukas M, Konecny M, Zboril V: Rifaximin in patients with mild to moderate activity of ulcerative colitis: an open label study. Gastroenterology 2002;122(suppl 1):A434.

27   Guslandi M, Giollo P, Testoni PA: Corticosteroid-sparing effect of rifaximin, a nonabsorbable oral antibiotic, in active ulcerative colitis: preliminary clinical experience. Cur Ther Res 2004;65: 292–296.

28   Gionchetti P, Rizzello F, Venturi A, Ugolini F, Rossi M, Brigidi P, Johansson R, Ferrieri A, Poggioli G, Campieri M: Antibiotic combination therapy in patients with chronic, treatment-resistant pouchitis. Aliment Pharmacol Ther 1999;13:713–718.

29   Present DH: How to do without steroids in inflammatory bowel disease. Inflamm Bowel Dis I 2000;6:48–57.

30   Blichfeldt P, Blomhoff JP, Myhre E, Gjone E: Metronidazole in Crohn's disease. A double-blind cross-over clinical trial. Scand J Gastroenterol 1978;13:123–127.

31   Ursing B, Alm T, Barany F, Bergelin I, Ganrot-Norlin K, Hoevels J, Huitfeldt B, Jarnerot G, Krause U, Krook A, Lindstrom B, Nordle O, Rosen A: A comparative study of metronidazole and sulfasalazine for active Crohn's disease: the cooperative Crohn's disease study in Sweden. II. Result. Gastroenterology 1982;83:550–562.

32   Ambrose NS, Allan RN, Keighley MR, Burdon DW, Youngs D, Lennard-Jones JE: Antibiotic therapy for treatment in relapse of intestinal Crohn's disease. A prospective randomized study. Dis Colon Rectum 1985;28:81–85.

33   Sutherland LR, Singleton J, Sessions J, Hanauer S, Krawitt E, Rankin G, Summers R, Mekhjian H, Greenberg N, Kelly M: Double-blind, placebo-controlled trial of metronidazole in Crohn's disease. Gut 1991;32:1071–1075.

34   Prantera C, Zannoni F, Scribano ML, Berto E, Andreoli A, Kohn A, Luzzi C: An antibiotic regimen for the treatment of active Crohn's disease: a randomized controlled clinical trial of metronidazole plus ciprofloxacin. Am J Gastroenterol 1996;91:328–332.

35 Steinhart AH, Feagan BG, Wong CJ, Vandervoort M, Mikolainins S, Croitoru K, Seidmand E, Leddin DJ, Bitton A, Drouin E, Cohen A, Greemberg GR: Combined budesonide and antibiotic therapy for active Crohn's disease: a randomized controlled trial. Gastroenterology 2002;123: 33–40.

36 Colombel JF, Lemann M, Cassagnou M, Bouhnik Y, Duclols B, Dupas JL, Notteghem B, Mary JY: A controlled trial comparing ciprofloxacin with mesalazine for the treatment of active Crohn's disease. Am J Gastroenterol 1999;94:674–678.

37 Arnold GL, Beaves MR, Prydun VO, Mook WJ: Preliminary study of ciprofloxacin in active Crohn's disease. Inflamm Bowel Dis 2002;8:10–15.

38 Leiper K, Morris AI, Rhodes JM: Open label trial of oral clarithromycin in active Crohn's disease. Aliment Pharmacol Ther 2000;14:801–806.

39 Shafran I, Johnson L: An open-label evaluation of rifaximin in the treatment of active Crohn's disease. Curr Med Res Opin 2005;21:1165–1169.

40 Rutgeerts P, Hiele M, Geboes K, Peeters M, Penninckx F, Aerts R, Kerremans R: Controlled trial of metronidazole treatment for prevention of Crohn's recurrence after ileal resection. Gastroenterology 1995;108:1617–1621.

41 Rutgeerts P, Van Assche G, D'Haens G, Baert F, Norman M, Aerden I, Geboes K, D'Hoore A, Penninckx F: Ornidazole for prophylaxis of postoperative Crohn's disease: final results of a double-blind placebo controlled trial. Gastroenterology 2002;122:A80.

42 Campieri M, Rizzello F, Venturi A, Poggioli G, Ugolini F, Helwig U, Amadini C, Romboli E, Gionchetti P: Combination of antibiotic and probiotic treatment is efficacious in prophylaxis of post-operative recurrence of Crohn's disease: a randomized controlled study vs. mesalamine. Gastroenterology 2000;118:A781.

43 Hulten K, Almashhrawi A, El-Zaatari FA, Graham DY: Antibacterial therapy for Crohn's disease: a review emphasizing therapy directed against mycobacteria. Dig Dis Sci 2000;45: 445–456.

44 Greenstein RJ: Is Crohn's disease caused by a mycobacterium? Comparisons with leprosy, tuberculosis, and Johne's disease. Lancet Infect Dis 2003;3:507–514.

45 Borgaonkar MR, MacIntosh DG, Fardy JM: A meta-analysis of antimycobacterial therapy for Crohn's disease. Am J Gastroenterol 2000;95:725–729.

46 Schwartz DA, Pemberton JH, Sandborn WJ: Diagnosis and treatment of perianal fistulas in Crohn's disease. Ann Intern Med 2001;135:906–918.

47 Bernstein LH, Frank MS, Brandt LJ, Boley SJ: Healing of perianal Crohn's disease with metronidazole. Gastroenterology 1980;79:357–365.

48 Brandt LJ, Bernstein LH, Boley SJ: Metronidazole therapy for perianal Crohn's disease: a follow-up study. Gastroenterology 1982;83:383–387.

49 Solomon MR, McLeod R: Combination ciprofloxacin and metronidazole in severe perianal Crohn's disease. Can J Gastroenterol 1993;7:571–573.

50 Sandborn WJ, McLeod, Jewell DP: Medical therapy for induction and maintenance of remission in pouchitis. A systematic review. Inflamm Bowel Dis 1999;5:33–39.

51 Hurst RD, Molinari M, Chung P, Rubin M, Michelassi F: Prospective study of the incidence, timing and treatment of pouchitis in 104 consecutive patients after restorative proctocolectomy. Arch Surg 1996;131:497–502.

52 Madden M, McIntyre A, Nicholls RJ: Double-blind cross-over trial of metronidazole versus placebo in chronic unremitting pouchitis. Dig Dis Sci 1994;39:1193–1196.

53 Shen B, Achkar JP, Lashner BA, Ormsby AH, Remzi FH, Brzenzinski A, Bevins CL, Bambrick ML, Seidner DL, Fazio VW: A randomized clinical trial of ciprofloxacin and metronidazole to treat acute pouchitis. Inflamm Bowel Dis 2001;7:301–305.

54 Gionchetti P, Amadini C, Rizzello F, Venturi A, Poggioli G, Campieri M: Diagnosis and treatment of pouchitis. Best Pract Res Clin Gastroenterol 2003;17:75–87.

55 Sandborn WJ, Pardi DS: Clinical management of pouchitis. Gastroenterology 2004;127: 1809–1814.

56 Gionchetti P, Rizzello F, Ferrieri A, Venturi A, Brignola C, Ferretti M, Peruzzo S, Miglioli M, Campieri M: Rifaximin in patients with moderate or severe ulcerative colitis refractory to steroid-treatment: a double-blind, placebo-controlled trial. Dig Dis Sci 1999;44:1220–1221.

57   Mimura T, Rizzello F, Helwig U, Poggioli G, Schreiber S, Talbot IC, Nicholls RJ, Gionchetti P, Campieri M, Kamm MA: Four week open-label trial of metronidazole and ciprofloxacin for the treatment of recurrent or refractory pouchitis. Aliment Pharmacol Ther 2002;16:909–917.
58   Abdelrazeq AS, Kelly SM, Lund JN, Leveson SH: Rifaximin-ciprofloxacin combination therapy is effective in chronic active refractory pouchitis. Colorectal Dis 2005;7:182–186.

Note Added in Proof

After submission of this paper some authors reported at the meeting of the *American College of Gastroenterology* in Honolulu (Hawaii, USA) their experience with rifaximin in IBD. The steroid-sparing activity of this poorly absorbed antibiotic was confirmed not only in CD [1, 2] but also in UC [2]. The drug proved to be effective – as an add-on medication – in patients with mild to moderately active CD with 75% of them achieving a complete (67%) or partial (33%) response in a median time of 21 (14–30) days [3]. Of those who did not respond to antibiotic treatment, the majority had ileocolic CD.

References

1   Blonski W, Kundu R, Lichtenstein GR: Efficacy of rifaximin in steroid-dependent Crohn's disease. Am J Gastroentererol 2005;100 (suppl):S241–S242.
2   Feldman D, Baradarian R, Iswara K, Li JJ, Tenner S: Rifaximin as a steroid-sparing medication in the management of patients with inflammatory bowel disease. Am J Gastroenterol 2005; 100(suppl):S307.
3   Baidoo L, Blonski W, Kundu R, Lichtenstein GR: Rifaximin for mild to moderately active Crohn's disease. Am J Gastroenterol 2005;100(suppl):S319–S320.

Paolo Gionchetti, MD
Department of Internal Medicine and Gastroenterology
Policlinico S. Orsola, Via Massarenti 9
IT–40138 Bologna (Italy)
Tel. +39 051 636 4122, Fax +39 051 392 538, E-Mail paolo@med.unibo.it

This chapter should be cited as follows:

Gionchetti P, Rizzello F, Lammers KM, Morselli C, Tambasco R, Campieri M: Antimicrobials in the Management of Inflammatory Bowel Disease. Digestion 2006;73(suppl 1):77–85.

Scarpignato C, Lanas Á (eds): Bacterial Flora in Digestive Disease.
Focus on Rifaximin.

....

Hepatic Encephalopathy: From Pathophysiology to Treatment

Antoni Mas

Liver Unit, Institute of Digestive and Metabolic Diseases, IDIBAPS, Hospital Clinic, University of Barcelona, Barcelona, Spain

Abstract

Hepatic encephalopathy (HE) is a neuropsychiatric syndrome due to hepatic dysfunction and porto-systemic shunting of the intestinal blood. Cirrhosis is the most frequent liver disease causing HE. On most occasions, HE appears due to a superimposed precipitating factor (gastrointestinal bleeding, infections, renal and electrolyte disturbances, etc.). Ammonia produced in colon by intestinal bacteria is the main toxic substance implicated in the pathogenesis of HE. Other mechanisms, such as changes in the GABA-benzodiazepine system, accumulation of manganese into the basal ganglia of the brain, changes in blood-brain barrier and neurotransmission disturbances are also present. Clinical manifestations of HE may vary widely, from minimal neurologic changes, only detected with specific tests, to deep coma. Treatment of HE should be directed to controlling the precipitating factors, as well as therapies aimed at correcting the above-mentioned pathophysiological changes, mainly reduction of blood ammonia levels. Artificial liver support systems may play a role in the future. Liver transplantation should be evaluated as a definitive therapy in all cases of HE.

Patients with liver diseases frequently develop neurological problems. The most specific is hepatic encephalopathy (HE), a neuropsychiatric syndrome caused by two main mechanisms: the presence of important hepatic dysfunction and the diversion of the portal blood to the systemic circulation, without having been purified of toxic intestinal substances by the liver (porto-systemic shunts) [1]. The relative proportion of both features varies greatly from one clinical situation to another. This paper briefly reviews the main mechanisms implicated in the development of HE, its clinical presentation and the different therapeutic approaches based on the above-mentioned pathophysiology.

Table 1. Classification of HE (from Ferenci et al. [2])

Type A	HE associated with **A**cute liver failure
Type B	HE associated with portal-systemic **B**ypass, no intrinsic hepatocellular disease
Type C	HE associated with **C**irrhosis and portal hypertension or portal-systemic shunts:
	– Episodic HE: precipitated, spontaneous, recurrent
	– Persistent HE: mild, severe, treatment-dependent
	– Minimal HE

Definitions and Nomenclature

A consensus conference on this entity was held in Vienna in 1998. The experts decided to classify HE into three types – A, B, and C [2]. The main characteristics of these three types are given in table 1. The most frequent is type C, which is associated with cirrhosis, and the present review will deal nearly exclusively with this topic, with the occasional mention of type A, i.e. HE associated with acute liver failure.

Pathophysiology

At present, the main substances considered to be implicated in the development of HE are ammonia and other intestinal neurotoxins, manganese and the benzodiazepine-GABA system [1]. Neurotransmission changes induced by these compounds play a major role in the development of the neurologic disturbances presented by the patients [3, 4]. The cellular basis of most of the changes that occur in HE is the astrocyte, the only cerebral cell capable of metabolizing ammonia [5]. In the past, other hypotheses on the pathophysiology of HE were proposed. The false neurotransmitter theory, very popular some decades ago, has practically been abandoned today, due to the inconsistence of its basis.

Ammonia and Other Intestinal Neurotoxins
For many years, ammonia was considered as the key molecule implicated in the pathophysiology of HE. The fact that in many cases blood ammonia levels may not correlate with the presence and degree of HE, and the interest of other mechanism(s) by some investigators, led the ammonia theory to lose importance in the field of HE, especially in the 1970s and 1980s. However, more recently, ammonia has re-emerged as the main neurotoxin implicated in the pathogenesis

of HE [1, 4]. Many reasons may explain this: ammonia is produced mainly in the colon by the intestinal flora, its portal concentration is high and is efficiently extracted by the liver (in individuals with normal hepatic function more than 90% of portal ammonia is metabolized by the liver), the majority of factors causing HE in a cirrhotic patient increase blood ammonia, and most of the therapeutic measures used in HE cause a decrease in ammonia levels [1].

The reasons explaining the low correlation between arterial or venous ammonia concentrations and the presence and degree of HE observed in many cases are multiple: on one hand, some authors have suggested the use of the partial pressure of ammonia (pNH_3) rather that its blood concentration. Arterial pNH_3 correlated more closely than total ammonia with the grade and the neurophysiological abnormalities in HE [6]. However, the main cause of the discrepancies between ammonia levels and HE is probably related to a difference in the brain uptake of ammonia, which is increased in patients with HE, independently of blood ammonia levels [7]. Glutamine concentrations in the CSF fluid, which reflect the degree of intracerebral ammonia metabolism, have a good correlation with HE in cirrhosis [8]. Cerebral micro-circulation and blood-brain barrier abnormalities may account for the different ammonia uptake by the brain in this situation.

Many reasons may explain why ammonia produces changes in the cerebral function, with the most well known relating ammonia to cerebral energy failure and to changes in neurotransmission by different ways, including an agonistic effect on GABAergic transmission, causing inhibition of neurotransmission [1, 4, 9].

In the last decade, some investigators have tried to correlate the presence of *Helicobacter pylori* infection and HE in cirrhotics. Urease activity of this bacteria causes a release of ammonia in the stomach, and therefore may account for an increase in its levels due to intestinal absorption. The results of different studies are conflicting, but most of the data did not confirm this hypothesis. We performed a study in 62 cirrhotic patients with mild liver impairment and absence of overt signs of HE. *H. pylori* infection was detected in 52% of cases, with no differences in ammonia levels and in other data suggesting minimal HE in positive and negative individuals. Furthermore, no changes in the above-mentioned parameters were observed after eradication of the microorganism [10].

Many other substances originating in the gut have been identified as possible additional neurotoxins in HE having a synergistic effect with ammonia: mercaptans (one of them, methanethiol seems to be the cause of *fetor hepaticus*, a unique odor that can be detected in some patients with HE), short and medium chain fatty acids and phenols. The role of these compounds in HE remains unclear because of the lack of consistent data and knowledge of the mechanisms affecting brain function [11].

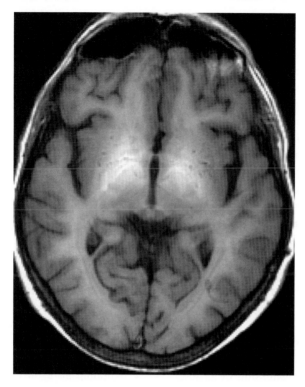

Fig. 1. MRI of a patient's brain with HE. An increase in the T_1 signal in the globus pallidus is seen.

Benzodiazepines and GABAergic Tone

An increase of 'endogenous' benzodiazepines and other compounds (neurosteroids) has been described in HE, both being modulators of the GABA receptor complex (GRC), a potent inhibitor of neurotransmission. Alterations of constituents of GRC have also been found in cases of HE [12]. Benzodiazepines can be produced in the brain, favored by some precursors present in the intestinal flora. Brain GABA content is also increased in HE, due to increased GABA uptake caused by an altered permeability of the blood-brain barrier. As stated previously, the GABA system inhibits neurotransmission, and therefore some manifestations of HE may be due to a higher GABAergic tone [1, 3, 11, 12].

Manganese

Many cirrhotics exhibit an increase in the T_1 signal in the basal ganglia of the brain (globus pallidus), detected by magnetic resonance imaging (MRI) [13], which disappears after liver transplantation (fig. 1). This abnormality is considered to be caused by accumulation of manganese in the brain. Increased cerebral concentrations of manganese have been found in cirrhotics dying with hepatic coma. Although there are no good correlations between plasma manganese levels and HE, the similarity between the clinical manifestations of manganese intoxication and the extrapyramidal signs present in some patients with HE suggests that these may be due to the accumulation of manganese in the brain [1, 13].

Neurotransmission in HE

The false neurotransmitters theory is now considered obsolete. However, alterations in neurotransmission are probably the main cause of HE. Glutamatergic tone is altered in HE, as it is GABAergic tone, as previously discussed [1, 4, 9]. Ammonia possibly plays a major role in these abnormalities. At present, it is difficult to ascribe changes in other neurotransmission systems that have been detected in HE to the clinical manifestations of this syndrome [11].

Pathology and Neuroimaging in HE

Astrocytes control the concentration of many substances in the interstitial compartment of the brain, and play a crucial role in neuronal function. Although HE is a functional syndrome, the most common pathological finding in patients with advanced or persistent HE is the presence of the so-called Alzheimer's type II astrocytosis. Astrocytes undergo this change because of an increase in intracellular water that is produced by the hyperammonemia. The increase in astrocyte water is due to the osmotic effect of glutamine synthesis brought about by the intracellular metabolism of ammonia. There are convincing data that swelling of the astrocytes plays a major role in cerebral edema in acute liver failure. In fact, ammonia concentrations correlate with the risk of brain herniation in this situation [14]. In cirrhosis the degree of cerebral edema is usually much less important, probably due to the activation of osmoregulatory mechanisms, mainly the release of myoinositol from the cells. On magnetic resonance spectroscopy (MRS), the cerebral concentrations of glutamine are high and those of myoinositol low, reflecting the activation of the osmoregulation. Alterations in astrocyte function due to the above-mentioned changes seem to be very important in neuronal function, thereby contributing to the neurological manifestations of HE [1, 5].

The role of neuroimaging in the study of HE is stressed by the finding of the previously mentioned changes in MRI (fig. 1) or MRS. Positron emission tomography (PET) has also been used in the study of the pathophysiological mechanisms of HE. An excellent review on this topic has recently been published by Butterworth [15], who also analyses the complex problem of the changes in the expression of genes coding for key brain proteins in HE.

Table 2. Classification of HE (from Ferenci et al. [2])

Grade I	Trivial lack of awareness Euphoria or anxiety Shortened attention span
Grade II	Lethargy or apathy Minimal disorientation for time or place Subtle personality change Inappropriate behavior
Grade III	Somnolence to semistupor Confusion Gross disorientation
Grade IV	Coma (no response to verbal or noxious stimuli)

Clinical Manifestations of HE

Signs and symptoms of HE may vary widely, oscillating from minimal HE, only manifested by some neuro-psychological tests or on performing actions which re-quire relatively complex neuromuscular and psychological activities (i.e. minimal encephalopathy) such as driving, to a deep coma. HE may appear acutely in a patient without previous neurological problems and disappear rapidly, or may be chronic, with repeated episodes separated by periods of neuropsychiatric normality or presented as permanent HE (table 1).

The clinical manifestations of overt HE are related to mental status (from nearly normal to deep coma), neuromuscular changes (the most common and frequent being flapping tremor), as well as modifications in mood and behavior (some times very peculiar and bizarre in a previously normal individual). The consensus conference on the nomenclature of HE suggested that the classical West Haven classification be maintained as four degrees, especially useful in acute HE (table 2). In patients in grade IV HE (i.e. hepatic coma), subclassification according to the Glasgow Coma Scale was recommended [2]. In cases of chronic permanent HE, the classification is less useful and other neurological disturbances, which are infrequent in acute HE, may appear, such as extrapyramidal changes and dementia. In rare cases, myelopathy may be present [1, 11].

The diagnosis of HE is based on the clinical data with very few complementary exams being really useful. Ammonia levels (preferably arterial) may have a very poor correlation with the presence and severity of HE, as previously discussed. EEG changes are very common and relatively typical, especially the so-called 'triphasic' waves. However, they are not specific for HE and may appear in other metabolic encephalopathies. Neuropsychological tests are especially used in clinical research, but their clinical usefulness is very slight. The

Psychometric Hepatic Encephalopathy Score (PHES), a standardized test battery including five different tests – number connection A and B, digit-symbol, line-tracing and serial-dotting tests – has been described in recent years although its use is restricted to the study of mild and minimal HE. 1 Apart from EEG, other neurophysiologic studies include evoked potentials, particularly the study of the P300 wave, which are also used in research and only exceptionally in the clinical setting [1, 2, 11]. The role of brain imaging techniques in the study of HE has been discussed previously. CT scan may detect some degree of cerebral edema, but the clinical usefulness of this technique lays mainly in the detection of structural changes in the brain, such as hemorrhage or tumors, which can cause neurological changes in cirrhotic patients that are obviously not due to HE. Differential diagnosis is based on the exclusion of those lesions, as well as other metabolic, toxicological or infectious causes. In exceptional cases HE may be the first manifestation of liver failure. This occurs in hyperacute hepatic failure cases (neurological changes appearing before jaundice in a previously healthy individual) or in patients with well-compensated cirrhosis and having large spontaneous porto-systemic shunts.

With the aim of providing a more objective index of HE, Conn et al. [16] proposed many years ago the use of the Porto-Systemic Encephalopathy (PSE) Index. It includes five different parameters: mental status, according to the classical classification from I to IV (considered to have a potency of 3), intensity of flapping tremor, levels of ammonia, number connection test type A and the mean frequency of EEG waves. This index was very popular in research on HE during many years but has now been almost abandoned because it is considered too artificial.

The Pathophysiological Basis of HE Therapy

From a very simple point of view, the most useful therapy of HE should include the cure of the liver insufficiency and/or the closing of the porto-systemic shunts. In fact, the first approach is exceptionally achieved in cirrhosis without liver transplantation. In patients with acute liver failure who survive with conventional measures, HE and signs of cerebral edema disappear rapidly when liver improvement is achieved. In cirrhotics, the possibility of a transient aggravation of liver dysfunction (called 'acute-on-chronic') is relatively frequent: HE may also be transient in these cases. The main causes of this 'acute-on-chronic' are alcoholic hepatitis, gastrointestinal bleeding or infections. However, the presence of HE in a cirrhotic patient, regardless of the degree of HE and the factors causing the episode, carries a very bad prognosis. In a study performed in our unit, survival probability after the first episode of HE was 42

Table 3. Precipitating factors of HE (from Córdoba and Blei [1] and Blei [11])

Gastrointestinal bleeding
Infections/systemic inflammatory response syndrome
Renal failure/electrolyte disturbances
Psychotropic drugs
Increase of protein intake
Constipation
Unknown in 20–30% of cases

and 23% at 1 and 3 years respectively [17]. This means that HE should be an indication for evaluation and listing for liver transplantation (if no contraindications are present) in every cirrhotic patient.

It has been repeatedly mentioned that HE usually appears when an event, previously not present, occurs during the course of a cirrhosis without neurological impairment. These are called 'precipitating factors', the main ones being listed in table 3. As stated beforehand, most of these factors cause an increase in the ammonia levels, apart from the possible aggravation of liver function (the above-mentioned 'acute-on-chronic'). Gastrointestinal bleeding, excessive protein intake and constipation increase ammonia due to the higher absorption of nitrogenous compounds from the gut and renal failure or hydroelectrolytic abnormalities, often due to diuretics, provoke increased renal ammonia production or reabsorption. In fact, in the recent years a new view of the pathophysiology of HE takes four organs into account in which the traffic of ammonia may result in increases of this substance in the brain: the liver, the gut, the kidney and the muscle [18]. In cases of HE induced by the intake of benzodiazepines, it is obvious that this compounds plays a major causative role. Recently, the pathophysiology of HE induced by one of the most common precipitating factors (i.e. infection) has been clarified. The systemic inflammatory response syndrome (SIRS) and its mediators (nitric oxide and pro-inflammatory cytokines such as interleukin-6, interleukin-β1 and tumor necrosis factor-α) present during infection in patients with cirrhosis cause significant deterioration of neuropsychological test scores following induced hyperammonemia, but not after its resolution [19]. Therefore, inflammation and its mediators may modulate the cerebral effect of ammonia in these cases. Likewise, aggravation of HE in acute liver failure when SIRS develops has also been described [20].

The prompt correction of the precipitating factors constitutes the most important therapeutic feature in HE [1, 11]. Some authors consider that this is the only therapy that should be instituted, the remaining procedures not being

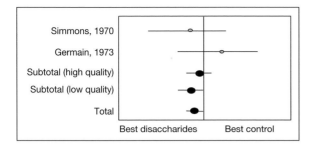

Fig. 2. Meta-analysis of the treatment of HE with non-absorbable disaccharides. Conclusions: (a) few high-quality studies; (b) insufficient evidence of disaccharide efficacy, and (c) non-absorbable antibiotics, better than disaccharides (from Als-Nielsen et al. [24]).

useful or even being dangerous [21]. However, in a significant proportion of cases, no precipitating factor can be detected.

According to the different mechanisms involved in the pathophysiology of HE, therapy should be directed to correct the following abnormalities [1, 5, 11]:

(1) *Lower intestinal absorption of ammonia and other neurotoxins*: This is achieved by reducing the amount of nitrogen in the diet, by oral administration of non-absorbable disaccharides (lactulose, lactitol, lactose in lactose-intolerant individuals) or by enema, and by the administration of non-absorbable or poorly absorbable antibiotics, e.g. neomycin, paromomycin, and more recently rifaximin [22, 23]. In a recent meta-analysis, antibiotics showed a better efficacy in HE in comparison with non-absorbable disaccharides (fig. 2) [24]. Since the pathophysiological and clinical value of these therapies are discussed elsewhere, the most important aspect to stress here is the fact that a restrictive protein diet worsens the nutritional status of the patients, does not improve the outcome of HE and can actually lead to an increase in ammonia due to reduction in the muscular removal of this substance [18]. In this connection, a recent study has shown that a normoproteic diet can be safely administered to patients with acute HE (fig. 3) [25]. Vegetable-based diets are used in cases of chronic HE with intolerance to normal diet and seem to be useful in this selected group of patients.

From a clinical point of view, the different procedures discussed in this point are the most commonly used [26].

(2) *Manipulation of the intestinal production of ammonia*: Apart from the changes in the gut flora caused by non-absorbable disaccharides and antibiotics, another approach is to modify colonic bacteria by administering high doses of urease-negative bacteria (*Lactobacillus acidophilus, Enterococus faecium* SF 68) [27]. These therapies require further investigation.

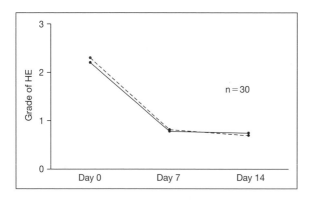

Fig. 3. Effects of a hypoproteic diet (----, 0 g × 3 days, progressive increase) vs. a nor-moproteic diet (——, 1.2 g/kg/day from the first day) in acute HE (from Córdoba et al. [25]).

(3) *Drugs acting on the urea cycle*: This includes the administration of ornithine-aspartate, which provides substrates for urea and glutamine synthesis [28], zinc supplements, since zinc is a cofactor for many enzymes of the urea cycle [29], or sodium benzoate, a compound used in children with urea cycle diseases. A study published in 1992 [30] showed that this drug improves HE in a manner similar to that of lactulose.

(4) *Benzodiazepine antagonists*: The use of flumazenil in HE not induced by the administration of external benzodiazepines results in a transient improvement in mental status in a small number of patients. Therefore, the real efficacy of this drug is poor [31]. Probably, the usefulness of flumazenil in HE is to rule out the possible previous administration of benzodiazepines as a cause of the neurologic impairment.

(5) *Dopaminergic agonists*: The use of bromocriptine or L-dopa is restricted to cases of chronic HE with important extrapyramidal signs. A recently published meta-analysis did not provide evidence that these drugs are of benefit in this setting, although it seems that there is also insufficient data to exclude a potential beneficial effect [32]. Since the extrapyramidal signs that some patients with chronic HE present have been related to brain manganese accumulation, chelation of this substance could be an option; however, up to now no studies have been performed to explore this possibility.

(6) *Diets enriched with branched chain amino acids*: The use of intravenous solutions of branched chain amino acids based on the 'false-neurotransmitters' theory was very common some years ago as a treatment of acute HE. This procedure is now rarely employed, although oral supplements of branched chain amino acids continue to be used as a complementary therapy in cases of protein-intolerant patients with chronic HE. Administration of branched chain

keto analogues have also been studied in small trials with conflicting results [1, 11, 33].

(7) *Surgery or angiographic techniques*: In cases of chronic HE the reduction or obliteration of large spontaneous porto-systemic anastomoses, or shunts previously done by surgery or TIPSS (transjugular percutaneous porto-systemic shunt), can be a therapeutic option. The risk of bleeding due to the increase in portal pressure after performing these procedures is obvious. Splenic artery embolization or total colectomy are other possibilities that have been used in highly selected patients with chronic HE resistant to other less aggressive therapies [1, 11].

(8) *Artificial and bioartificial liver support in HE*: In recent years different extracorporeal systems have been developed with the aim of substituting liver function. Some of these systems consist in non-biological procedures (i.e. artificial), similar to hemodialysis used in renal insufficiency, while others contain active liver cells in the circuit (i.e. bioartificial) [34]. The possible efficacy of these procedures in HE has been investigated either in acute liver failure or cirrhosis.

MARS (molecular adsorbent recirculating system) is based on albumin dialysis. The rationale of this system is to remove the toxins bound to albumin, as well as other water-soluble substances. In HE, MARS has been used in different circumstances. It seems to reduce cerebral edema in acute liver failure with improvement in mental status in some cases. In cirrhosis with HE, MARS has shown a reduction in the degree of encephalopathy in non-controlled studies. In a recent clinical trial carried out in the USA, this system was found to significantly improve HE in comparison with controls [35]. MARS, therefore, seems to be a useful tool in cases of severe acute HE, especially if rapid improvement is not achieved with conventional measures.

Bioartificial liver support systems, based on different types of hepatocytes (porcine, human immortalized, human non-manipulated), have also been used in HE, especially in acute liver failure. The most important study of these systems, using the HepatAssist device, has recently been published. Unfortunately, however, no data is given on the outcome of HE [36]. In a previous publication using the same system, the Glasgow Coma Scale as well as intracranial pressure significantly decreased after treatment with this system [37].

According to a meta-analysis published in 2004, the positive effects, including improvement in HE of the artificial and bioartificial liver support systems in patients with liver failure, seemed to be restricted to the 'acute-on-chronic' situation, while their efficacy in patients with acute liver failure remained doubtful [38].

(9) *Liver transplantation*: Substitution of the sick liver by a new organ is obviously the most radical therapy for improving the manifestations of hepatic failure. As stated previously, any patient who has presented an episode of HE should be evaluated for this procedure [17]. In cases of chronic HE, improvement in neurological signs after liver transplantation may not occur, or recovery may

be only partial. This is also an argument to proceed with early liver transplantation, before the development of important organic brain lesions develop on sustained HE.

References

1   Cordoba J, Blei AT: Hepatic encephalopathy; in Schiff ER, Sorrell MF, Maddrey WC (eds): Schiff's Diseases of the Liver. Philadelphia, Lippincott Williams & Wilkins, 2003, pp 595–623.
2   Ferenci P, Lockwood A, Mullen K, Terter R, Weissenborn K, Blei AT, et al: Hepatic encephalopathy – definition, nomenclature, diagnosis, and quantification. Final Report of the Working Party at the 11th World Congresses of Gastroenterology, Vienna 1998. Hepatology 2002;35:716–721.
3   Butterworth RF: The neurobiology of hepatic encephalopathy. Semin Liver Dis 1996;16:235–244.
4   Jones EA: Ammonia, the GABA neurotransmitter system, and hepatic encephalopathy. Metab Brain Dis 2002;17:275–281.
5   Haussinger D, Kircheis G, Fischer R, Schliess F, vom Dahl S: Hepatic encephalopathy in chronic liver disease: a clinical manifestation of astrocyte swelling and low-grade cerebral edema? J Hepatol 2000;32:1035–1038.
6   Kramer L, Tribl B, Gendo A, Zauner C, Schneider B, Ferenci P, et al: Partial pressure of ammonia versus ammonia in hepatic encephalopathy. Hepatology 2000;31:30–34.
7   Lockwood AH, McDonald JM, Rieman RE, Gelbard AS, Laughlin JS, Duffy TE et al: The dynamics of ammonia metabolism in man. Effects of liver disease and hyperammonemia. J Clin Invest 1979;63:449–460.
8   Watanabe A, Takei N, Higashi T, Shiota T, Nakatsukasa H, Fujiwara M, et al: Glutamic acid and glutamine levels in serum and cerebrospinal fluid in hepatic encephalopathy. Biochem Med 1984;32:225–231.
9   Butterworth RF: Hepatic encephalopathy: a neuropsychiatric disorder involving multiple neurotransmitter systems. Curr Opin Neurol 2000;13:721–727.
10 Vasconez C, Elizalde JI, Llach J, Ginès A, de la Rosa C, Fernández RM et al: *Helicobacter pylori*, hyperammonemia and subclinical porto-systemic encephalopathy: effects of eradication. J Hepatol 1999;30:260–264.
11 Blei AT: Hepatic encephalopathy; in Bircher J, Benhamou JP, McIntyre N, Rizzetto M, Rodés J (eds): Oxford Textbook of Clinical Hepatology, ed 2. Oxford, Oxford Medical, 1999, pp 765–783.
12 Ahboucha S, Butterworth RF: Pathophysiology of hepatic encephalopathy: a new look at GABA from the molecular standpoint. Metab Brain Dis 2004;19:331–343.
13 Córdoba J, Sanpedro F, Alonso J, Rovira A: ^{1}H-magnetic resonance in the study of hepatic encephalopathy in humans. Metab Brain Dis 2002;17:415–429.
14 Clemmesen JO, Larsen FS, Kondrup J, Hansen BE, Ott P: Cerebral herniation in patients with acute liver failure is correlated with arterial ammonia concentration. Hepatology 1999;29:648–653.
15 Butterworth RF: Pathogenesis of hepatic encephalopathy: new insights from neuroimaging and molecular studies. J Hepatol 2003;39:278–285.
16 Conn HO, Leevy CM, Vhlacevic ZR, Rodgers JB, Maddrey WB, Seeff L, et al: Comparison of lactulose and neomycin in the treatment of chronic portal-systemic encephalopathy. A double-blind controlled trial. Gastroenterology 1977;72:573–583.
17 Bustamante J, Rimola A, Ventura PJ, Navasa M, Cirera I, Reggiardo V, et al: Prognostic significance of hepatic encephalopathy in patients with cirrhosis. J Hepatol 1999;30:890–895.
18 Vaquero J, Chung C, Cahill ME, Blei AT: Pathogenesis of hepatic encephalopathy in acute liver failure. Semin Liver Dis 2003;23:259–269.
19 Shawcross DL, Davies NA, Williams R, Jalan R: Systemic inflammatory response exacerbates the neuropsychological effects of induced hyperammonemia in cirrhosis. J Hepatol 2004;40:247–254.
20 Rolando N, Wade J, Davalos M, Wendon J, Philpott-Howard J, Williams R: The systemic inflammatory response syndrome in acute liver failure. Hepatology 2000;32:734–739.

21 Blanc P, Daurès JP, Liautard J, Buttigieg R, Desprez D, Pageaux G, et al: Association lactulose-néomycine versus placebo dans le traitement de l'encéphalopathie hépatique aiguë. Résultats d'un essai contrôlé randomisé. Gastroentérol Clin Biol 1994;18:1063–1068.

22 Scarpignato C, Pelosini I: Rifaximin, a poorly absorbed antibiotic: pharmacology and clinical potential. Chemotherapy 2005;51(suppl 1):36–66.

23 Zeneroli ML, Avallone R, Corsi L, Venturini I, Baraldi C, Baraldi M: Management of hepatic encephalopathy; role of rifaximin. Chemotherapy 2005;51(suppl 1):90–95.

24 Als-Nielsen B, Gluud LL, Gluud C: Non-absorbable disaccharides for hepatic encephalopathy: systematic review of randomised trials. BMJ 2004;328:1046–1051.

25 Córdoba J, López-Hellín J, Planas M, Sabín P, Sanpedro F, Castro F: Normal diet for episodic hepatic encephalopathy: results of a randomized study. J Hepatol 2004;41:38–43.

26 Blei AT, Córdoba J: Practice Parameters Committee of the American College of Gastroenterology. Hepatic encephalopathy. Am J Gastroenterol 2001;96:1968–1976.

27 García-Tsao G: Gut microflora in the pathogenesis of the complications of cirrhosis. Best Pract Res Clin Gastroenterol 2004;18:353–372.

28 Kircheis G, Wettstein M, Dahl S, Hausinger D: Clinical efficacy of L-ornithine-L-aspartate in the management of hepatic encephalopathy. Metab Brain Dis 2002;17:453–462.

29 Marchesini G, Fabbri A, Bianchi G, Brizi M, Zoli M: Zinc supplementation and amino acid-nitrogen metabolism in patients with advanced cirrhosis. Hepatology 1996;23:1084–1092.

30 Sushma S, Dasarathy S, Tandon RK, Jain S, Gupta S, Bhist MS: Sodium benzoate in the treatment of acute hepatic encephalopathy: a double-blind randomised trial. Hepatology 1992;16:138–144.

31 Als-Nielsen B, Kjaergard LL, Gluud C: Benzo-diazepine receptor antagonists for acute and chronic hepatic encephalopathy. Cochrane Database Syst Rev 2001;4:CD002798.

32 Als-Nielsen B, Gluud L, Gluud C: Dopaminergic agonists for hepatic encephalopathy. Cochrane Database Syst Rev 2004;4:CD003047.

33 Als-Nielsen B, Koretz RL, Kjaergard LL, Gluud C: Branched-chain amino acids for hepatic encephalopathy. Cochrane Database Syst Rev 2003;2:CD001939.

34 Jalan R, Sen S, Williams R: Prospects for extracorporeal liver support. Gut 2004;53:890–898.

35 Hassanein T, Tofteng F, Brown RS Jr, McGuire BM, Lynch P, Mehta R, et al: Efficacy of albumin dialysis (MARS) in patients with cirrhosis and advanced grades of hepatic encephalopathy: a prospective, controlled, randomized multicenter trial. Hepatology 2004;40 (suppl 1):726A–727A.

36 Demetriou AA, Brown RS Jr, Busuttil RW, Fair J, McGuire BM, Rosenthal P, et al: Prospective, randomized, multicenter, controlled trial of a bioartificial liver in treating acute liver failure. Ann Surg 2004;239:660–667.

37 Samuel D, Ichai P, Feray C, Saliba F, Azoulay D, Arulnaden JL, et al: Neurological improvement during bioartificial liver sessions in patients with acute liver failure awaiting transplantation. Transplantation 2002;73:257–264.

38 Kjaergard LL, Liu J, Als-Nielsen B, Gluud C: Artificial and bioartificial support systems for acute and acute-on-chronic liver failure: a systematic review. JAMA 2003;289:217–222.

Antoni Mas, MD
Liver Unit, Hospital Clinic
Villarroel 170
ES–08036 Barcelona (Spain)
Tel. +34 93 227 5400, ext. 3329
Fax +34 93 227 9348
E-Mail amas@clinic.ub.es

This chapter should be cited as follows:

Mas A: Hepatic Encephalopathy: From Pathophysiology to Treatment. Digestion 2006;73(suppl 1):86–93.

Scarpignato C, Lanas Á (eds): Bacterial Flora in Digestive Disease.
Focus on Rifaximin.

....

Management of Hepatic Encephalopathy: Focus on Antibiotic Therapy

Davide Festi, Amanda Vestito, Giuseppe Mazzella, Enrico Roda,
Antonio Colecchia

Department of Internal Medicine and Gastroenterology, University of Bologna,
Bologna, Italy

Abstract

Hepatic encephalopathy (HE) is a major neuropsychiatric complication of both acute
and chronic liver failure. Symptoms of HE include attention deficits, alterations of sleep patterns and muscular incoordination progressing to stupor and coma. The pathogenesis of HE
is still unknown, although ammonia-induced alterations of cerebral neurotransmitter balance, especially at the astrocyte-neurone interface, may play a major role. Treatment of HE is
therefore directed at reducing the production and absorption of gut-derived neurotoxic substances, especially ammonia. The non-absorbable disaccharides lactulose and lactitol were
long considered as a first-line pharmacological treatment of HE, but a recent systematic
review questioned their efficacy, pointing out that there is insufficient high-quality evidence
to support their use. Oral antibiotics are regarded as a suitable therapeutic alternative.
However, the prolonged use of antimicrobials is precluded by the possible occurrence of
adverse events. Rifaximin, a synthetic antibiotic structurally related to rifamycin, displays a
wide spectrum of antibacterial activity against Gram-negative and Gram-positive bacteria,
both aerobic and anaerobic, and a very low rate of systemic absorption. Available evidence
suggests that rifaximin – thanks to its efficacy and remarkable safety – has the highest benefit-
risk ratio in the overall treatment of HE.

Introduction

Hepatic encephalopathy (HE) is a potential reversible, or progressive, neuropsychiatric syndrome characterized by changes in cognitive function, behaviour,
and personality, as well as by transient neurological symptoms and characteristic

Table 1. Predisposing factors for HE development (from Mullen et al. [3] and Ferenci et al. [4])

Nitrogen products	Metabolic alteration	Drugs	Others
Gastrointestinal bleeding	Hypokalaemia	Opiates	Infections
Hyperazotaemia	Alkalosis	Benzodiazepines	Surgery
Constipation	Hypoxia	Diuretics	Renal failure
High-protein diet	Hyponatraemia	Sedatives	Short fatty acids
H. pylori	Hyperkalaemia	Phenol	
Uraemia	Dehydration		

electroencephalographic patterns associated with acute and chronic liver failure [1]. The clinical spectrum of this syndrome ranges from minor signs of altered brain function to deep coma [2, 3].

Recently, to overcome the lack of established terminology and diagnostic criteria for HE in humans, a consensus terminology has been proposed [4] to normalize the identification of the different clinical presentations of HE [5]. As a neuropsychiatric disorder, HE involves cognitive, affective and/or emotional, behavioural, and bioregulatory domains; definition of HE is, therefore, multi-dimensional.

The most distinctive presentation of HE is the development of an acute confusional state that can evolve into coma (acute encephalopathy). Patients with fulminant hepatic failure and subjects with liver cirrhosis can present with acute encephalopathy. In patients with cirrhosis, acute encephalopathy is most commonly associated with a precipitating factor that triggers the change in mental state (table 1).

In cirrhosis, recurrent episodes of an altered mental state may occur in the absence of precipitating factors (recurrent encephalopathy) and neurological deficits may not be completely reversible (persistent encephalopathy). The most frequent neurological disturbances are not evident on clinical examination: mild cognitive abnormalities are only recognizable with psychometric or neuro-physiologic tests (minimal or subclinical encephalopathy).

Quantification of the degree of HE is mainly based on the West Haven Criteria [5], which grades HE from I to IV. An additional instrument is the Glasgow Coma Scale (table 2) [6] which, measuring the response to eye opening, verbal behaviour, and motor responsiveness, quantifies neurological impairment and is less subject to observer variability than the evaluation of consciousness; however, it has not been rigorously evaluated in patients with HE.

Table 2. Glasgow Coma Scale: level of consciousness
(from Teasdale et al. [6])

Eyes open	
Spontaneously	4
To command	3
To pain	2
No response	1
Best motor response	
Obeys verbal orders	6
Localizes painful stimuli	5
Painful stimulus, flexion	3
Painful stimulus, extension	2
No response	1
Best verbal response	
Oriented, conversant	5
Disoriented, conversant	4
Inappropriate words	3
Inappropriate sounds	2
No response	1

Table 3. Toxins likely involved in the pathogenesis of HE

Ammonia
GABA/benzodiazepine
Multiple synergistic toxins
False neurotransmitters/plasma amino acid imbalance
True neurotransmitters
  (i.e. glutamate, dopamine, norepinephrine, etc.)
Serotonin/tryptophan
Manganese
Endogenous opioids

Pathophysiology of Hepatic Encephalopathy

From a pathophysiological point of view, it is widely accepted that in chronic liver dysfunction the cause of HE is due to the failure of hepatic clearance of toxic products from the gut. Different toxins have been suggested to have a pathogenic role in HE development (table 3); however, the scientific debate continues about which toxin, alone or in concert with other noxious agents, mediates HE [7]. A detailed and complete description of the experimental and clinical evidence of the role of each putative toxin is beyond the aim of this paper. However, two hypotheses (i.e. the ammonia hypothesis and the GABA$_A$/benzodiazepine hypothesis) will be discussed since they represent the rationale upon which current treatments are based [7, 8].

Ammonia remains the key gut-derived neurotoxin implicated in the pathogenesis of HE [9, 10]. It is released from several tissues (kidney, muscle), but the highest concentrations are found in the portal vein. Portal ammonia, which is the key substrate for the synthesis of urea and glutamine in the liver, is derived from both the urease activity of colonic bacteria and deamination of glutamine in the small bowel. The blood-brain barrier permeability to ammonia is increased in patients with HE [11].

Several studies [12–14] have evaluated the structural and neurochemical changes in the brain exposed to ammonia. This toxin induces type 2 astroglial changes, contributes to cell swelling through increases in intracellular glutamine, causes alterations in the blood-brain barrier, influences glutamatergic neurotransmission, and increases neuronal nitric oxide synthase (iNOS) expression. Furthermore, ammonia has been linked to abnormalities in GABAergic neurotransmission through its direct action on the GABA$_A$/benzodiazepine receptor complex and its ability to increase the density of the peripheral-type benzodiazepine (BZ) receptor. This is followed by enhancement of neurosteroid production, which in turn acts on the GABA$_A$/benzodiazepine receptor complex [7, 15, 16]. Despite this pathophysiological background, studies on the correlation between blood ammonia levels and severity of HE have provided conflicting results [12, 17].

Other gut-derived toxins have been proposed. BZ-like substances have been postulated to arise from a specific bacterial population in the colon (e.g. *Acinetobacter lwoffi*) [18–20]. Other products of colonic bacterial metabolism [21], such as neurotoxic short- and medium-chain fatty acids, phenols, and mercaptans, may interact with ammonia and result in additional neurochemical changes [1]. In addition, a manganese deposit could occur in basal ganglia and induce extrapyramidal symptomatology [22]. The GABA$_A$/benzodiazepine hypothesis suggests that endogenous or natural (found in the food cycle) BZs accumulate in the brain and cause HE by a mechanism similar to that triggered by exogenous BZ drugs. These BZs may derive either from occult ingestion of prescription drugs or from dietary and endogenous (i.e. synthesized by gut bacteria) sources [18, 19, 23]. Correlation of the levels of BZ with the severity of HE has been reported by some investigators [24], but not by others [20]. Flumazenil, a potent BZ receptor antagonist, is able to reverse HE only in a subset of cirrhotic patients [25]. These results and the findings showing that ammonia modulates GABA$_A$/benzodiazepine receptor complex [15, 16] suggest that a combination treatment of HE directed towards *both* ammonia and BZ-like substances could be more effective than the pharmacological approach specifically addressing one single toxin.

Treatment of Hepatic Encephalopathy

According to recent guidelines [1, 4], the treatment goals of HE are the provision of supportive care, the identification and removal of precipitating factors, the reduction of nitrogenous load from the gut and the assessment of the need for long-term therapy.

Different treatment strategies have been proposed to achieve these objectives: nutritional management, non-absorbable disaccharides and/or antibiotics to reduce the nitrogenous load arising from the gut, drugs affecting neurotransmission, antidopaminergic drugs, branched-chain amino acids (BCAA) to resolve the imbalance between aromatic and BCAA, radiological and/or surgical procedure to manage portal-systemic shunts. All these approaches have been discussed in another paper of this issue [5]. This review will specifically address antimicrobial use in the management of HE.

Antimicrobials

Given the primary role of gut-derived ammonia in HE, most therapeutic approaches are directed at reducing bacterial production of ammonia and enhancing its elimination [11]. Therapeutic management consists primarily of control of precipitating factors, restriction of dietary protein, bowel cleansing, and administration of disaccharides [26–29].

Antibiotic therapy was the first approach proposed for the treatment of HE, even on the basis of non-controlled clinical studies [30]. Suppression of intestinal flora and its metabolic activities will translate into decrease of production of ammonia and other bacteria-derived toxins. Conversely from antimicrobials, lactulose lowers the colonic pH as a result the production of organic acids by bacterial fermentation. The decrease in pH creates an environment that is hostile to the survival of urease-producing intestinal bacteria and may promote the growth of non-urease-producing lactobacilli, resulting in a reduced production of ammonia in the colonic lumen [29].

Different antibiotics have been tested, both in open and controlled studies. The aminoglycoside neomycin has been reported to be as effective as the non-absorbable disaccharide lactulose [31, 32]. Similar evidence has been achieved using different antimicrobials, such as paromomycin, ampicillin, metronidazole [33–37] (table 4).

The non-absorbable disaccharides lactulose and lactitol have long been considered as a first-line pharmacological treatment of HE [1], despite the lack

Table 4. Oral antibiotic therapy for HE (see text for references)

Drug	Antibacterial activity	Regimen g/day	Potential adverse effects	Efficacy
Ampicillin	Wide spectrum	4	Resistant strains	Good
Paromomycin	Wide spectrum	4	Nephro/ototoxicity	Good
Neomycin	Aerobic bacteria	4–6	Nephro/ototoxicity	Good
Metronidazole	Anaerobic bacteria	0.8	Neurotoxicity	Good
Rifaximin	Wide spectrum	1.2	Not reported	Good

of good clinical evidence. In fact, a recent Cochrane systematic review on the available clinical studies [38] questioned the benefit of non-absorbable disaccharides and highlighted that there are insufficient high-quality trials to support this treatment. The same review concluded that antibiotics appeared to be superior to non-absorbable disaccharides in improving HE, but it was unclear whether this difference in treatment effect is clinically relevant.

The potential adverse events associated with the use of currently available antibiotics preclude their first-line use for HE [27]. Although neomycin, vancomycin, and paromomycin are generally poorly absorbed, they may reach the systemic circulation in amounts sufficient to cause serious adverse effects, including hearing loss and renal damage [39–41]. Like lactulose, these antibiotics may also cause diarrhoea and intestinal malabsorption [39–41]. Because of its adverse tolerability profile in patients with HE, the absorbed antibiotic metronidazole is not recommended for longer than 2 weeks in these patients [26, 42–44]. Metronidazole must be used cautiously in patients with neuropsychiatric diseases including HE because of its potential to cause neurotoxicity. Furthermore, the dosage of metronidazole requires adjustment in patients with severe liver disease. Patients using alcohol concomitantly with metronidazole or within 3 days after therapy with metronidazole may experience an Antabuse-like reaction characterized by abdominal discomfort, vomiting, flushing, and headache. Metronidazole has also been reported to cause dose-dependent peripheral neuropathy.

Rifaximin in the Treatment of HE

Rifaximin is a poorly absorbed rifamycin derivative whose wide spectrum of antibacterial action covers both aerobes and anaerobes, either Gram-positive and Gram-negative [45, 46]. Due to the lack of absorption this antibiotic is remarkably safe also in the long term [45, 46]. Its antimicrobial efficacy and

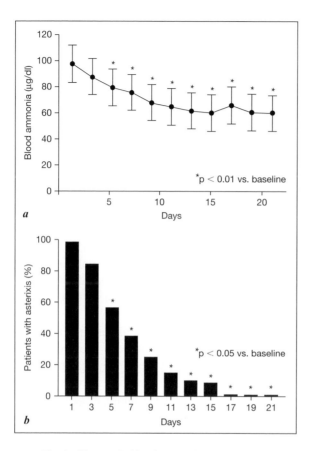

Fig. 1. Changes in blood ammonia (*a*) and incidence of asterixis (*b*) during open-label administration of rifaximin to 80 patients with grade I HE (from Festi et al. [47]).

safety make it the ideal agent to reduce the ammonia-producing bacterial load. Indeed, the drug proved to be very effective both in reducing blood ammonia and improving clinical status in patients with HE (fig. 1) [47]. The clinical experience with rifaximin has been thoroughly examined in two recent reviews [48, 49], which the reader is referred to.

The effectiveness of rifaximin in the treatment of HE has been assessed in 16 clinical trials [47, 50–64]. Overall, 809 patients were involved, of whom 521 were treated with rifaximin, while 176 received disaccharides (lactulose or lactitol) and 113 with other antibiotics (neomycin, paromomycin) employed as reference drug. Two recent studies [61, 62], performed in accordance with the Good Clinical Practice (GCP) guidelines, are particularly interesting and will be discussed in detail. The first investigation [61] was a dose-finding study

Table 5. Change in PSE index of cirrhotic patients between baseline (day 1) and day 7 of treatment with rifaximin (from Williams et al. [61])

Dosage group	Time	PSE index, %				95% CI for mean
		n	mean ± SD	minimum	maximum	
600 mg	Day 1	14	37.8 ± 11.4	25.0	64.3	
	Day 7 or withdrawal	17	31.9 ± 16.9	3.6	67.9	
	Change	14	−6.4 ± 13.7	−25.0	25.0	−14.0, 1.2
1,200 mg	Day 1	16	38.4 ± 13.8	21.4	75.0	
	Day 7 or withdrawal	16	28.2 ± 18.9	7.1	82.1	
	Change	16	−10.3 ± 13.7	−28.6	32.1	−17.4, 3.1
2,400 mg	Day 1	16	41.7 ± 8.5	17.9	50.0	
	Day 7 or withdrawal	16	31.0 ± 14.2	7.1	57.1	
	Change	16	−10.7 ± 14.9	39.3	14.3	−17.8, −3.6

n = Number of patients for whom data were available.

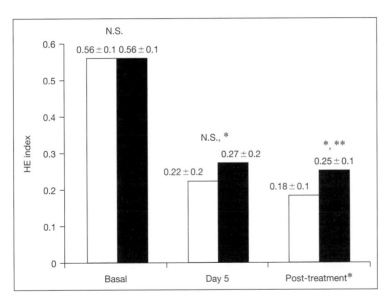

Fig. 2. Changes occurring in the PSE index in cirrhotic patients with grade I–III HE following 5–10 days treatment with rifaximin (□, 1,200 mg/day) or lactitol (■, 60 g/day). Values are expressed as mean grade (SD); N.S. = p ≥ 0.05; *p values vs. basal mean values, p = 0.0000 in both groups; **significant comparison between groups, p = 0.0103 in favour of the rifaximin group (from Mas et al. [62]).

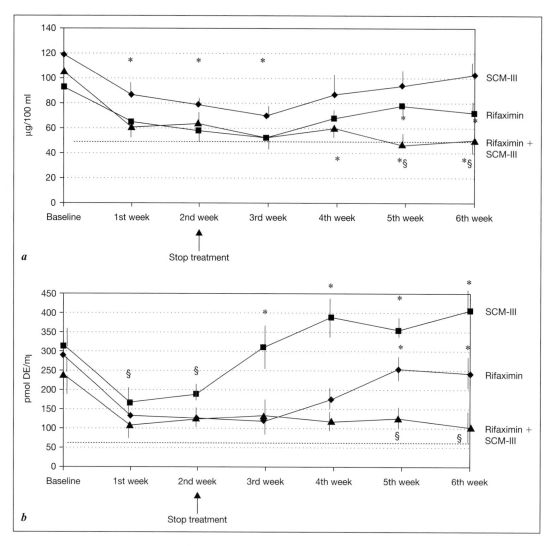

Fig. 3. Blood levels of ammonia (*a*) and benzodiazepine-like substances (*b*) in compensated cirrhotic patients: effect of rifaximin alone and in association with a symbiotic preparation (SCM-III: *L. acidophilus*, *Lactobacillus helveticus* and Bifidobacteria in an ion- and vitamin-enriched medium). *$p < 0.05$ vs. pre-treatment values; $^{§}p < 0.05$, rifaximin + SCM-III vs. other groups; dotted line: normal value (from Lighthouse et al. [68]).

where 54 patients with grade I–III HE, three daily dosages (600, 1,200 and 2,400 mg) were assessed. The main objective parameters were the portal-systemic encephalopathy (PSE) index, the Reitan test, the EEG, and the blood ammonia concentrations. The clinical status improved at all dose levels, but a clear relationship with dose was not detected (table 5). In addition, the negligible systemic absorption of rifaximin was confirmed and no significative side effect was documented.

The second study was a large multicentre trial performed in Spain according to a double-blind, double-dummy design [62]. One-hundred and three patients with grade I–III acute HE were enrolled: 50 patients received rifaximin and 53 the disaccharide lactitol. The efficacy and safety endpoints of the study were the same of previous study [61]. The global efficacy of both therapies was similar: 81.6% of the patients in the rifaximin group and 80.43% in the lactitol group showed improvement or total regression of the episode. A significant better evolution of the PSE index was observed in the rifaximin group (fig. 2), due to a greater effect of rifaximin on blood ammonia levels and EEG abnormalities.

The results of these two studies [60, 61] indicate that rifaximin administration is a useful alternative to disaccharides for the treatment of grade I–III encephalopathy.

The early clinical studies [47, 50–60], although not performed in GCP, have all demonstrated the good clinical efficacy and excellent tolerability of rifaximin in patients with HE, giving further support to its use in this clinical condition. A recent clinical study [63] has actually shown the efficacy of rifaximin administration in patients intolerant or non-responsive to a previous treatment with non-absorbable disaccharides.

In addition to its ammonia-lowering effect, rifaximin is able to reduce blood concentrations of BZ-like compounds in patients with liver cirrhosis [65]. While these results are consistent with hypothesis that intestinal bacteria are, at least partially, a source of endogenous BZ [65–67], they suggest that this antibiotic – administered cyclically – could prevent the accumulation of both pathogenetic (i.e. ammonia) and precipitating (i.e. BZ) factors. In this connection, a recent paper [68] – while confirming the ability of rifaximin to reduce both ammonia and BZ level – did show a significant reduction of plasma endotoxin concentration. Furthermore, it did show that – after stopping rifaximin – subsequent treatment with a probiotic mixture achieves a sustained reduction of all the above toxic substances (fig. 3).

Conclusions

The available evidence clearly shows that antibiotics are effective in the management of HE. Their role needs to reappraised especially in the lack of evidence supporting the use of disaccharides. Among the poorly absorbed antimicrobials, rifaximin seems to be the drug of choice thanks to its efficacy and remarkable safety even in the long term.

References

1   Blei AT, Cordoba J: Hepatic encephalopathy. Am J Gastroenterol 2001;96:1968–1976.
2   Hofnagle JH, Carithers RL Jr, Shapiro C, Ascher N: Fulminant hepatic failure: summary of a workshop. Hepatology 1995;21:240–252.
3   Mullen KD, Dasarathy S: Hepatic encephalopathy; in Schiff ER, Sorrell ME, Maddney WC (eds): Schiff's Diseases of the Liver, vol I. Philadelphia, Lippincott-Raven, 1999, pp 545–581.
4   Ferenci P, Lockwood A, Mullen K, Tarter R, Weissenborn K, Blei A: Hepatic encephalopathy – Definition, nomenclature, diagnosis, and quantification: final report of the Working Party at the 11th World Congress of Gastroenterology, Vienna 1998. Hepatology 2002;35:716–721.
5   Mas A: Hepatic encephalopathy: from pathophysiology to treatment. Digestion 2005;73(suppl 1): 78–85.
6   Teasdale G, Knill-Jones R, van der Sande J: Observer variability in assessing impaired consciousness and coma. J Neurol Neurosurg Psychiatry 1978;41:603–610.
7   Ong JP, Mullen KD: Hepatic encephalopathy. Eur J Gastroenterol Hepatol 2001;13:325–334.
8   Lizardi-Cervera J, Almeda P, Guevara L, Uribe M: Hepatic encephalopathy: a review. Ann Hepatol 2003;2:122–130.
9   Butterworth RF: The neurobiology of hepatic encephalopathy. Semin Liver Dis 1996;16:235–244.
10 Norenberg MD: Astrocytic-ammonia interactions in hepatic encephalopathy. Semin Liver Dis1996;16:245–253.
11 Lockwood AH, Yap EW, Wong WH: Cerebral ammonia metabolism in patients with severe liver disease and minimal hepatic encephalopathy. J Cereb Blood Flow Metab 1991;11:337–341.
12 Butterworth RE, Giguere JF, Michaud J, Lavoie J, Layragues GP. Ammonia: a key factor in the pathogenesis of hepatic encephalopathy. Neurochem Pathol 1987;6:1–12.
13 Norenberg MD: Astroglial dysfunction in hepatic encephalopathy. Metab Brain Dis 1998;13:319–335.
14 Rao VL, Butterworth RE: Neuronal nitric oxide synthase and hepatic encephalopathy. Metab Brain Dis 1998;13:175–189.
15 Ha JH, Basile AS: Modulation of ligand binding to components of the $GABA_A$ receptor complex by ammonia: implications for the pathogenesis of hyperammonemic syndromes. Brain Res 1996;720:35–44.
16 Basile AS, Jones EA: Ammonia and GABAergic neurotransmission: interrelated factors in the pathogenesis of hepatic encephalopathy. Hepatology 1997;25:1303–1305.
17 Mullen KD: Benzodiazepine compounds and hepatic encephalopathy. N Engl J Med 1991; 325:509–511.
18 Mullen KD, Jones EA: Natural benzodiazepines and hepatic encephalopathy. Semin Liver Dis 1996;16:225–264.
19 Yurdaydin C, Walsh TJ, Engler HD, Ha JH, Li Y, Jones EA, Basile AS: Gut bacteria provide precursor of benzodiazepine receptor ligands in a rat model of hepatic encephalopathy. Brain Res 1995;679:42–48.
20 Avallone R, Zeneroli ML, Venturini I, Corsi L, Schreier P, Kleinschnitz M, Ferrarese C, Farina F, Baraldi C, Pecora N, Frigo M, Baraldi M: Endogenous benzodiazepine-like compounds and diazepam binding inhibitor in serum of patients with liver cirrhosis with and without overt encephalopathy. Gut 1998;42:861–867.
21 Zieve L, Doizaki WM, Zieve J: Synergism between mercaptans and ammonia or fatty acids in the production of coma: a possible role for mercaptans in the pathogenesis of hepatic coma. J Lab Clin Med 1974;83:16–28.
22 Rose C, Butterworth RF, Zayed J: Manganese deposition in basal ganglia structures results from both portal-systemic shunting and liver dysfunction. Gastroenterology 1999;117:640–644.
23 Aronson LR, Gacad RC, Kaminsky-Russ K, Gregory CR, Mullen KD: Endogenous benzodiazepine activity in the peripheral and portal blood of dogs with congenital portosystemic shunts. Vet Sug 1997;26:189–194.
24 Hernandez-Avila CA, Shoemaker WJ, Ortega-Soto HA: Plasma concentrations of endogenous benzodiazepine-receptor ligands in patients with hepatic encephalopathy: a comparative study. J Psychiatry Neurosci 1998;23:217–222.

25   Barbaro G, Di Lorenzo G, Soldini M, Marziali M, Bellomo G, Belloni G: Flumazenil for hepatic encephalopthy grade III and IVa in patients with cirrhosis: an Italian multicenter double-blind, placebo-controlled, cross-over study. Hepatology 1998;28:374–378.
26   Abou-Assi S, Vlahcevic ZR: Hepatic encephalopathy: metabolic consequence of cirrhosis often is reversible. Postgrad Med 2001;109:52–70.
27   Córdoba J, Blei AT: Treatment of hepatic encephalopathy. Am J Gastroenterol 1997;92:1429–1439.
28   Morgan MY: The treatment of chronic hepatic encephalopathy. Hepatogastroenterology 1991;38: 377–387.
29   Riordan SM, Williams R: Treatment of hepatic encephalopathy. N Engl J Med 1997;337:473–479.
30   Fast BB, Wolfe SJ, Stormont JM, Davidson CS: Antibiotic therapy in the management of hepatic coma. AMA Arch Intern Med 1958;101:467–475.
31   Conn HO, Leavy CM, Vlahcevic ZR, Rodgers JB, Maddrey WB, Seeff L: Comparison of lactulose and neomycin in the treatment of chronic portal-systemic encephalopathy. A double-blind controlled trial. Gastroenterology 1977;72:573–583.
32   Orlandi F, Freddara U, Candelaresi MT, Morettini A, Corazza GR, Di Simone A: Comparison between neomycin and lactulose in 173 patients with hepatic encephalopathy: a randomized clinical study. Dig Dis Sci 1981;26:498–506.
33   Koshy A, Ayyagari A, Bharati G, Goyal AK, Kaur U: Relative efficacy of neomycin and ampicillin against urease producing organisms. Indian J Med Res 1981;74:486–488.
34   Meyers S, Lieber CS: Reduction of gastric ammonia by ampicillin in normal and azotemic subjects. Gastroenterology 1976;70:244–247.
35   AlexanderT, Thomas K, CherianAM, Kanakasabapathy: Effect of three antibacterial drugs in lowering blood and stool ammonia production in hepatic encephalopathy. Indian J Med Res 1992;96:292–296.
36   Tromm A, Griga T, Greving I, Hilden H, Huppe D, Schwegler U, Micklefield GH, May B: Orthograde whole gut irrigation with mannite versus paromomycine + lactulose as prophylaxis of hepatic encephalopathy in patients with cirrhosis and upper gastrointestinal bleeding: results of a controlled randomized trial. Hepatogastroenterology 2000;47:473–477.
37   Morgan MH, Read AE, Speller DC: Treatment of hepatic encephalopathy with metronidazole. Gut 1982;23:1–7.
38   Als-Nielsen B, Gluud LL, Gluud C: Non-absorbable disaccharides for hepatic encephalopathy: systematic review of randomized trials. Br Med J 2004;328:1046–1052.
39   Chambers JF, Sande MA: The aminoglycosides; in Hardman JG, Limbird LE, Molinoff PB, et al (eds): Goodman and Gilman's the Pharmacological Basis of Therapeutics, ed 9. New York, McGraw-Hill, 1995, pp 1103–1121.
40   Green PHR, Tall AR: Drugs, alcohol and malabsorption. Am J Med 1979;67:1066–1076.
41   Faloon WW: Metabolic effects of nonabsorbable antibacterial agents. Am J Clin Nutr 1970;23: 645–651.
42   Tracy JW, Webster LT: Drugs used in the chemotherapy of protozoal infections; in Hardman JG, Limbird LE (eds): Goodman & Gilman's the Pharmacological Basis of Therapeutics, ed 10. New York, McGraw-Hill, 2001, pp 1097–1120.
43   Uhl MD, Riely CA: Metronidazole in treating portosystemic encephalopathy. Ann Intern Med 1996;124:455.
44   Kim KH, Choi JW, Lee JY, Kim TD, Paek JH, Lee EJ, Oh HA, Kim JH, Jang BI, Kim TN, Chung MK, Lee HJ, Byun WM: Two cases of metronidazole-induced encephalopathy (in Korean). Korean J Gastroenterol 2005;45:195–200.
45   Scarpignato C, Pelosini I: Rifaximin, a poorly absorbed antibiotic: pharmacology and clinical potential. Chemotherapy 2005;51(suppl 1):36–66.
46   Baker DE: Rifaximin: a nonabsorbed oral antibiotic. Rev Gastroenterol Disord 2005;5:19–30.
47   Festi D, Mazzella G, Orsini M, Sottili S, Sangermano A, Li Bassi S, Parini P, Ferrieri A, Falcucci M, Grossi L, Marzio L, Roda E: Rifaximin in the treatment of chronic hepatic encephalopathy: results of a multicenter study of efficacy and safety. Curr Ther Res 1993;54:598–609.
48   Williams R, Bass N: Rifaximin, a nonabsorbed oral antibiotic, in the treatment of hepatic encephalopathy: antimicrobial activity, efficacy, and safety. Rev Gastroenterol Disord 2005;5 (suppl 1): 10–18.

49   Zeneroli ML, Avallone R, Corsi L, Venturini I, Baraldi C, Baraldi M: Management of hepatic encephalopathy: role of rifaximin. Chemotherapy 2005;51(suppl 1):90–95.

50   De Marco F, Santamaria Amato P, D'Arienzo A: Rifaximin in collateral treatment of portal-systemic encephalopathy: a preliminary report. Curr Ther Res 1984;36:668–674.

51   Testa R, Eftimiadi C, Sukkar GS, De Leo C, Rovida S, Schito GC, Celle G: A non-absorbable rifamycin for treatment of hepatic encephalopathy. Drugs Exp Clin Res 1985;11: 387–392.

52   Di Piazza S, Filippazzo MG, Valenza LM, Morello S, Pastore L, Conti A, Cottone S, Pagliaro L: Rifaximin versus neomycin in the treatment of portosystemic encephalopathy. Ital J Gastroenterol 1991;23:403–407.

53   Pedretti G, Calzetti C, Missale G, Fiaccadori F: Rifaximin versus neomycin on hyperammoniemia in chronic portal systemic encephalopathy of cirrhotics. A double-blind, randomized trial. Ital J Gastroenterol 1991;23:175–178.

54   Parini P, Cipolla A, Ronchi M, Salzetta A, Mazzella G, Roda E: Effect of rifaximin in the treatment of portal-systemic encephalopathy. Curr Ther Res 1992;52:34–39.

55   Fera G, Agostinacchio F, Nigro M, Schiraldi O, Ferrieri A: Rifaximin in the treatment of hepatic encephalopathy. Eur J Clin Res 1993;4:57–66.

56   Bucci L, Calmieri GC: Double-blind, double-dummy comparison between treatment with rifaximin and lactulose in patients with medium to severe degree hepatic encephalopathy. Curr Med Res Opin 1993;13:109–118.

57   Massa P, Vallerino E, Dodero M: Treatment of hepatic encephalopathy with rifaximin: double-blind, double-dummy study versus lactulose. Eur J Clin Res 1993;4:7–18.

58   Puxeddu A, Quartini M, Massinetti A, Ferrieri A: Rifaximin in the treatment of chronic hepatic encephalopathy. A double-blind randomised trial. Curr Med Res Opin 1995;13:274–281.

59   Miglio F, Valpiani D, Rosselli SR, Ferrieri A: Rifaximin, a non-absorbable rifamycin, for hepatic encephalopathy. A double-blind randomised trial. Curr Med Res Opin 1997;13:593–601.

60   Loguercio C, Federico A, De Girolamo V, Ferrieri A, Del Vecchio Blanco C: Cyclic treatment of chronic hepatic encephalopathy with rifaximin. Min Gastroenterol Dietol 2003;49:53–62.

61   Williams R, James O, Warnes TW, Morgan MY: Evaluation of the efficacy and safety of rifaximin in the treatment of hepatic encephalopathy: a double-blind, randomized, dose-finding multi-centre study. Eur J Gastroenterol Hepatol 2000;12:203–208.

62   Mas A, Rodes J, Sunyer L, Rodrigo L, Planas R, Vargas V, Castells L, Rodriguez-Martinez D, Fernandez-Rodriguez C, Coll I, Pardo A: Comparison of rifaximin and lactitol in the treatment of acute hepatic encephalopathy: results of a randomized, double-blind, double-dummy, controlled clinical trial. J Hepatol 2003;38:51–58.

63   Sama C, Morselli-Labate AM, Pianta P, Lambertini L, Berardi S, Martini G: Clinical effects of rifaximin in patients with encephalopathy intolerant or non-responsive to previous lactulose treatment: an open-label, pilot study. Cur Ther Res 2004;65:413–422.

64   Paik YH, Lee KS, Han KH, Song KH, Kim MH, Moon BS, Ahn SH, Lee SJ, Park HJ, Lee DK, Chon CY, Lee SI, Moon YM: Comparison of rifaximin and lactulose for the treatment of hepatic encephalopathy: a prospective randomized study. Yonsei Med J 2005;46:399–407.

65   Zeneroli ML, Venturini I, Stefanelli S, Farina F, Cosenza R, Miglioli L, Minelli E, Amedei R, Ferrieri A, Avallone R, Baraldi M: Antibacterial activity of rifaximin reduces the levels of benzodiazepine-like compounds in patients with liver cirrhosis. Pharmacol Res 1997;35: 557–600.

66   Unseld E, Klotz U: Benzodiazepines: are they of natural origin? Pharmacol Res 1989;6:1–3.

67   Yurdaydin C, Walsh TJ, Howard DE, Ha J, Li Y, Jones EA, Basile AS: Gut bacteria provide precursors of benzodiazepine receptor ligands in a rat model of hepatic encephalopathy. Brain Res 1995;679:42–48.

68   Lighthouse J, Naito Y, Helmy A, Hotten P, Fuji H, Min CH, Yoshioka M, Marotta F: Endotoxinemia and benzodiazepine-like substances in compensated cirrhotic patients: a randomized study comparing the effect of rifaximin alone and association with a symbiotic preparation. Hepatol Res 2004;28:155–160.

Note Added in Proof

A recent retrospective study [1] pointed out the superiority of antibiotic therapy over treatment with disaccharides in the management of HE. In this study, 145 patients received lactulose (30 ml b.i.d.) for $\geq$ 6 months, followed by rifaximin (400 mg t.i.d.) for $\geq$ 6 months. Charts were then reviewed to compare the patients' last 6 months on disaccharide and first 6 months on antibiotic. The number of hospitalizations was significantly lower during the period of rifaximin therapy compared with lactulose (mean 0.5 vs. 1.6, respectively, $p < 0.001$). During the rifaximin therapy period, patients spent significantly less time in the hospital (mean time 3.1 days) than during the lactulose period (mean time 12.5 days, $p < 0.001$). Compared with the lactulose therapy period, HE grade was significantly lowered following rifaximin therapy ($p < 0.001$). On the contrary, medication compliance was significantly higher with rifaximin therapy compared with lactulose ($p < 0.001$). Using Health Care Cost Utilization Project (H-CUP) data, the reductions in occurrences and duration of hospitalizations achieved with rifaximin therapy resulted in an average cost savings of USD 67,559 per patient. These results show that treatment of HE with rifaximin is not only more effective than treatment with lactulose but represents also a cost-saving approach.

Reference

1   Leevy CB, Philips JA: A crossover retrospective chart review evaluating hospitalization associated with the use of rifaximin vs. lactulose in the management of patients with hepatic encephalopathy. Am J Gastroenterol 2005;100(suppl):S134.

Prof. Davide Festi, MD
Dipartimento di Medicina Interna e Gastroenterologia
Università di Bologna, Policlinico S. Orsola-Malpighi
Via Massarenti 9, IT–40138 Bologna (Italy)
Tel./Fax +39 051 636 4123, E-Mail festi@med.unibo.it

This chapter should be cited as follows:

Festi D, Vestito A, Mazzella G, Roda E, Colecchia A: Management of Hepatic Encephalopathy: Focus on Antibiotic Therapy. Digestion 2006;73(suppl 1):94–101.

Scarpignato C, Lanas Á (eds): Bacterial Flora in Digestive Disease.
Focus on Rifaximin.

....

Epidemiology, Etiology and Pathophysiology of Traveler's Diarrhea

Joaquim Gascón

Secció Medicina Tropical, Centre de Salut Internacional de l'Hospital
Clínic de Barcelona, IDIBAPS, Barcelona, Spain

Abstract

Traveler's diarrhea (TD) is the most frequent health problem in travelers to developing countries. Several personal and environmental risk factors are at the basis of TD acquisition and are discussed in this paper. TD is caused by a wide range of infectious organisms, ETEC and EAEC bacteria strains being the main enteropathogens incriminated in TD. Other causative bacteria are: *Shigella* spp., *Campylobacter* spp., *Vibrio* spp., *Aeromonas* spp., *Salmonella* spp., and *Plesiomonas* spp. Parasite species are also included: *Cyclospora cayetanensis, Giardia lamblia, Crystosporidium, Entamoeba histolytica*, as well as viruses: rotavirus, adenovirus, Norwalk virus. Due to the great diversity of pathogens incriminated, several pathophysiological mechanisms have been described and some of them are still poorly understood. The clinical symptoms present are also quite variable, although inflammatory and non-inflammatory diarrhea have been established as a classical and basic classification of diarrhea.

Introduction

Traveler's diarrhea (TD) is the most frequent health problem in travelers to developing countries. Its prevalence varies according to different authors, and different geographical areas with different sanitary conditions, being estimated between 13 and 60% [1, 2]. TD has been defined as the passing of ≥3 watery stools per day with or without other symptoms, or as the occurrence of unformed stools accompanied by some of the following: abdominal cramps, tenesmus, vomiting, nausea, fever, chills or prostration [3]. However, a significant number of travelers experience an intestinal disturbance with only 1–2 loose stools per day [4].

According with this variety of clinical symptoms, Passaro and Parsonnet [5] proposed a four-stage classification of TD ranging from minimal TD (1–2 loose stools with no other enteric symptoms or only moderate cramping), mild TD (≥3 loose stools without enteric symptoms), moderate TD (corresponding to Merson's criteria [3]), until severe TD (≥3 loose stools with incapacitating symptoms or dysentery).

TD is usually self-limited, lasting 1–5 days, but in an epidemiologic study from Spain, 15% of affected travelers experienced a persisting diarrhea, 20% needed to take to bed during the trip and 1% needed to be hospitalized [1]. Other studies show that at least 2% of TD progresses into a situation of chronic diarrhea [6].

TD has a short incubation time and the onset most often occurs in two different peaks, the first is early during the trip (first 3–4 days) [4] and the second one is around the 10th day. However, TD can occur at anytime during the trip [7] and the attack rate for TD is higher the longer the trip is [8]. In the International Health Clinics in Europe, people consulting because of TD (approximately 12% of all TD occur in returned travelers) [9] usually start to have diarrhea during the last days of the trip or have suffered a persistent/chronic diarrhea, often despite having been self-treated.

Risk Factors

Travelers' behavior as well as the public health measures in the country being visited are the main determinant factors to acquire TD. The lack of hygiene and poor general sanitation in tropical countries cause a high environmental contamination. Therefore, the destination is one of the main risk factors for TD, as industrialized countries are areas with the least risk and tropical countries the areas with a high risk for TD (fig. 1) [10–12]. The incidence of TD is increased by other factors related to the quality, type and location of food consumption [13, 14]. There also are some personal factors that can play a key role in the susceptibility of travelers to acquire TD: immunodeficiency and decreased gastric acidity. Travelers with diminished gastric secretion or taking acid lowering drugs have a higher probability for acquiring TD [15].

In the majority of studies on TD, children and young adults have more diarrheal episodes than other age groups, the latter probably due to a more adventurous type of travel that includes a variety of dietary habits [1, 15]. The modality of the trip is also a risk factor. Even if the adventurous trips have potentially a higher risk for TD, some high-level trips in luxury hotels as well as

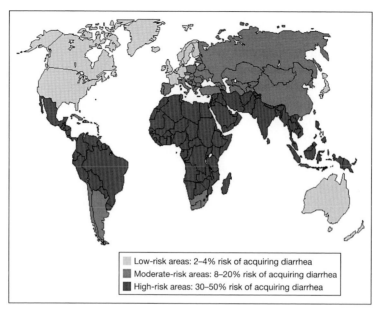

Fig. 1. Incidence of TD by geographical area (from DuPont [12]).

cruises on the Nile (Egypt) and Rio Negro (Brazil) have been described as risk factors probably due to the food storage conditions for a prolonged period [1, 8]. Belonging to a higher socio-economic status seems to carry a significant risk to develop TD when people visit a high-risk area [16]. Season is also a factor that influences not only the risk of acquiring TD [8] but also the etiology. *Cyclospora cayetanensis* infection is, for instance, more frequent during the rainy season in Nepal [17]. *Campylobacter jejuni* was more frequently isolated in Finnish tourists visiting Morocco during the winter compared to those who travelled during the summer [18].

Etiology

TD is caused by a wide range of infectious organisms. A study on Spanish travelers to tropical countries showed an etiological bacterial agent in 61% of patients and a protozoan in 17% of them [19]. These results are similar to those obtained by other groups. Usually in 25–50% of TD cases, no enteropathogen is isolated, but not all the studies have used all available techniques for bacterial or viral detection.

Table 1. Common enteropathogens causing TD, with some pathogenic mechanisms and minimum inoculum necessary to induce diarrhea

	Pathogenic mechanisms	Inoculum
Bacteria		
Aeromonas spp.	Enterotoxins (Ast, Alt), cytotoxin (aerolysin) and invasion	10^4
Campylobacter spp.	Unclear: enterotoxin (CJT), cytotoxin, invasion	500–1,000 microorganisms
Enteroaggregative *E. coli* (EAEC)	Enterotoxin (EAST-1, Pet, Shet-1, Shet-2), mucus biofilm, cytotoxic effects on mucosa (Sat, CDT)	$>10^8$
Enterotoxigenic *E. coli* (ETEC)	Enterotoxins (ST/LT), LPS	$>10^8$
Salmonella spp.	Unclear: enterotoxin (Stn), cytotoxin, invasion	10^5–10^8
Shigella spp.	Enterotoxins (Shet-1, Shet-2, EAST), cytotoxin (Shiga, Sat, SepA), invasion	10–100 bacteria
Vibrio parahemolyticus	Hemolysin (TDH)	10^5–10^8
Yersinia spp.	Enterotoxin (YST), invasion	10^9
Parasites		
Cryptosporidium parvum	Unknown	10–1,000
Cyclospora cayetanensis	Invasion (upper small intestine) but mechanism for diarrhoea unknown	oocysts
Entamoeba histolytica	Invasion, proteases, phagocytose	10–100
Giardia lamblia	Adherence to the mucosa	10–25 cysts
Viruses		
Adenovirus	Interference with the brush border function, and malabsorption	
Norwalk virus	Lysis of enterocytes and enterotoxin	10–100 viral particles
Rotavirus	NSP4 (rotavirus)	10^2–10^3 virus particles

Bacteria are the enteropathogens more frequently incriminated (50–80%) as a cause of TD (table 1). Strains of *Escherichia coli* are the most isolated bacteria in travelers with TD. Among them, enterotoxigenic *E. coli* (ETEC) continues to be the most frequently isolated strain [20]. Other *E. coli* (enteropathogenic (EPEC), enterohemorrhagic (EHEC) and enteroinvasive (EIEC)) strains have also been isolated (although less frequently) and the enteroaggregative (EAEC) strains have been increasingly incriminated in cases of travelers with diarrhea [21–23].

Table 1 shows other bacteria as *Aeromonas* spp., *C. jejuni, Salmonella* spp., *Shigella* spp., or *Vibrio* species that have also been described as a cause of TD [20, 24, 25]. The percentage of each pathogen varies greatly following several studies, mainly due to the different techniques used for microbial identification, and the seasonal variations and geographical areas studied.

Viruses have been less studied except for the easily diagnosed rotavirus with a wide spectrum of prevalence (0–36%) in different series [26]. The prevalence is generally low in most studies even in those involving children [27]. Other viruses described as a cause of diarrhea have been detected in other studies (table 1) [20].

Giardia lamblia and *Entamoeba histolytica* are a less frequent cause of TD. *Giardia* is a very common pathogen in some places [28], although it is a cosmopolitan protozoa. The diagnostic of *E. histolytica* is still problematic due to the fact that microscopically it is indistinguishable from the non-pathogenic *Entamoeba dispar*, and probably the diagnosis of amebiasis in travelers is overestimated. In recent years, *C. cayetanensis* has emerged as a causative organism of diarrhea [29] affecting travelers [30, 31]. Together with *Cyclospora* and *Criptosporidium* species, *Giardia* is often the cause of persistent diarrhea in the returned traveler [32].

Among non-infectious causes, ciguatoxin is prominent as an intoxication in travelers to the Caribbean and the Pacific areas [33, 34]. Destination, season and especially alimentary behavior have a great influence on its presence. Ciguatera poisoning causes early diarrhea followed by neurological and less frequently cardiovascular symptoms.

Pathophysiology

Because TD is mainly caused by microbial agents or toxins, the fecal-oral route is the way through which TD is acquired when people ingest contaminated food or water. The incubation period and the mechanisms potentially responsible for TD depend on the microbiological agent causing it (table 2). The proposed pathophysiology of bacterial gastroenteritis includes the elaboration of enterotoxins by toxigenic pathogens, the action of lipopolysaccharide endotoxin, the invasion of intestinal mucosa by invasive pathogens and the release of cytotoxins. Previously, all bacteria need to colonize intestinal mucosa. Various colonization factors (motility, fimbriae, pili and non-fimbrial adhesins) have been detected, playing an initial key role for bacteria attachment to the intestinal mucosa. Bacteria can then release toxins.

Enterotoxins are released by bacteria colonizing the upper small intestine in the majority of cases. Enterotoxins bind a specific cellular receptor to penetrate into the cells, and thus deregulate the cellular adenylate cyclase regulatory system, increasing the levels of cAMP, and inducing a secretory fluid mechanism. ETEC (ST and LT enterotoxins) [35] and *Vibrio cholerae* (cholera toxin) are the prototypes of bacteria exhibiting these properties. The diarrhea caused by these enteropathogens is non-inflammatory and watery.

Table 2. Incubation period and type of diarrhea for some enteropathogens causing TD

Enteropathogen	Incubation period	Type of diarrhea	Persistent/chronic diarrhea
ETEC	10–48 h	Non-inflammatory watery diarrhea	−
EAEC	8–48 h	Watery and inflammatory diarrhea	++
Shigella spp.	1–3 days	Watery diarrhea, dysentery	−
Campylobacter jejuni	2–4 days	Watery diarrhea, dysentery	+*
Salmonella spp.	12–24 h	Watery diarrhea, dysentery	+*
Aeromonas spp.	1–2 days	Watery diarrhea, inflammatory diarrhea	+*
Vibrio parahemolyticus	2–48 h	Watery diarrhea	−
Yersinia enterocolitica	2–10 days	Watery and inflammatory diarrhea	±*
Rotavirus	1–3 days	Watery and osmotic diarrhea	−
Adenovirus	7–10 days	Watery diarrhea	−
Giardia lamblia	3–40 days	Non-inflammatory, chronic and intermittent diarrhea	+++
Cyclospora cayetanensis	2–11 days	Watery and chronic intermittent diarrhea	+++

*Mostly acute diarrhea.

Other enterotoxins operate through the cGMP pathway, also causing a watery diarrhea. ST enterotoxin from ETEC strains as well as lipopolysaccharide endotoxin use this mechanism [36]. Other toxins like the ciguatera toxin use the calcium-dependent pathways [37] and recently a nitric oxide pathway has been described for *Shigella* [38]. All these mechanisms induce an increase of fluid secretion and watery diarrhea.

Osmotic mechanism is another way to induce non-inflammatory diarrhea. Osmotic diarrhea is due to the presence of poorly absorbable solute exerting an osmotic pressure across the intestinal mucosa. This type of mechanism is seen mainly in chronic diarrhea and in rotavirus infection.

Bacteria causing inflammatory diarrhea usually colonize the distal ileum and the colon where they invade the mucosa inducing a dysenteric illness. Moreover, some enteropathogens release cytotoxins that disrupt intestinal mucosa. Cytotoxins kill target cells through two different mechanisms: acting at the intracellular level inhibiting the cellular protein synthesis or inhibiting the actin filament formation. *Shigella dysenteriae* type 1 is the prototype of bacteria causing inflammatory diarrhea through the inhibition of cellular protein synthesis (shiga toxin). Other kinds of cytotoxins act forming pores in the cell membrane (hemolysins). *Vibrio parahemolyticus* is an example of enteropathogen acting through one hemolysin (TDH).

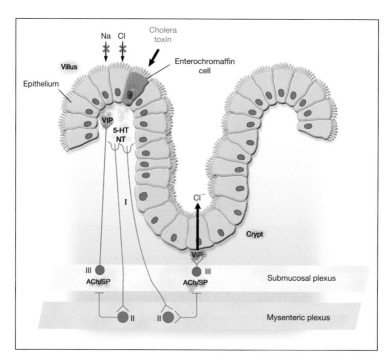

Fig. 2. Activation of an intramural neural reflex from cholera toxin (CT) secretion. 5-HT = Serotonin; ACh = acetylcholine; NT = neurotensin; SP = substance P; VIP = vasoactive intestinal peptide (from Field [45]).

Some bacteria may exhibit both capacities, i.e. to release enterotoxins and cytotoxins. *C. jejuni*, which has an invasive capacity, releases an enterotoxin similar to cholera toxin and a cytotoxin that may play a role in the inflammatory diarrhea [39]. *Salmonella* spp. and *Aeromonas* spp. [40], both with invasive capacity, can also induce both types of diarrheal mechanisms (secretory and inflammatory).

Sometimes, diarrheogenic agents use several mechanisms which are not always well understood. Enteroaggregative *E. coli* strains (EAEC), e.g. are able to form a mucus biofilm, but also induce a shortening of the villi, hemorrhagic necrosis of the villous tips, exfoliation of enterocytes and a mild inflammatory response [41, 42]. Some strains are also able to release an enterotoxin (EAST1). Heterogeneity has been established for the role of some virulent factors present in some bacterial EAEC strains. These are potentially related to diarrhea as a plasmid-encoded protein that has enterotoxin secretory properties as well as the capacity to induce changes in the cellular cytoskeleton [43].

Aside from the described pathways for some enterotoxins, there is some evidence that LT/ST from ETEC strains and CT from *V. cholerae* could induce diarrhea through activation of neural reflexes (fig. 2) [44, 45]. Concerning the viral agents, these mechanisms include osmotic and secretory mechanisms through the interference with the brush border function leading to carbohydrate malabsorption, the action of protein-like enterotoxins (NSP4 for rotavirus) and lysis of enterocytes [46–48].

E. histolytica is an invasive protozoa with several well-identified virulence factors: contact-dependent cytolysis, proteases, toxins adhesion molecules and phagocytic activity [49]. Intestinal ulceration is the rule and progression of illness can lead to intestinal perforation. From the intestinal world, *E. histolytica* can spread to other body organs, the liver being the most affected one.

For some protozoa like *Giardia* that adheres to the mucosa in the small intestine, no specific virulence factors have been identified. *C. cayetanensis* is able to invade enterocytes and to promote a mucosal inflammation with mild reduction in villous height, intraepithelial lymphocyte infiltration and some vacuolization in the surface epithelium; however, specific virulence factors have not been identified to date [50, 51].

Clinical Symptoms

Although several studies have attempted to correlate specific enteropathogens with clinical presentation, the wide range of symptoms and the possibility for bacteria to express several mechanisms make this impossible for the majority of cases. However, some common generalities have been established. Patients with acute non-inflammatory diarrhea affecting the small intestine typically present with high-volume watery stools and dehydration is frequent. Children and the elderly are the age groups most affected by dehydration. The number of stools varies greatly and diarrhea could be accompanied by other symptoms like cramps, borborygmi, bloating, nausea, low-grade fever and less frequently vomiting. Accompanying symptoms are sometimes so severe to confine patients to bed.

Patients with an inflammatory bowel illness involving the large intestine usually present with small-volume stool and tenesmus. Dysentery presents with blood and mucus in the stools. Moreover, invasive pathogens may cause fever and abdominal pain which is occasionally severe. Bacteria with the capacity to produce enterotoxins and also invasion may cause a sequential clinical picture.

Parasites and sometimes certain bacteria (EAEC and to a lesser extent *Salmonella* or *Campylobacter* strains) can cause persistent (>14 days) or chronic diarrhea (>30 days). Nausea, vomiting, dyspepsia, and asthenia are usual symptoms for *G. lamblia* and *C. cayetanensis*. Often, symptoms are intermittent and weight loss is common [21]. A number of patients with TD present gastrointestinal chronic symptoms months after the trip and in one study, 11% of them met the Rome II criteria for irritable bowel syndrome [52]. More long-term follow-up studies are needed to determine the incidence of post-infectious complications of TD.

Extraintestinal symptoms can follow an infection for an invasive microorganism. Hemolytic-uremic syndrome is the most severe complication for some bacteria like *Shigella* or EHEC strains (unusual in travelers). Guillain-Barré syndrome and Reiter's syndrome are also well-known complications [53]. Finally, *Salmonella* can invade several sites in the organism and cause endocarditis, osteomyelitis, arthritis and other complications. *E. histolytica* can spread to the liver through the portal circulation, causing single or multiple amebic hepatic abscesses. *E. histolytica* can also affect other body tissues causing a high diversity of clinical illnesses, mainly thoracic and less frequently in the CNS and dermatological localizations.

Conclusions and Perspectives for the Future

TD reflects one of the most important public health (diarrheal disease) issues worldwide causing 2.5 million deaths annually and mainly in children from low-income countries. Even though TD is one of the widest studied health problems in travelers, some questions still remain unresolved. The intestine is an ecological set-up where a mixture of bacterial strains exchange genes related to virulent factors and sensitivity/resistance to antibiotics. Epidemiological surveillance and monitoring the geographical migrations of certain strains and their level of antibiotic resistance over time is needed in the present era of globalization. Basic studies to understand the pathophysiological mechanisms are also needed in order to provide new tools (vaccines or other strategies) against the most virulent strains causing diarrhea. Travelers and children from underdeveloped countries will certainly benefit from such advances.

References

1   Gascón J, Ruiz L, Canela J, Mallart M, Corachán M: Epidemiología de la diarrea del viajero en turistas españoles a países en desarrollo. Med Clin (Barc) 1993;100:365–367.
2   Von Sonnenburg F, Tornieporth N, Waiyaki P, Lowe B, Peruski LF, DuPont HL, Mathewson JJ: Risk and aetiology of diarrhoea at various tourist destinations. Lancet 2000;356:133–134.
3   Merson MH, Morris GK, Sack DA, Wells JG, Feeley JC, Sack RB, Creech WB, Kapikian AZ, Gangarosa EJ: Travelers' diarrhea in Mexico: a prospective study of physicians and family members attending a congress. N Engl J 1976;294:1299–1305.

4   Steffen R, Van der Linde F, Gyr K, Schar M: Epidemiology of diarrhea in travelers. JAMA 1983;249:1176–1180.

5   Passaro DJ, Parsonnet J: Advances in the prevention and management of travelers' diarrhea. Curr Clin Top Infect Dis 1998;18:217–236.

6   DuPont H, Khan FM: Travelers' diarrhea: epidemiology, microbiology, prevention and therapy. J Travel Med 1994;1:84–93.

7   Bouchaud O, Cabie A, Coulaud JP: Epidémiologie, physiopathologie et traitement de la diarrhée du voyageur. Ann Med Intern 1995;146:431–437.

8   Kollaritsch H: Traveler's diarrhea among Austrian tourists in warm climate countries. I. Epidemiology. Eur J Epidemiol 1989;5:74–81.

9   DuPont HL, Ericsson CD: Travelers' diarrhea: approaches to prevention and treatment. Clin Infect Dis 1993;16:616–626.

10 Ryder RW, Wells JG, Gangarosa EJ: A study of travelers' diarrhea in foreign visitors to the United States. J Infect Dis 1977;136:605–607.

11 Black RE: Epidemiology of travelers' diarrhea and relative importance of various pathogens. Rev Infect Dis 1990;12(suppl):S73–S79.

12 DuPont HL: Traveler's diarrhea: antimicrobial therapy and chemoprevention. Gastroenterol Hepatol 2005;2:191–198.

13 Tjoa WS, DuPont HL, Sullivan P, Pickering LK, Holguin AH, Olarte J, Evans DG, Evans DJ: Location of food consumption in the prevention of travelers' diarrhea in Mexico. Am J Epidemiol 1977;106:61–66.

14 Kozicki M, Steffen R, Schar M: 'Boil it, cook it, peel it or forget it': does this rule prevent travelers' diarrhea? Int J Epidemiol 1985;14:169–172.

15 Gobelens GFJ, Leentvaar-Kuijpers A, Kleijnen J, Countinho RA: Incidence and risk factors of diarrhoea in Dutch travellers: consequences for priorities in pre-travel health advice. Trop Med Int Health 1998;3:896–903.

16 Ryder RW, Oquist CA, Greenberg H, Taylor DN, Orskov F, Orskov I, Kapikian AZ, Sack RB: Travelers' diarrhea in panamian tourist in Mexico. J Infect Dis 1981;144:442–448.

17 Shlim DR, Hoge CW, Rajah R, Scott RM, Pandy P, Echeverria P: Persistent high risk of diarrhea among foreigners in Nepal during the first two years of residence. Clin Infect Dis 1999;29:613–616.

18 Mattila L, Siitonen A, Kyronseppa H, Simula I, Oksanen P, Stenvik M, Salo P, Peltola H: Seasonal variation in etiology of travelers' diarrhea. J Infect Dis 1992;165:385–388.

19 Gascón J, Vila J, Valls ME, Ruiz L, Vidal J, Corachán M, Prats G, Jiménez de Anta MT: Etiology of travellers diarrhea in Spanish travellers to developing countries. Eur J Epidemiol 1993;9:217–223.

20 Jiang ZD, Lowe B, Verenkar MP, Ashley D, Steffen R, Tornieporth N, von Sonnenburg F, Waiyaki P, DuPont HL: Prevalence of enteric pathogens among international travelers with diarrhea acquired in Kenya (Mombasa), India (Goa) or Jamaica (Montego Bay). J Infect Dis 2002;185:497–502.

21 Gascón J, Vargas M, Quintó L, Corachán M, Jiménez de Anta MT, Vila J: Enteroaggregative Escherichia coli strains as a cause of traveler's diarrhea: a case-control study. J Infect Dis 1998;177:1409–1412.

22 Huang DB, Okhuysen PC, Jiang ZD, DuPont HL: Enteroaggregative Escherichia coli: an emerging enteric pathogen. Am J Gastroenterol 2004;99:383–389.

23 Infante RM, Ericsson CD, Jiang ZD, Ke S, Steffen R, Riopel L, Sack DA, DuPont HL: Enteroaggregative Escherichia coli diarrhoea in travellers: response to rifaximin therapy. Clin Gastroenterol Hepatol 2004;2:135–138.

24 Vila J, Ruiz J, Gallardo F, Vargas M, Soler L, Figueras MJ, Gascón J: Aeromonas spp. and traveler's diarrhea: clinical features and antimicrobial resistance. Emerg Infect Dis 2003;9:552–555.

25 Gallardo F, Gascón J, Ruiz J, Corachán M, Jiménez de Anta MT, Vila J: Campylobacter jejuni as a cause of traveler's diarrhea: clinical features and antimicrobial susceptibility. J Trav Med 1998;5:23–26.

26 Black RE: Pathogens that cause travelers' diarrhea in Latin America and Africa. Rev Infect Dis 1986;8(suppl):S131–S135.

27 Essers B, Burnens AP, Lanfranchini FM, Somaruga SG, von Vigier RO, Schaad UB, Aebi C, Bianchetti MG: Acute community-acquired diarrhea requiring hospital admission in Swiss children. Clin Infect Dis 2000;31:192–196.

28 Egorov A, Paulauskis J, Petrova L, Tereschenko A, Drizhd N, Ford T: Contamination of water supplies with *Cryptosporidium parvum* and *Giardia lamblia* and diarrheal illness in selected Russian cities. Int J Hyg Environ Health 2002;205:281–289.

29 Ortega YR, Sterling CR, Gilman RH, Cama VA, Diaz F: *Cyclospora cayetanensis*: a new protozoan pathogen of humans. Am J Trop Med Hyg 1992;47(suppl):210, abstr 289.

30 Shlim DR, Cohen MT, Eaton M, Rajah R, Long EG, Ungar BL: An alga-like organism associated with an outbreak of prolonged diarrhea among foreigners in Nepal. Am J Trop Med Hyg 1991;45: 383–389.

31 Gascón J, Valls ME, Corachán M, Gené A, Bombi JA: Cyanobacteria-like body in travellers with diarrhea. Scand J Infect Dis 1993;25:253–257.

32 Sanders JW, Tribble DR: Diarrhea in the returned traveler. Curr Gastroenterol Rep 2001; 3:304–314.

33 Bavastrelli M, Bertucci P, Midulla M, Giardini O, Sanguigni S: Ciguatera fish poisoning: an emerging syndrome in Italian travellers. J Travel Med 2001;8:139–142.

34 Gascón J, Macià M, Oliveira I, Corachán M: Intoxicación por ciguatera en viajeros. Med Clin (Barc) 2003;120:777–779.

35 Vila J, Gascón J, Gene A, Ruiz L, Corachán M, Jimenez de Anta MT: Caracteristicas epidemiológicas, clínicas y microbiológicas de *E. coli* enterotoxigénico como causante de la Diarrea del Viajero. Enf Inf Microbiol Clin 1992;10:148–151.

36 Closs EI, Enseleit F, Koesling D, Pfeilschifter JM, Schwarz PM, Forstermann U: Coexpression of inducible NO synthase and soluble guanylyl cyclase in colonic enterocytes: a pathophysiologic signaling pathway for the initiation of diarrhea by Gram-negative bacteria? FASEB J 1998; 12: 1643–1649.

37 Fasano A, Hokama Y, Russell R, Morris JG Jr: Diarrhea in ciguatera fish poisoning: preliminary evaluation of pathophysiological mechanisms. Gastroenterology 1991;100:471–476.

38 Fasano A: Toxins and the gut: role in human disease. Gut 2002;50(suppl 3):9–14.

39 Wassenaar TM: Toxin production by *Campylobacter* spp. Clin Microb Rev 1997;10:466–476.

40 Steinberg JR, Del Rio C: Otros bacilos gram-negativos; in Mandell, Douglas, Bennett (eds): Enfermedades Infecciosas, 5th Spanish edition. Buenos Aires, Panamericana, 2002, vol 2, pp 2989–2990.

41 Nataro JP, Steiner T, Guerrant RL: Enteroaggregative *Escherichia coli*. Emerg Infect Dis 1998;4:251–261.

42 Hicks S, Candy DCA, Phillips AD: Adhesion of enteroaggregative *Escherichia coli* to paediatric intestinal mucosa in vitro. Infect Immun 1996;64:4751–4760.

43 Nataro JP, Yikang D, Cookson S, Cravioto A, Savarino SJ, Guers LD, Levine MM, Tacket CO: Heterogeneity of enteroaggregative *Escherichia coli* virulence demonstrated in volunteers. J Infect Dis 1995;171:465–468.

44 Farthing M J: Enterotoxins and the enteric nervous system – a fatal attraction. Int J Med Microbiol 2000;290:491–496.

45 Field M: Intestinal ion transport and the pathophysiology of diarrhea. J Clin Invest 2003;111: 931–943.

46 Jourdan N, Brunet JP, Sapin C, Blais A, Cotte-Laffitte J, Forestier F, Quero AM, Trugnan G, Servin AL: Rotavirus infection reduces sucrase-isomaltase expression in human intestinal epithelial cells by perturbing protein targeting and organization of microvillar cytoskeleton. J Virol 1998;72:7228–7236.

47 Ball JM, Tian P, Zeng CQ, Morris AP, Estes MK: Age-dependent diarrhea induced by a rotaviral non-structural protein. Science 1996;272:101–104.

48 Perez JF, Chemello ME, Liprandi F, Ruiz MC, Michelangeli F: Oncosis in MA 104 cells is induced by rotavirus infection through an increase in intracellular Ca^{2+} concentrations. Virology 1998;252:17–27.

49 Farthing MJG, Cevallos AM, Kelly P: Intestinal protozoa; in Cook GC, Zumla A (eds): Manson's Tropical Diseases, ed 21. London, Saunders, 1996, pp 1373–1385.

50 Gascón J, Corachán M, Bombí J, Valls ME, Bordes JM: *Cyclospora* in patients with traveler's diarrhea. Scand J Infect Dis 1995;27:511–514.
51 Bendall RP, Lucas S, Moody A, Tovey G, Chiodini PL: Diarrhea associated with cyanobacterium-like bodies: a new coccidian enteritis of man. Lancet 1993;341:590–592.
52 Okhuysen PC, Jiang ZD, Carlin L, Forbes C, DuPont HL: Post-diarrhea chronic intestinal symptoms and irritable bowel syndrome in North American travelers to Mexico. Am J Gastroenterol 2004;99:1774–1778.
53 Rees JH, Soudain SE, Gregson NA, Hughes RA: *Campylobacter jejuni* infection and Guillain-Barré syndrome. N Engl J Med 1995;333:1374–1379.

Joaquim Gascón, MD
c/ Villarroel, 170
ES–08036 Barcelona (Spain)
Tel. +34 93 227 5400 ext. 2182
Fax +34 93 227 9853
E-Mail jgascon@clinic.ub.es

This chapter should be cited as follows:

Gascón J: Epidemiology, Etiology and Pathophysiology of Traveler's Diarrhea.
Digestion 2006;73(suppl 1):102–108.

Scarpignato C, Lanas Á (eds): Bacterial Flora in Digestive Disease.
Focus on Rifaximin.

....

Prevention and Treatment of Traveler's Diarrhea

Focus on Antimicrobial Agents

Francesco Castelli, Nuccia Saleri, Lina Rachele Tomasoni, Giampiero Carosi

Institute for Infectious and Tropical Diseases, School of Medicine and Dentistry,
University of Brescia, Brescia, Italy

Abstract

Diarrhea, mostly due to bacterial infection of the gut, is the most frequent health complaint
in the international traveler, affecting 20–70% of the traveling population depending on the destination and other factors. It is usually benign and self-limiting in nature, but symptoms may
occasionally be distressing causing modifications of normal activities and sometimes confinement to bed or hospitalization. Prevention of traveler's diarrhea should ideally be based on
dietary restrictions, but experience shows that this target is extremely difficult to achieve.
Antibiotic chemoprophylaxis should be restricted to selected groups of travelers at risk of severe
complications of diarrhea or when diarrhea-driven alterations of planned activities are highly
undesirable (critical trips). The effectiveness of alternative prophylactic approaches, such as vaccination orthe use of probiotics, still awaits confirmation. Treatment of mild diarrheal cases
without intestinal symptoms may be limited to rehydration with or without antimotility agents.
When antibiotic therapy is considered, non-absorbable antibiotics, such as rifaximin, may be
considered a valid alternative to systemic antibiotics to treat uncomplicated cases, leaving fluoroquinolones and/or azithromycin for use in more severe cases or when invasive pathogens are
suspected. Indeed, therapeutic use of doxycycline and trimethoprim-sulfamethoxazole (TMP-
SMX) is limited by widespread resistance of many enteropathogens. The addition of loperamide
or other antimotility agents usually provides symptom relief and further shortens the duration of
illness and may be therefore safely adopted in the healthy adult unless dysentery is present.

Epidemiology

There is little doubt that traveler's diarrhea (TD) is to be considered the
most frequent illness in international travelers, with a 2-week incidence rate

ranging from 20 to 70% according to various factors including age, provenance and destination, season of traveling, preexisting gastrointestinal disturbances leading to achlorhydria, previous travels to developing countries, number of dietary errors, mode of travel and standard of accommodation [for review, see 1]. Its nature is infectious in the large majority of cases, with *Escherichia coli* (EC)[1] accounting for 30–60% of TD cases with a surprising homogeneity across the continents. Other bacterial microorganisms isolated during TD studies are *Campylobacter jejuni, Salmonella* spp., *Shigella* spp., *Aeromonas hydrophila, Plesiomonas shigelloides* and non-choleric vibrios. More rarely, also viruses (*Rotaviruses, Caliciviruses* and *Enteroviruses*) and protozoa (*Entamoeba histolytica, Cryptosporidium parvum, Giardia lamblia* and *Cyclospora cayetanensis*) may be involved as causative agents of TD in international travelers. However, according to the different studies [2], no causative agent may be identified in as many as 40% of TD cases. As a general rule, the more severe the clinical presentation, the more likely that an invasive microorganism is the causative agent of the syndrome, although no reliable relationship could be established between symptoms and etiology. Among other non-infectious possible causes of TD, jet lag, increase in alcohol consumption, stress and modification of intestinal bacterial flora due to dietary changes are also to be considered.

TD is usually self-limiting in the healthy traveler, but more severe syndromes may be observed in young children, old patients and in subjects with underlying debilitating conditions (diabetes, chronic cardiac diseases, immunocompromised hosts, etc.). In these cases the illness may be incapacitating, cause confinement to bed and even hospitalization during and/or after the travel with significant (direct and indirect) costs [3]. Furthermore, the impact of TD on the income of destination countries may be devastating and cause a substantial damage to the national budget of many developing countries with limited resources and for whom touristic revenues are crucial.

Apart from its implications in international travelers, TD may be considered an indirect mirror of the far more important infectious diarrheal diseases of childhood in developing countries, i.e. the cause of more than 2 million deaths of children under 5 years of age each year.

Prevention of Traveler's Diarrhea

Given the dimension of the medical and social problem, the prevention of TD is of course one of the priority goals of travel medicine. While anybody

[1]Enterotoxigenic (ET)-EC, enteroadhesive (EA)-EC, enteroinvasive (EI)-EC and enteroaggregative (EA)-EC.

agrees on this statement, a lower degree of agreement exists on how to achieve this objective. Indeed an extremely large array of microbiological, geographical and travel/traveler-related variables may play a confounding role in developing preventive guidelines.

In this review we will try to present the available and most updated scientific information concerning the preventive strategies of diarrhea in the international traveler. A discussion of the far more relevant problem of childhood diarrhea in developing countries goes beyond the aims of this paper and will not be attempted here.

Alimentary Precautions

A large body of evidence indicates that most cases of TD are caused by ingested infectious agents – mainly bacteria – that the gut of the traveler had not encountered before and towards which mucosal immunity is lacking, leading to colonization, inflammation and diarrhea. This process is facilitated by gut flora modifications due to alimentary changes during travel.

Taking these data into account, it is evident that the higher the number of dietary errors, the higher the incidence rate of TD in the travelers. The famous aphorism '*boil it, cook it, peel it or forget it*' was then coined and became one of the cornerstones of pre-travel advice sessions all over the world as primary prevention of the diarrheal syndrome in the traveler.

What is really a dietary error? The number of precautions that should be taken by travelers to avoid ingesting enteropathogens is actually endless [for review, see 4].

- Drinking tap water should be avoided unless boiled for at least 3–5 min. Chlorination is a safe alternative to boiling, but protozoan cysts are not destroyed. Ice cubes made from tap water are also unsafe and should be avoided. Once boiled to make tea or coffee, water-derived beverages should be consumed when still piping hot to assure microbiological safety.
- Bottled beverages, especially if alcoholic and/or carbonated, are usually safe due to their lower pH.
- Raw or rare cooked food (fish, meat) and dietary products (creams, fresh cheese, milk and butter) may be an important source of enteric infection and should be avoided. On the contrary, well-cooked food and baked food such as bread are usually considered safe.
- Fresh vegetables (often infected by sewage-contaminated irrigation) and fruits (possibly contaminated by handling) should be avoided unless carefully washed and peeled personally.

In conclusion, while this approach is theoretically correct, it has been challenged since its full achievement appears almost impossible in the general traveling population. Already in 1986 a Swiss survey reported that as many as 98%

of travelers to East African destinations committed at least one alimentary mistake during the first 3 days of stay abroad [5]. This is largely, but not solely, due to the fact that only a limited proportion of the general traveling population usually has pre-travel contact with a health professional, as recently pointed out by a large airport KAP (Knowledge, Attitudes, and Practices) survey carried out in nine major European airports by the European Travel Health Advisory Board (ETHAB) [6]. The same survey showed that as many as 94.5% of the 2,695 respondents waiting to leave for high TD incidence destinations were ready to adopt at least one alimentary behavior at risk for TD [7].

These data confirm that TD prevention by the sole means of health education would require that a substantially higher proportion of travelers have access to pre-travel health advice, provided a significant prevention is to be achieved.

Vaccination

TD is a syndrome with multiple possible etiologies. This fact makes the development of a preventive vaccine difficult. Organisms that have been targeted for the development of a vaccine include ETEC, *Salmonella typhi, Shigella* and rotaviruses. ETEC, mostly heat-labile toxin (LT)-producing strains, has been claimed to be responsible of as many as 30–60% of all cases of TD [8]. LT-ETEC toxin B-subunit is structurally related to cholera toxin B-subunit, for which a vaccine exists (whole cell/recombinant B subunit vaccine – WC/rBS), raising the hope that cross-protection could be achieved against LT-ETEC. Phase III clinical trials have demonstrated 67% protection against LT-ETEC in a Bangladeshi population [9] and 50% protection against ETEC in US students traveling in Mexico [10], but the effect was shortlived. Live-attenuated *E. coli* vaccine [11] as well as vaccine targeting various ETEC colonization factors are also under early investigation [12]. Despite considerable effort and progress, however, adequate vaccine protection against *all* TD microbiological causes is still difficult to achieve.

Chemoprophylaxis

Being TD is mostly an infectious syndrome, it has been suggested that chemoprophylaxis could decrease its incidence rate in the international traveler. Since the 1980s, several studies have demonstrated the preventive efficacy of neomycin [13], doxycycline [14], trimethoprim-sulfamethoxazole (TMP-SMX) [15] and fluoroquinolones [16] in reducing the incidence rate of TD in different parts of the world. A recent investigation [17] performed on US students traveling to Mexico did show a remarkable efficacy of the poorly absorbed antibiotic, rifaximin, thus confirming the effectiveness of 'topical' antimicrobials [for review, see 18]. This drug provided 72% protection against TD and all the drug regimens tested (i.e. 200 mg once, twice or three times

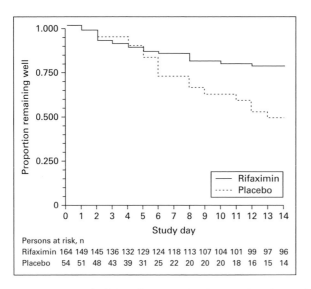

Fig. 1. Probability of not experiencing diarrhea during the first 2 weeks in Mexico in participants taking 200 mg of rifaximin once, twice, or three times daily (three groups combined) compared with placebo (from DuPont et al. [17]).

daily) were significantly better than placebo (fig. 1). In addition, rifaximin was very well tolerated, the rate of untoward reactions being comparable to that of placebo. In the above study [17] the major enteropathogens isolated from stool cultures were ETEC and EAEC. To establish whether rifaximin will be able to protect the traveler against invasive bacteria a specifically designed study has been planned in Asia, where pathogens like *Shigella, Salmonella* and *Campylobacter* species are important causes of diarrhea. In this connection, a clinical pharmacological study [19] did show that this antibiotic proved to be capable of preventing diarrhea in healthy volunteers challenged with *Shigella flexneri* 2a.

The preventive efficacy of antidiarrheal chemoprophylaxis has ranged from 71 to 95% [for reviews, see 17, 18, 20] according to the area of destination and the antibiotic class used, being lower than 60% with TMP-SMX combination and higher than 80% with fluoroquinolones [21, 22].

Despite their proved efficacy, the widespread use of antimicrobials to prevent has several limitations:

Adverse Effects. Most antibiotics used to prevent diarrhea pose the traveler at risk for untoward effects. Doxycycline may engender phototoxic reactions and, altering microbic flora, may lead to vaginal candidiasis and diarrhea. In addition, this drug cannot be used in infancy and pregnancy. The use of

TMP-SMX has been associated to rashes, mild to severe hypersensitivity reactions, bone marrow depression and gastrointestinal adverse reactions. Fluoroquinolones, even if generally well tolerated, may cause rashes, gastrointestinal disturbances, tendon lesions and central nervous system complaints. Their use too is contraindicated in infancy and pregnancy. Azithromycin is better tolerated than erythromycin but it can occasionally lead to ear and liver disturbances regardless of the dose. The poorly absorbed antibiotic rifaximin is generally well tolerated. Although serious adverse effects of any antibiotic occur in 0.01% of subjects, minor untoward effects present in 3% of drug recipients [21]. Since TD is usually a self-limiting condition in the majority of travelers, the benefit of prevention should always outweigh the risk connected with the drug treatment. As rifaximin is well tolerated at any dose level [23], its benefit-risk ratio is very favorable.

Drug Resistance. The possible emergence of drug-resistant enteropathogen strains is a very important issue limiting the widespread use of antibiotic prophylaxis. First, when it involves molecules included in the Country Essential Drug List, as it is generally the case for doxycycline and TMP-SMX, it further reduces the scarce therapeutic armamentarium of resources-limited countries. Secondly, it makes diarrheal syndrome difficult to treat with alternative drugs. Increasing resistance of ETEC to tetracyclines and TMP-SMX has been reported almost everywhere in developing countries [3] and fluoroquinolone-resistant *Campylobacter* strains from South-East Asia have been described frequently [24]. The available data concerning rifaximin use in the short term show the lack of emergence of drug-resistant Gram-positive and Gram-negative organisms [25]. Provided these results are confirmed in longer trials, this antibiotic could represent the ideal drug for TD chemoprophylaxis.

Cost. A reliable cost-benefit analysis of the prophylactic strategy against early treatment strategy is very difficult to perform since it is affected to a large extent by the estimated cost of hospitalization and incapacitation that are considered. Obviously, results may change over time with the changing cost of antibiotics and the changing pattern of resistance in a given area. When attempted, the prophylactic option gave more favorable cost-benefit results than the treatment option [26].

Risk Behavior. Chemoprophylaxis reduces but does not eliminate the risk of suffering from diarrheal syndromes caused by resistant enteropathogens or of contracting protozoan or viral diseases such as amebiasis or viral hepatitis A or E. Some travelers receiving chemoprophylaxis may feel a false sense of safety and complacently adopt a risky behavior leading to potentially severe systemic diseases.

The complex of such issues has been analyzed by a panel of experts during a Consensus Conference held at the National Institutes of Health (NIH) in 1985.

Table 1. Candidates for chemoprophylaxis of TD

High-risk travelers
  Immunosuppressed travelers, including HIV-infected subjects
  Travelers with autoimmune disorders
  Travelers with diabetes and/or chronic cardiac conditions
  Travelers with impaired gastric acid secretion
  Travelers with inflammatory bowel disease
Short-term critical trips
  Diplomats
  Athletes
  Any other trip whose interruption is deemed highly
  detrimental by the traveler

The final conclusion of the Consensus [27] was that chemoprophylaxis of TD should be discouraged unless specific conditions posing the traveler at particular risk do occur (table 1). The same conclusion was reached by a German-speaking panel of experts [22].

Should a cheap, extremely safe and non-resistance-prone antimicrobial be available (a very difficult task indeed), widespread TD chemoprophylaxis could become reality. However, at the present time, the recommendations of the 1985 NIH Consensus Conference on Traveler's Diarrhea may still be considered valid. In case antibiotic chemoprophylaxis is deemed advisable, non-absorbed rifaximin might be considered the safest alternative to fluoroquinolones.

Other Preventive Approaches to Traveler's Diarrhea

Various other preventive approaches to TD have been considered. Among those, the use of probiotics and of bismuth subsalicylate.

Probiotics. The use of probiotics as TD-preventive agents has long been advocated on the basis of their ability of preventing enteropathogen colonization. However, results of the available clinical trials are conflicting [28] and modest benefit has been shown only by some – but not all – trials using *Lactobacillus GG* [29] or *Saccharomyces boulardii* [30]. Probiotics are safe, but available data are not robust enough at the present time to recommend their use as the sole prophylactic agents of TD.

Bismuth Subsalicylate. The use of bismuth subsalicylate has been associated with about 65% reduction in the incidence rate of TD [31]. Since it is virtually not absorbed when administered orally, its use is devoid from adverse events. However, the need for frequent dosing (4 times daily), the possible appearance of tinnitus, the blackening of the tongue caused by chewing the drug and its relatively modest preventive efficacy do not facilitate compliance [18].

Table 2. Composition of WHO/UNICEF and home-made oral rehydration solutions (modified from Scarpignato and Rampal [18])

WHO/UNICEF oral rehydration solution		Home-made solution	
Water	1 liter	Water	1 liter
Glucose (anhydrous)	20 g	Sucrose	5 spoons of ordinary sugar
Sodium chloride	3.5 g	Sodium chloride	1 coffee-spoon of ordinary salt
Sodium bicarbonate *or*	2.5 g	Potassium	fruit juices
Trisodium citrate	2.9 g		
Potassium chloride	1.5 g		

Treatment

While chemoprophylaxis is not universally accepted, consensus exists on the need for *early* treatment of TD to shorten its duration, limit discomfort and confinement to bed and prevent its potentially severe consequences [32]. Oral rehydration, symptomatic therapy and antimicrobial therapy represent the cornerstones of treatment of infectious diarrhea.

Oral Rehydration Therapy
Although TD is seldom a dehydrating syndrome, rehydration is always suggested to restore hydric and electrolytic balance and to prevent possible complications, especially in those patients with underlying diseases, in young children and in the elderly. In this connection the large ETHAB survey has pointed out that as many as 8.8% of travelers are over 60 years of age. This proportion was even higher in the subset of travelers from specific countries (e.g. 22.3% in European travelers from Stockholm) [6]. Early refeeding is also advocated, especially if antidiarrheal treatment limits the duration of the syndrome to 1–2 days.

Oral rehydration solutions are best prepared with optimal concentrations of glucose, which facilitate the absorption of sodium and water, and of bicarbonates to correct diarrheal-related acidosis. Table 2 provides the composition of the WHO/UNICEF formula used to rehydrate young children with diarrheal diseases in developing countries and of a possible 'home-made solution' that can be used in the outpatient treatment of TD [18].

Despite the consensus on the need for rehydration during diarrheal illnesses, a surprisingly low proportion of travelers (as low as <5% of Finnish travelers with diarrhea!) do in reality increase the amount of liquid intake while suffering from TD, underlying the need of a better health education [33].

Symptomatic Therapy

The two most studied agents used to alleviate symptoms of diarrhea are bismuth subsalicylate preparation and loperamide [18]. Both decrease the number of unformed stools, but loperamide acts more rapidly by exerting an anti-motility action. Loperamide should be avoided in young children, due to the reported risk of intussusception, and when invasive enteropathogens are suspected because of the risk of their prolonged retention. However, when concomitant antibiotic treatment is administered, this fear was not confirmed [34] while a significant benefit in the treatment of *Shigella* infection compared to antibiotic treatment alone was reported [35].

Other 'purely antisecretory' agents for treatment of TD include zaldaride maleate (a potent and selective calmodulin inhibitor) [36] and racecadotril (an enkepha-linase inhibitor) [37]. Both these compounds are devoid of any effect on gastrointestinal motility and their use is not followed by treatment-related rebound constipation.

Antimicrobial Treatment

Being an infectious disease, antimicrobial therapy represents the 'logical' treatment of TD. The high success rate of the empirical (i.e. without susceptibility testing) antimicrobial treatment further confirms the infectious etiology of TD. Although rational, antibiotic use in the treatment of TD should always take into consideration the following issues:

- Uncomplicated watery TD is usually a self-limiting disease in the healthy traveler and symptomatic agents may easily control symptoms.
- TD is a syndrome and no specific microbial isolation is usually available when therapeutical decision is to be taken, making susceptibility-driven choice of antibiotic practically unfeasible.
- The use of systemic antibiotics may be associated with untoward effects.
- Taking into account the epidemiology and drug susceptibility of those bacteria usually involved as the causative agents of TD, the following antimicrobial agents have been adopted for its treatment:

Trimethoprim-Sulfamethoxazole

Historically, TMP-SMX was the first antimicrobial agent used to treat diarrhea in the traveler with preliminary excellent results [38]. However, resistant ETEC strains soon became prevalent in most developing countries [39] and *C. jejuni* – generally non-susceptible to the drug [40] – was recognized as the cause of a significant proportion of TD. These findings, together with the significant incidence of untoward effects, has led to a general dismissal of the drug as first-line treatment of diarrhea in the traveler apart from central Mexico where it retained a satisfactory degree of activity against *E. coli* until recently [41].

Doxycycline

The drug was successfully used during the 1970s and 1980s before significant *E. coli* resistance to the drug became the rule [42]. This fact, together with the possible occurrence of untoward effects (candidiasis, intestinal dismicrobism, skin sun reactions) has relegated this drug to a second choice treatment [43].

Fluoroquinolones

After their introduction in the clinical practice, fluoroquinolones soon became the first-line drug for the treatment of TD due to their excellent efficacy against enteropathogens and their favorable safety profile. Their pharmacokinetic properties allow peak tissue levels to be reached quickly. Ciprofloxacin has been extensively studied as a therapeutic agent of TD and has proved effective even in single dose in particular conditions (young male otherwise healthy soldiers) [44]. However, virtually any member of the family (norfloxacin, ofloxacin, levofloxacin, gatifloxacin, lomefloxacin, moxifloxacin) has been satisfactorily used to treat diarrheal syndromes [for review, see 43]. Fluoroquinolones are usually well tolerated, but occasionally untoward effects occur (rashes, gastro-intestinal disturbances, tendon lesions and central nervous system complaints) and they should not be used in childhood and pregnancy. Furthermore, *Campylobacter* isolates, especially from South-East Asia, increasingly show a reduced susceptibility to fluoroquinolones [45, 46].

Azithromycin

This macrolide antibiotic exerted similar efficacy when compared to levofloxacin for the treatment of acute TD in Mexico [47]. It has recently been considered as possible first-line antidiarrheal drug in those areas where fluoroquinolone-resistant strains of *C. jejuni* have been increasingly reported, such as Thailand and other South-East Asian countries [24]. Its gastrointestinal untoward effects are milder than those exerted by erythromycin, but hearing and liver disturbances occasionally do occur.

Rifaximin and Other Poorly Absorbed Antibiotics

Lack of absorption was once considered to weigh against the predicted efficacy of an antibiotic in the treatment of bacterial diarrhea. Haltalin et al. [48] many years ago compared the efficacy of ampicillin with a non-absorbable aminoglycoside in the treatment of shigellosis. When the patients in the aminoglycoside arm failed to respond as those treated with ampicillin, the authors concluded that only an absorbable drug should be used in the treatment of bacterial diarrhea. It was later realized that poorly absorbed antimicrobials could be of value in the treatment of enteric infections. Indeed, early trials assessing the efficacy and safety profile of bicozamycin and aztreonam were promising [49, 50], but those drugs did not undergo further development. Recently a rifamycin

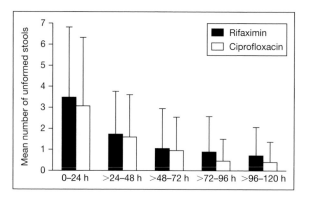

Fig. 2. Mean number of unformed stools passed per day of study by subjects with TD taking rifaximin (400 mg twice daily) or ciprofloxacin (500 mg twice daily). The mean values for the two treatment groups were comparable for each day of the study (from DuPont et al. [61]).

derivative, rifaximin, has shown comparable effectiveness as fluoroquinolones in uncomplicated infectious diarrhea [reviewed in 23, 51–54] and has been approved for the treatment of TD by the US Food and Drug Administration (FDA).

Rifaximin is virtually non-absorbed (<0.4%) when administered orally and has a wide antimicrobial spectrum against most enteropathogens, even if activity against Gram-negative bacteria is somehow lower than against Gram-positive ones [reviewed in 55–57]. On the contrary, its activity against *C. jejuni* is rather low [58]. However, it should be pointed out that stool concentrations of the drug are 250–500 times higher than the MIC_{90} values [59] which makes in vitro differences of activity against the various pathogens meaningless from a clinical standpoint.

Rifaximin compared favorably with TMP-SMX in the treatment of TD in Mexico [60] and was as effective as ciprofloxacin when tested in a randomized, double-blind clinical trial in Jamaica and Mexico [61] (fig. 2), with limited adverse events. When a double-blind, placebo-controlled study of rifaximin 600 or 1,200 mg/day was carried out in various countries (Kenya, Guatemala, Mexico), rifaximin proved effective at the dose of 600 mg/day or higher without relevant untoward effects [62]. A recent study [63] confirmed rifaximin effectiveness in treatment of diarrhea in travelers to Mexico and Kenya and showed that the antibiotic shortened the duration of the illness also in patients with EAEC diarrhea. A synopsis of the available studies with rifaximin in the treatment of TD is shown in table 3.

Concerns have been raised about the possible induction of drug resistance following the use of the rifamycin derivative, rifaximin. According to recent data, however, rifaximin differs from related rifampicin in this respect and has a low potential for inducing resistance in Gram-negative and Gram-positive

Table 3. Clinical studies assessing rifaximin efficacy in the treatment of TD (modified from Al-Abri et al. [51])

Reference	Type of study	Patients	Destination	Origin of travelers	Duration of treatment days	Intervention: rifaximin vs. comparator	Median time to last unformed stool, h	p
DuPont et al. [60]	Randomized, double-blind	72	Mexico	USA	5	Rifaximin Cotrimoxazole	35 47	0.001
DuPont et al. [61]	Randomized, double-blind	187	Mexico, Jamaica	USA	3	Rifaximin Ciprofloxacin	25.7 25	0.199
Steffen et al. [62]	Randomized, double-blind	380	Mexico, Guatemala, Kenya	Inter-national	3	Rifaximin 200 mg 3 × daily Rifaximin 400 mg 3 × daily Placebo	32.5 32.9 60.0	0.0001
Infante et al. [63]	Randomized, placebo-controlled (effect on EAEC)	380	Mexico, Guatemala, Kenya	Inter-national	3	Rifaximin 200 mg 3 × daily Placebo	22 72	0.003

intestinal flora during therapy [25, 56, 57]. Since rifaximin does not affect the activity of CYP_{450} isoenzymes [57, 64, 65], the potential of drug-to-drug inter-action is virtually absent. Therefore, the pharmacokinetic and pharmacody-namic of concomitant drugs (e.g. antimalarials) will not be affected by the administration of this antibiotic.

Being effective and safe, rifaximin can then be considered an alternative first-line drug to treat uncomplicated TD. This therapeutic strategy would leave fluoroquinolones and/or azithromycin – whose restricted use will limit the development of resistance – for those cases, where the clinical picture suggests the presence of invasive pathogens.

Guidelines for Treatment of Traveler's Diarrhea

Early treatment of TD, including adequate intake of fluids, offers today the best option to limit discomfort and prevent potentially severe complications, limiting chemoprophylaxis to selected cases of at-risk travelers.

Mild diarrheal cases without intestinal symptoms may well be exclusively treated with rehydration and/or bismuth subsalicylate, where available. When antibiotic therapy (table 4) is considered, poorly absorbed antibiotics, such

Table 4. Recommended antimicrobial regimens to treat TD (modified from Vila et al. [42])

	Dose	Remarks
Fluoroquinolones		
Ciprofloxacin	500 mg p.o. b.i.d. × 1–3 days	
Norfloxacin	400 mg p.o. b.i.d. × 1–3 days	
Ofloxacin	400 mg p.o. b.i.d. × 1–3 days	
Levofloxacin	500 mg p.o. q.d. × 1–3 days	
Gatifloxacin	400 mg p.o. q.d. × 1–3 days	
Lomefloxacin	400 mg p.o. q.d. × 1–3 days	
Moxifloxacin	400 mg p.o. q.d. × 1–3 days	
Macrolides		
Azithromycin	500 mg p.o. b.i.d. × 3 days	Consider first-line for countries with quinolone-resistant *Campylobacter* (e.g. Thailand)
Rifamycin derivatives		
Rifaximin	400 mg p.o. b.i.d. × 3 days	

Table 5. Guidelines for treatment of TD (from Ericsson [3])

Clinical symptoms	Recommended therapy	Comments
Mild diarrhea (1–2 stools/24 h) with mild or absent symptoms	Bismuth subsalicylate *or* Attapulgite *or* nothing	Long-term travelers should consider not treating mild diarrhea with an antibiotic to build some immunity
Mild to moderate classic diarrhea (≥3 stools/24 h) with no distressing symptoms	Loperamide *or* bismuth subsalicylate	Business travelers or others on a short, critical trip might consider addition of an antibiotic
Diarrhea with distressing frequency or symptoms	Loperamide *plus* fluoroquinolone[a], *or* azithromycin *or* rifaximin	Reassess symptoms after 24 h; single dose antibiotic usually suffices
Severe diarrhea or diarrhea with fever or passage of bloody stools	Fluoroquinolone[a], azithromycin, *or* rifaximin, with *or* without loperamide	Take full 3 days of antibiotic. Loperamide can be added for severe cramps or fluid losses. Its use in dysentery is controversial

[a]Azithromycin or rifaximin preferred in South-East Asia where fluoroquinolone-resistant organisms are common.

as rifaximin, may be considered a valid alternative to systemic antimicrobials to treat uncomplicated cases, reserving fluoroquinolones and/or azithromycin to more severe cases or when invasive pathogens are suspected (table 5), where the use of systemic drugs is mandatory. This approach will preserve fluoroquinolones and azithromycin from developing drug resistance also for their other extraintestinal use (e.g. respiratory tract infections). Loperamide or other antimotility agents usually provide symptom relief and may be safely adopted in the healthy adult if no signs or symptoms of dysentery are present. Loperamide, however, should be avoided in young children.

Conclusions

TD, an infectious intestinal syndrome, is and will probably continue to be the most frequent health complaint of the traveling population in the future. If dietary restrictions are probably critical to prevent the ingestion of enteropathogens, their adoption in reality is far from being optimal. Pharmacodynamic and safety considerations limit chemoprophylaxis to selected categories of travelers and early treatment is presently considered the best option to limit discomfort and prevent complications. If treatment of mild diarrheal cases without intestinal symptoms may be limited to rehydration and/or symptomatic agents, antibiotics are effective in reducing severity and duration of symptoms in more severe cases. When antibiotic therapy is considered worthwhile, poorly absorbed antibiotics, such as rifaximin, should be preferred to treat uncomplicated cases, leaving systemic antibiotics (i.e., fluoroquinolones and/or azithromycin) for use in more severe cases or when invasive pathogens are suspected.

References

1 Castelli F, Pezzoli C, Tomasoni L: Epidemiology of travelers' diarrhea. J Trav Med 2001;8(suppl 2): S26–S30.
2 Peltola H, Gorbach SL: Travelers' diarrhea: epidemiology and clinical aspects; in DuPont HL, Steffen R (eds): Textbook of Travel Medicine and Health. Hamilton/London, BC, Decker, 2001, pp 151–159.
3 Ericsson CD: Travelers' diarrhea. Int J Antimicrob Agents 2003;21:116–124.
4 Castelli F, Carosi G: Epidemiology of travelers' diarrhea. Chemotherapy 1995;41(suppl 1):20–32.
5 Kozicki M, Steffen R, Schar M: '*Boil it, cook* I *it, peel it or forget it*': does this rule prevent travelers' diarrhea? Int J Epidemiol 1985;14: 169–172.
6 Van Herck K, Castelli F, Zuckerman J, Nothdurft H, Van Damme P, Dahlgren A, Gargalianos P, Lopez-Velez R, Overbosh D, Caumes E, Walker E, Gisler S, Steffen R: Knowledge, attitude and practices in travel-related infectious diseases: the European Airport Survey. J Trav Med 2004; 11:3–8.
7 Castelli F: Human mobility and diseases: a global challenge. J Trav Med 2004;11:1–2.
8 Gascon J, Vargas M, Quinto L, Corachan M, Jimenez de Anta MT, Vila J: Enteroaggregative *Escherichia coli* strains as cause of travelers' diarrhea: a case-control study. J Infect Dis 1998; 177:1409–1412.
9 Peltola H, Siitonen A, Kyronseppa H, Simula I, Mattila L, Oksanen P, Kataja MJ, Cadoz M: Prevention of travelers' diarrhea by oral B-subunit/whole cell cholera vaccine. Lancet 1991;338: 1285–1289.

10   Scerpella EG, Sanchez JL, Mathewson II JJ, et al: Safety, immunogenicity and protective efficacy of the whole-cell/recombinant B subunit (WC/rBS) oral cholera vaccina against travelers' diarrhea. J Trav Med 1995;2:22–27.

11   Turner A, Terry T, Sack DA, Londono-Archila P, Darsley MJ: Construction and characterization of genetically defined aro omp mutants of enterotoxinogenic *Escherichia coli* and preliminary studies of safety and immunogenicity in humans. Infect Immun 2001;69:4969–4979.

12   Katz D, DeLorimier A, Wolf M, Hall ER, Cassels FJ, van Hamont JE, Newcomer RL, Davachi MA, Taylor DN, McQueen CE: Oral immunization of adult volunteers with micro-encapsulated enterotoxinogenic *Escherichia coli* (ETEC) CS6 antigen. Vaccine 2003;21:341–346.

13   Kean BH: Travelers' diarrhea: an overview. Rev Infect Dis 1986;8(suppl 2):S111–S116.

14   Sack DA, Kaminsky DC, Sack JN, Itiotia RR, Arthur AZ, Kapikian F, Orskov F, Orskov I: Prophylactic doxycycline for travelers' diarrhea: results of a prospective double-blind study of Peace Corps volunteers in Kenya. N Engl J Med 1978;298:758–763.

15   DuPont HL, Evans DG, Rios N, Cabada FJ, Evans DJ, DuPont MW: Prevention of travelers' diarrhea with trimethoprim-sulphametoxazole. Rev Infect Dis 1982;4:533–539.

16   Parry H, Howard AJ, Galpin OH, Hassan SP: The prophylaxis of travelers' diarrhea: a double-blind placebo-controlled trial of ciprofloxacin during a Himalayan expedition. J Infect 1994;28:337–338.

17   DuPont HL, Jiang ZD, Okhuysen PC, Ericsson CD, de la Cabada F, Ke S, DuPont MW, Martinez-Sandoval F: A randomized, double-blind, placebo-controlled trial of rifaximin to prevent travelers' diarrhea. Ann Intern Med 2005;142:805–812.

18   Scarpignato C, Rampal P: Prevention and treatment of travelers' diarrhea: a clinical pharmacological approach. Chemotherapy 1995;41(suppl 1):48–81.

19   Taylor DN, Mckenzie R, Durbin A, Carpenter C, Atzinger CB, Haake R, Bourgeois AL: Double-blind, placebo-controlled trial to evaluate the use of rifaximin to prevent diarrhea in volunteers challenged with *Shigella flexneri*. 53rd Meeting of the American Society of Tropical Medicine and Hygiene, Miami, Nov 7–11, 2004.

20   Ostrosky-Zeichner L, Ericsson C: Prevention of travelers' diarrhea; in Keystone J, Kozarsky P, Freedman DO, Nothdurft H, Connor BA (eds): Travel Medicine. Edinburgh, Mosby Elsevier, 2004, pp 185–190.

21   Ericsson CD: Travelers' diarrhea. Epidemiology, prevention and self-treatment. Infect Dis Clin North Am 1998;12:285–303.

22   Steffen R, Kollaritsch H, Fleischer K: Travelers' diarrhea in the new millennium: consensus among experts from German-speaking countries. J Trav Med 2003;10:38–45.

23   Ericsson CD, DuPont HL: Rifaximin in the treatment of infectious diarrhea. Chemotherapy 2005;51(suppl 1):73–80.

24   Kuschner RA, Trofa AF, Thomas RJ, Hoge CW, Pitarangsi C, Amato S, Olafson RP, Echeverria P, Sadoff JC, Taylor DN: Use of azithromycin for the treatment of *Campylobacter enteritis* in travelers to Thailand, an area where ciprofloxacin resistance is prevalent. Clin Infect Dis 1995; 21:536–541.

25   DuPont HL, Jiang ZD: Influence of rifaximin treatment on susceptibility of intestinal Gram-negative flora and enterococci. Clin Microbiol Infect 2004;10:1009–1011.

26   Reves RR, Johnson PC, Ericsson CD, DuPont HL: A cost-effectiveness comparison of the use of antimicrobial agents for treatment or prophylaxis of travelers' diarrhea. Arch Intern Med 1988;148:2421–2427.

27   Gorbach SL, Edelman R: Travelers' diarrhea: National Institutes of Health Consensus Development Conference. Rev Infect Dis 1986;8(suppl 2):S109–S233.

28   Katelaris PH, Salam I, Farthing MJ: Lactobacilli to prevent traveler's diarrhea? N Engl J Med 1995;333:1360–1361.

29   Marteau PR, de Vrese M, Cellier CJ, Schrezenmeier J: Protection from gastrointestinal diseases with the use of probiotics. Am J Clin Nutr 2001;73(suppl 2):S430–S435.

30   D'Souza AL, Rajkumar C, Cooke J, Bullpit CJ: Probiotic in prevention of antibiotic-associated diarrhea: meta-analysis. BMJ 2002;324:1361.

31   DuPont HL, Ericsson CD, Johnson PC, Bitsura JAM, DuPont MW, de la Cabada FJ: Prevention of travelers diarrhea by the tablet formulation of bismuth subsalicylate. JAMA 1987;257:1347–1350.

32   Connor BA, Landzberg BR: Prevention and treatment of acute traveler's diarrhea. Infect Med 2004;21:18–19.

33   Meuris B: Observational study of traveler's diarrhea. J Trav Med 1995;2:11–15.

34   Ericsson CD, DuPont HL, Mathewson JJ, West MS, Johnson PC, Bitsura JA: Treatment of traveler's diarrhea with sulfamethoxazole and trimethoprim and loperamide. JAMA 1990;263: 257–261.

35   Murphy GS, Bodhidatta L, Echeverria P, et al: Ciprofloxacin and loperamide in the treatment of bacillary dysentery. Ann Intern Med 1993;118:582–586.

36   Okhuysen PC, DuPont HL, Ericsson CD, Marani S, Martinez-Sandoval FG, Olesen MA, Ravelli GP: Zaldaride maleate (a new calmodulin antagonist) versus loperamide in the treatment of traveler's diarrhea: randomized, placebo-controlled trial. Clin Infect Dis 1995;21:341–344.

37   Wang HH, Shieh MJ, Liao KF: A blind, randomized comparison of racecadotril and loperamide for stopping acute diarrhea in adults. World J Gastroenterol 2005;11:1540–1543.

38   DuPont HL, Reves R, Galindo R, Sullivan P, Wood L, Mendiola J: Treatment of travelers' diarrhea with trimethoprim-sulphametoxazole and with trimethoprim alone. N Engl J Med 1982;307: 841–844.

39   Echeverria P, Verhaert L, Ulyangco CV, Komalarini S, Ho MT, Orskov F, Orskov I: Antimicrobial resistance and enterotoxin production among isolates of *Escherichia coli* in the Far East. Lancet 1978;ii:589–592.

40   Sack RB, Rahman M, Yunus M, Khan EH: Antimicrobial resistance in organisms causing diarrheal diseases. Clin Infect Dis 1997;24(suppl 1):S102–S105.

41   Bandres J, Mathewson J, Ericsson CD, DuPont HL: Trimethoprim-sulphametoxazole remains active against enterotoxigenic *Escherichia coli* and *Shigella* spp. in Guadalajara, Mexico. Am J Med Sci 1992;303:289–291.

42   Vila J, Vargas M, Ruiz J, Corachan M, Jimenez De Anta MT, Gascon J: Quinolone resistance in enterotoxigenic *Escherichia coli* causing diarrhea in travelers to India in comparison with other geographical areas. Antimicrob Agents Chemother 2000;44:1731–1733.

43   Loescher T, Connor BA: Clinical presentation and treatment of travelers' diarrhea; in Keystone J, Kozarsky P, Freedman DO, Nothdurft H, Connor BA (eds): Travel Medicine. Edinburgh, Mosby Elsevier, 2004, pp 191–199.

44   Salam I, Katelaris P, Leigh-Smith S, Farthing MJ: Randomised trial of single-dose ciprofloxacin for travellers' diarrhoea. Lancet 1994;344:1537–1539.

45   Piddock LJ: Quinolone resistance and *Campylobacter* spp. J Antimicrob Chemother 1995; 36:891–898.

46   Hoge CW, Gambel JM, Srijan A, Pitarangsi C, Echeverria P: Trends in antibiotic resistance among diarrheal pathogens isolated in Thailand over 15 years. Clin Infect Dis 1998;26:341–345.

47   Adachi JA, Ericsson CD, Jiang ZD, DuPont MW, Martinez-Sandoval F, Knirsch C, DuPont HL: Azithromycin found to be comparable to levofloxacin for the treatment of US travelers with acute diarrhea acquired in Mexico. Clin Infect Dis 2003;37:1165–1171.

48   Haltalin KC, Nelson JD, Hinton LV, Kusmiesz HT, Sladoje M: Comparison of orally absorbable and nonabsorbable antibiotics in shigellosis. A double-blind study with ampicillin and neomycin. J Pediatr 1968;72:708–720.

49   Ericsson CD, DuPont HL, Sullivan P, Galindo E, Evans DG, Evans DJ: Bicozamycin, a poorly absorbable antibiotic, effectively treats diarrhea. Ann Intern Med 1983;98:20–25.

50   DuPont HL, Ericsson CD, Mathewson JJ, de la Cabada FJ, Conrad D: Oral aztreonam, a poorly absorbed yet effective therapy for bacterial diarrhea in US travelers to Mexico. JAMA 1992; 267:1932–1935.

51   Al-Abri SS, Beeching NJ, Nye FJ: Traveller's diarrhoea. Lancet Infect Dis 2005;5:349–360.

52   Gerard L, Garey KW, DuPont HL: Rifaximin: a nonabsorbable rifamycin antibiotic for use in non-systemic gastrointestinal infections. Expert Rev Anti Infect Ther 2005;3:201–211.

53   Robins GW, Wellington K: Rifaximin. Drugs 2005;65:1697–1713.

54   Huang DB, DuPont HL: Rifaximin – a novel antimicrobial for enteric infections. J Infect 2005;50:97–106.

55   Gillis JC, Brogden RN: Rifaximin: a review of its antibacterial activity, pharmacokinetic properties and therapeutical potential in conditions mediated by gastrointestinal bacteria. Drugs 1995; 49:467–484.

56 Jiang ZD, DuPont HL: Rifaximin: in vitro and in vivo antibacterial activity – a review. Chemotherapy 2005;51(suppl 1):67–72.

57 Scarpignato C, Pelosini I: Rifaximin, a poorly absorbed antibiotic: pharmacology and clinical potential. Chemotherapy 2005;51(suppl 1):36–66.

58 Ripa S, Mignini F, Prenna M, Falcioni E: In vitro antibacterial activity of rifaximin against *Clostridium difficile, Campylobacter jejunii and Yersinia* spp. Drugs Exp Clin Res 1987;13: 483–488.

59 Jiang ZD, Ke S, Palazzini E, Riopel L, Dupont H: In vitro activity and fecal concentration of rifaximin after oral administration. Antimicrob Agents Chemother 2000;44:2205–2206.

60 DuPont HL, Ericsson CD, Mathewson JJ, Palazzini E, DuPont MW, Jiang ZD, Mosavi A, de la Cabada FJ: Rifaximin: a nonabsorbed antimicrobial in the therapy of travelers' diarrhea. Digestion 1998;59:708–714.

61 DuPont HL, Jiang ZD, Ericsson CD, Adachi JA, Mathewson JJ, DuPont MW, Palazzini E, Riopel LM, Ashley D, Martinez-Sandoval F: Rifaximin versus ciprofloxacin for the treatment of traveler's diarrhea: a randomized, double-blind clinical trial. Clin Infect Dis 2001;33:1807–1815.

62 Steffen R, Sack DA, Riopel L, Jianh ZD, Sturchler M, Ericsson CD, Lowe B, Phil M, Waiyaki P, White P, DuPont HL: Therapy of travelers' diarrhea with rifaximin on various continents. Am J Gastroenterol 2003;98:1073–1078.

63 Infante RM, Ericsson CD, Jiang ZD, Ke S, Steffen R, Riopel L, Sack DA, DuPont HL: Entero-aggregative *Escherichia coli* diarrhea in travelers: response to rifaximin therapy. Clin Gastroenterol Hepatol 2004;2:135–138.

64 King A, Marshall O, Connolly M, Kamm A, Boxenbaum H, Kastrissios H, Trapnell C: The effect of rifaximin on the pharmacokinetics of a single dose of ethinyl estradiol and norgestimate in healthy female volunteers. Clin Pharmacol Ther 2004;75:P96.

65 King A, Laurie R, Connolly M, Kamm A, Boxenbaum H, Kastrissios H, Trapnell C: The effect of rifaximin on the pharmacokinetics of single doses of intravenous and oral midazolam in healthy volunteers. Clin Pharmacol Ther 2004;75:P66.

Prof. Francesco Castelli, MD, PhD
Institute for Infectious and Tropical Diseases, University of Brescia
Piazza Spedali Civili, 1, IT–25123 Brescia (Italy)
Tel. +39 030 399 5664, Fax +39 030 303 061
E-Mail castelli@med.unibs.it

This chapter should be cited as follows:

Castelli F, Saleri N, Tomasoni LR, Carosi G: Prevention and Treatment of Traveler's Diarrhea. Focus on Antimicrobial Agents. Digestion 2006;73(suppl 1):109–118.

Scarpignato C, Lanas Á (eds): Bacterial Flora in Digestive Disease.
Focus on Rifaximin.

....

Helicobacter pylori Infection: Treatment Options

Xavier Calvet

Digestive Diseases Unit, Hospital de Sabadell, Institut Universitari Parc
Taulí, Universitat Autònoma de Barcelona, Barcelona, Spain

Abstract

After two decades of progress the best current approach to treatment of *Helicobacter pylori* infection is a strategy that combines two consecutive complementary treatments. Current guidelines recommend a first-line triple therapy – 7–10 days of a proton-pump inhibitor (PPI), clarithromycin and amoxicillin – followed by a quadruple therapy combining a PPI, metronidazole, tetracycline and a bismuth salt for treatment failures. Regrettably, present cure rates for first-line triple therapy are below 80%, and many patients require second-line treatment with further testing and control visits. Although most compliant patients are cured by the second-line treatment, patients often do not complete the full process and, as a result, final cure rates for the whole strategy often fall below 90%. This means that more effective first-line therapies are required. Promising recent developments include using quadruple therapy as first-line therapy, the use of adjuvant lactoferrin with triple therapy and a newly devised combination of a PPI, clarithromycin, amoxicillin and metronidazole, known as sequential treatment. Additional future developments will require the incorporation of new antibiotic weapons in the anti-*H. pylori* arsenal. The new quinolones and rifamycin derivates have recently demonstrated their efficacy in the treatment of *H. pylori* infection.

Copyright © 2006 S. Karger AG, Basel

Introduction

Antibacterial treatment for peptic ulcer preceded the discovery of *Helicobacter pylori*. For decades, patients preferred antacids (aluminum and/or magnesium containing compounds) or mucosal coating agents (bismuth-containing compounds and sucralfate), due to the apparent effectiveness of these drugs. The first report of antibiotic treatment for peptic ulcer disease was a monograph published in 1951 in which Solano [1] reported his experience treating ulcer patients with penicillin and convalescent patient serum. Ten years later, John Lykoudis [2], a Greek practitioner, patented Elgano, an antibacterial combination of streptomycin and oxyquinolines, among other components. The combination produced notable improvements in ulcer patients' symptoms. He treated more than 30,000 patients for two decades despite the lack of official approval, since no comparative trials of the compound were ever performed.

The first 'official' *H. pylori* treatment was serendipitously performed by Marshall [3] in 1983. A patient included in a trial comparing the anti-ulcer effect of bismuth salts and cimetidine developed a periodontal disease while receiving bismuth and received a 5-day metronidazole treatment. *H. pylori* was not found in the subsequent control endoscopy. Marshall later used this combination in many patients, including himself. The first reliable therapy was triple therapy combining bismuth, tetracycline and metronidazole which was very effective, though it had a complicated schedule and frequent side effects [4]. Dual therapies combining omeprazole and amoxicillin or clarithromycin had a short burst of popularity due to their simplicity and tolerability, but because of their lack of efficacy they were soon abandoned [5]. In 1993, Bell et al. [6] first reported the high efficacy of a triple therapy combining a proton-pump inhibitor (PPI), amoxicillin and metronidazole. Shortly afterwards, Bazzoli [7, 8] described a triple therapy combining a PPI, clarithromycin and metronidazole. The 'Italian' triple therapy was rapidly followed by the 'French' triple therapy which replaced metronidazole with amoxicillin. Triple therapy combined simplicity, tolerability and efficacy and was quickly accepted as a standard after many large multicentre trials had demonstrated cure rates of around 90% [9–11].

H. pylori Treatment: Current Status and Guidelines

After multiple studies a series of meta-analyses demonstrated that triple therapy works better if the proton pump is used twice a day [12], and when full doses of clarithromycin are administered [13]. All different PPIs seem to obtain similar results [14]. The ideal duration of treatment is still under discussion. All agree that it should not be less than 7 days [15], but the relative merits of 7- and 10-day regimens are still debated (see below).

In 2000, de Boer and Tytgat [16] published an influential review in *British Medical Journal* illustrating the concept of treatment strategy. The concept is simple: as there is no single 100% effective therapy, the approach for treating *H. pylori* infection should include two consecutive treatments. These treatments should ensure that resistances after initial failure do not interfere with rescue therapy. The initial recommendation was to use a clarithromycin-based regimen as

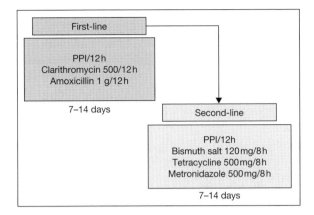

Fig. 1. Current recommended treatment strategy for *H. pylori* infection. PPI = Proton-pump inhibitor (adapted from Gisbert et al. [18]).

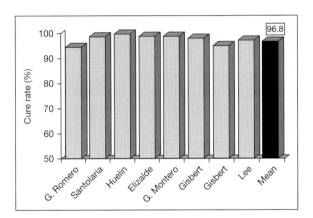

Fig. 2. Published efficacy of the strategy combining triple first-line with quadruple rescue therapy (from Gisbert et al. [18]).

first-line and a metronidazole-based second-line treatment. Importantly, combining clarithromycin and metronidazole was discouraged because no valid rescue regimen was available if this particular combination failed.

Many of the current *H. pylori* treatment guidelines implicitly or explicitly incorporate both these data and the concept of therapeutic strategy [17, 18]. With small discrepancies, first-line and second-line treatments coincide with those shown in figure 1. Reported cure rates for this combination have approached 100% in many series (fig. 2) [18].

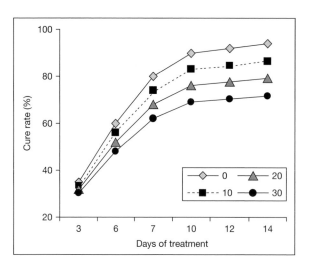

Fig. 3. Estimated effect of clarithromycin resistance on the efficacy of triple therapy. When the resistance rate rises above 20%, triple therapy achieves poor results regardless of treatment duration. Each curve refers to a given level of resistance.

H. pylori Treatment: Facing New Challenges and Scenarios

Changes in Antibiotic Resistances

Triple therapy efficacy is highly sensitive to antibiotic resistance. In vitro amoxicillin resistance is exceptional in *H. pylori* strains. However, clarithromycin resistance is frequent and has a strong impact on the efficacy of treatment. Cure rates with triple therapy fall to 20% in the presence of clarithromycin resistance [19]. It has been estimated that increases in the prevalence of clarithromycin resistance of over 20% will decrease triple therapy efficacy to unacceptably low levels, whatever the length of the treatment (fig. 3). Resistance to macrolides initially seemed to steadily increase but, fortunately, current reports suggest that the prevalence of resistant strains has stabilized at around 10% in recent years [20–22].

Broadening Eradication Indications

Until recently, the only uncontested indications for eradication were peptic ulcer and MALT lymphoma. However, many recent trials have shown that a 'test for *H. pylori* and treat' strategy is useful and safe for patients with uninvestigated dyspepsia [23–25] and that 5–10% of patients with functional

---

Calvet   194

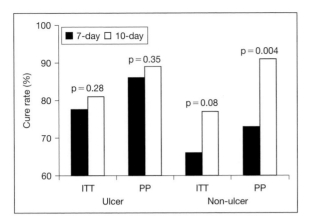

Fig. 4. Efficacy of 7- and 10-day triple therapies in patients with and without ulcer. Patients without ulcer showed markedly lower cure rates with 7-day therapy. ITT = Intention-to-treat analysis; PP = per protocol analysis (from Calvet et al. [32]).

dyspepsia benefit from eradication [26]. In addition, the clinical and biochemical link between *H. pylori* and stomach cancer has been firmly established and some preliminary data suggest that early cure of *H. pylori* infection may prevent gastric cancer development [27]. Many authors have therefore advocated beginning stomach cancer prevention programs by detecting and treating *H. pylori* infection in high-risk populations [28, 29]. This is important, as it means that many non-ulcer patients will receive eradication treatment. It is known that triple therapy is less effective in patients without ulcer disease [30, 31], especially for short triple therapies. In one recent study, cure rates with 7-day therapies were noticeably higher in patients with ulcer than in those without. In contrast, cure rates for 10-day therapies were very similar regardless of the underlying disease (fig. 4) [32].

Multi-Treated, Multi-Resistant Patients

Patients who have failed many treatments are increasingly seen in specialized gastroenterology clinics. They tend to harbour strains resistant to major antibiotics such as clarithromycin and metronidazole. Although comparative studies are scarce, devising adequate empirical treatment [33] has obtained similar or better results than the currently recommended strategy of using culture-driven rescue therapies [34, 35]. As secondary resistances are frequent and major antibiotics cannot be used, treatment of these patients requires new antimicrobials and atypical antibiotic combinations, and represents a challenge for the clinician.

H. pylori Treatment: Recent Developments

In addition to the different responses according to the underlying disease, there are geographical variations in the response to eradication treatment. These variations have been attributed to differences in the prevalence of antibiotic resistances and to genetic differences in the metabolism of PPIs [36]. However, to confront the new challenges of the expanding indications for eradication, a therapy with proven efficacy in all patients and settings is necessary. A striking finding in recent studies is that cure rates did not reach 80% even for 10-day triple therapies [37]. This does not seem to be a local trend. In a recent US study, Vakil et al. [37] observed cure rates of 77% for rabeprazole 10-day therapy and 73% for omeprazole 10-day triple therapy. In another recent multicentre study, eradication rates of 77% were achieved with a combination of esomeprazole 40 mg q.d., clarithromycin 500 mg b.d., and amoxicillin 1,000 mg b.d. administered for 10 days [38]. In three multicentre US trials with omeprazole 20 mg b.d. combined with amoxicillin 1,000 mg b.d. and clarithromycin 500 mg b.d. administered for 10 days in patients with duodenal ulcer, eradication rates ranged from 69 to 83%, with a combined eradication rate of 75% [39]. Many patients, therefore, will require second-line treatment with further testing and control visits. Although most compliant patients are cured by the second-line treatment [18], patients often do not complete the full course of therapy. In consequence, final cure rates of the whole strategy are often under 90% [40]. These data convincingly show that even using 10-day schedules, triple therapy achieves insufficient cure rates and that a more effective alternative must be sought. Three new alternatives deserve to be highlighted: the use of a quadruple therapy as first-line treatment, the addition of adjuvant compounds (mainly lactoferrin) to triple therapy, and a new 10-day sequential therapy.

Quadruple Therapy as First-Line Treatment

Quadruple therapy efficacy is not affected by resistance to clarithromycin and, if given at high metronidazole doses and for 7 days or more, is able to overcome in vitro resistance to metronidazole. In addition, it was very effective as rescue treatment [18] and as first-line therapy in pilot studies [41]. Recently, five randomized trials comparing triple vs. quadruple therapy as first-line treatment for *H. pylori* have been published [42–46]. The results have been summarized in a meta-analysis showing that the efficacy of the two approaches is similar (table 1) [47, 48]. It has also been shown that the strategy of using quadruple therapy as a first-line treatment and triple as rescue therapy is as effective as the combining of triple as first-line with quadruple for rescue. In addition, quadruple-first strategy was slightly less expensive and, in consequence, more cost-effective [40]. The minor differences between therapies

Table 1. Comparison of triple and quadruple therapy as first-line treatment for *H. pylori* eradication (from Mantzaris et al. [45])

Study	Triple n/N	Quadruple n/N	OR (95% CI random)	OR (95% CI random)
Calvet	132/171	130/166		
Gomollon	40/40	33/48		
Katelaris	104/134	110/134		
Laine	114/137	121/138		
Mantzaris	61/78	46/71		
Total (95% CI)	451/569	449/559		1.00 [0.64, 1.57]
Test for heterogeneity $\chi^2 = 8.75$, d.f. = 4, p = 0.068				
Test for overall effect z = 0.02, p = 1				

```
              0.1  0.2        1        5   10
           Favours quadruple      Favours triple
```

probably did not justify a generalized recommendation to shift first-line therapy from triple to quadruple. Quadruple therapy could, however, be useful in areas where the results of triple therapy are poor. In view of the evidence, the recent update of the Canadian guidelines for *H. pylori* treatment includes quadruple therapy as an alternative for first-line treatment [49].

Using Adjuvant Agents: Triple Therapy plus Lactoferrin

Lactoferrin, a milk protein that binds iron, has been shown to be effective against *H. pylori* in vitro, inhibiting *H. pylori* growth in culture and reducing both *H. pylori* intragastric density and adhesiveness to epithelial cells [50–52]. Although lactoferrin alone was ineffective for *H. pylori* treatment [53], its addition as adjuvant treatment to triple therapy has obtained excellent results. Thus, in a recent controlled trial, Di Mario et al. [54] observed that adding lactoferrin 200 mg twice a day to 7-day triple therapy combining a PPI, clarithromycin and tinidazole cure rates increased from 70 to 95% (fig. 5). It is worth mentioning however that when lactoferrin was added to a standard 7-day regimen combining esomeprazole (20 mg) with clarithromycin (500 mg) and amoxicillin (1g), all twice daily, no increase of eradication rate over the triple therapy alone has been observed [55]. These disappointing results were of course surprising but the reasons for the discrepancy between this and the previous Italian studies [54, 56] are not clear. Since a difference in the prevalence of primary bacterial resistance to clarithromycin could be reasonably ruled out, other causes must be sought. A possibility is that lactoferrin and tinidazole may exert a synergistic effect against *H. pylori*, while lactoferrin and amoxicillin do not. Such a hypothesis is supported by the observation that when lactoferrin is administered as monotherapy in the

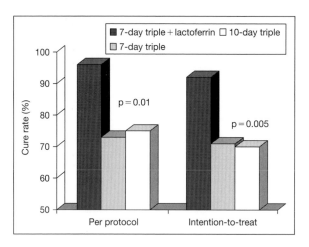

Fig. 5. Cure rates for first-line triple therapy with and without adjuvant lactoferrin (from Di Mario et al. [54]).

week before clarithromycin-tinidazole combination, it does not give any additive therapeutic effect [54]. Since lactoferrin can bind and disrupt some bacterial cell membranes [57], another possible explanation is that the antibacterial effect of lactoferrin, based on bacterial membrane damage of Gram-negative bacteria, could be marginalized when amoxicillin is simultaneously administered. Indeed, amoxicillin too mainly acts interfering with microbial membrane structure. On the contrary, such an effect of lactoferrin could be useful when tinidazole is administered, a different mechanism being exploited by such antimicrobial. Whatever the reason, further studies are needed before recommending lactoferrin as add-on medication to eradication regimens in clinical practice.

Sequential Therapy

Among the new promising alternatives to triple therapy, a 10-day sequential therapy combining a 5-day course of PPI with amoxicillin immediately followed by a second course of clarithromycin, metronidazole and a PPI for 5 additional days was recently described [58–62]. This treatment seems to be equally effective in patients with ulcer and in those without and achieves excellent cure rates even in patients with clarithromycin resistance [58–60]. Interestingly, it is the first alternative therapy that has proved superior to triple therapy in a large randomized trial. Zullo et al. [62] included more than 1,000 patients in a study comparing 7-day triple therapy with this new schedule. Cure rates were 92% for the sequential treatment and 74% for triple therapy ($p < 0.0001$, fig. 6). A possible disadvantage of this schedule is that it

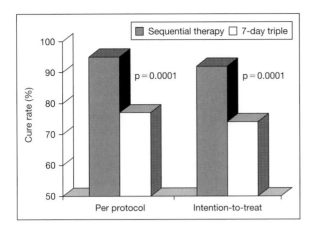

Fig. 6. Comparative efficacy of 7-day triple therapy and sequential therapy for *H. pylori* eradication (from Zullo et al. [62]).

combines clarithromycin and metronidazole, thus complicating the search for a rescue therapy. This fact, however, may no longer represent a problem, as new rescue combinations using quinolones or rifamycin derivatives are now available and ready for use. Currently, there is enough evidence to suggest that these new combinations are reliable for rescue therapy (see below).

New Drugs for Rescue (and Possibly First-Line) Therapy

The therapeutic arsenal for *H. pylori* infection has been very limited until recently. In addition to antibacterial bismuth compounds, four antibiotics have been the milestones of treatment: clarithromycin, tetracycline, metronidazole and amoxicillin. Furazolidone, a drug that has proved very effective, is not available in many Western countries. In recent years, the shortage of drugs has decreased somewhat with the incorporation of new antibiotic families. The two most interesting groups are the newly developed quinolones and the rifamycin derivates.

New Quinolones: Levofloxacin and Moxifloxacin

Levofloxacin and moxifloxacin have been tested both in vivo and in vitro for *H. pylori* treatment. In general, both in vitro sensitivities and in vivo effectiveness seem equal to or slightly better than clarithromycin. These quinolones have often been used in triple therapy, combined with metronidazole, clarithromycin or amoxicillin. Cure rates range from 70 to 94% for first-line cure rates and from 70 to 94% for rescue therapies (table 2) [63–76]. Neither the ideal dosages nor the ideal drug combination have yet been defined for the new

Table 2. Published studies evaluating new quinolone-based eradication treatments

Author	Indication	Days	Schedule	Cure rate, %
Cammarota [63]	First-line	7	Rabeprazole 20 mg/24 h Levofloxacin 500 mg/24 h Amoxicillin 1 g /12 h or Tinidazole 500 mg/12 h	90/92
Di Caro [64]	First-line	7	Lansoprazole 30 mg/24 h Moxifloxacin 400 mg/24 h Clarithromycin 500 mg/12 h	90
Di Caro [65]	First-line	7	Rabeprazole 20 mg/24 h Levofloxacin 500 mg/24 h Amoxicillin 1 g /12 h	90
Wong [66]	Second-line	7	Rabeprazole 20 mg/24 h Rifabutin 300 mg/24 h Levofloxacin 500 mg/24 h	91
Zullo [67]	Third-line	10	Rabeprazole 20 mg/12 h Levofloxacin 250 mg/12 h Amoxicillin 1 g /12 h	83
Nista [68]	Second-line	10	Rabeprazole 20 mg/12 h Levofloxacin 500 mg/24 h Amoxicillin 1 g /12 h or Tinidazole 500 mg/12 h	94/90
Perri [69]	Second-line	7	Pantoprazole 40 mg/12 h Amoxicillin 1 g /12 h Levofloxacin 500/24 h	85
Watanabe [70]	Second-line	7	Lansoprazole 30 mg/12 h Amoxicillin 1 g /12 h Levofloxacin 200 mg/12 h	70
Cammarota [71]	First-line	7	Rabeprazole 20 mg/24 h Levofloxacin 500 mg/24 h Clarithromycin 250 mg/12 h or Clarithromycin 500 mg/12 h	84/94
Bilardi [72]	Second- and third-line	10	Pantoprazole 40 mg/12 h Amoxicillin 1 g /12 h Levofloxacin 250 mg/12 h	70
Sharara [73]	First-line	7	Rabeprazole 40 mg/24 h Gatifloxacin 400 mg/24 h Amoxicillin 1 g /24 h	92
Iacopini [74]	First-line	7	Esomeprazole 20 mg/24 h Levofloxacin 500 mg/24 h Azithromycin 500 mg/24 h	70
Gatta [75]	Third-line	10	Proton-pump inhibitor/12 h Levofloxacin 250 mg/12 h Amoxicillin 1 g /12 h	85

Table 2. (continued)

Author	Indication	Days	Schedule	Cure rate, %
Nista [76]	First-line	7	Esomeprazole 20 mg/12 h Moxifloxacin 400 mg/24 h Clarithromycin 500 mg/12 h or Tinidazole 500 mg/12 h	89–92

quinolone treatments. It seems, however, that a 10-day triple therapy combining a PPI, amoxicillin and a new quinolone all twice a day is a reasonable approach.

Rifamycin Derivatives

Rifamycin derivates and specially rifabutin and the non-absorbable antibiotic rifaximin are highly effective against *H. pylori* in vitro [77]. Both drugs have been used as components of eradication regimens [77]. Rifabutin is currently employed as a salvage treatment for multi-resistant mycobacterial infections. It is an expensive antibiotic and carries a minimal risk of severe haematological adverse effects. For all these reasons it has been reserved for rescue therapy. It has been used at full doses (150 mg twice daily), mainly in triple therapy, usually associated with amoxicillin and a PPI, for 10–14 days. Even in the setting of patients who have failed multiple eradication attempts, cure rates are notably high, ranging from 70 to 85% [78–81].

Future Needs and Perspectives

The search for a 100% effective treatment for curing *H. pylori* infection is still underway and several very promising new alternatives are being developed. Either triple therapy with adjuvant lactoferrin or sequential therapy could become the new standard. However, a great deal of work remains to be done in order to define the best drugs and the ideal dosage and duration for these new alternatives. If first-line therapies change, the whole therapeutic strategy must be redesigned. New quinolones and rifamycin derivates have been incorporated to the reduced list of effective drugs for treating *H. pylori* infection and are gaining acceptance as a first-line or second-line therapies. Despite all these improvements, however, increasingly effective anti-*H. pylori* agents are still needed.

Acknowledgements

This study was supported by an educational grant from Bama-Geve and by a grant from the Instituto de Salud Carlos III (C03/02).

References

1 Solano Allende JA: La úlcera de estómago y su tratamiento por la asociación de suero de convale-ciente y penicilina. Gutenberg, Hijo de Ramirez-Guadalej ar, 1951.
2 Rigas B, Papavassiliou ED: John Lykoudis: the general practitioner in Greece who in 1958 dis-covered the etiology of, and a treatment for, peptic ulcer disease; in Marshall BJ (ed): *Helicobacter pylori* Pioneers. Carlton, Blackwell, 2002, pp 75–87.
3 Marshall BJ: The discovery that *Helicobacter pylori*, a spiral bacterium, caused peptic ulcer dis-ease; in Marshall BJ (ed): *Helicobacter pylori* Pioneers. Carlton, Blackwell, 2002, pp 165–202.
4 Borody TJ, Cole P, Noonan S, Morgan A, Lenne J, Hyland L, Brandl S, Borody EG, George LL: Recurrence of duodenal ulcer and *Campylobacter pylori* infection after eradication. Med J Aust 1989;151:431–435.
5 Calvet X, Lopez-Lorente M, Cubells M, Bare M, Galvez E, Molina E: Two-week dual vs. one-week triple therapy for cure of *Helicobacter pylori* infection in primary care: a multicentre, ran-domized trial. Aliment Pharmacol Ther 1999;13:781–786.
6 Bell GD, Powell KU, Burridge SM, Bowden AN, Rameh B, Bolton G, Purser K, Harrison G, Brown C, Gant PW, Jones PH, Trowell JE: *Helicobacter pylori* eradication: efficacy and side effect profile of a combination of omeprazole, amoxicillin, and metronidazole compared with four alternative regimens. Q J Med 1993;86:743–750.
7 Bazzoli F, Zagari RM, Fossi S, Pozzato P, I Roda A, Roda E: Efficacy and tolerability of a short-term, low-dose triple therapy for eradication of *Helicobacter pylori*. Gastroenterology 1993;104:A40.
8 Bazzoli F, Zagari RM, Fossi S, Pozzato P, Alampi G, Simoni P, Sottili S, Roda A, Roda E: Short-term low-dose triple therapy for the eradication of *Helicobacter pylori*. Eur J Gastroenterol Hepatol 1994;6:773–777.
9 Lind T, Veldhuyzen van Zanten, Unge P, Spiller R, Bayerdorffer E, O'Morain C, Bardhan KD, Bradette M, Chiba N, Wrangstadh M, Cederberg C, Idstrom JP: Eradication of *Helicobacter pylori* using one-week triple therapies combining omeprazole with two antimicrobials: the MACH I Study. Helicobacter 1996;1:138–144.
10 Malfertheiner P, Bayerdorffer E, Diete U, Gil J, Lind T, Misiuna P, O'Morain C, Sipponen P, Spiller RC, Stasiewicz J, Treichel H, Ujszaszy L, Unge P, Zanten SJ, Zeijlon L, The GU-MACH Study: The effect of 1-week omeprazole triple therapy on *Helicobacter pylori* infection in patients with gastric ulcer. Aliment Pharmacol Ther 1999;13:703–712.
11 Zanten SJ, Bradette M, Farley A, Leddin D, Lind T, Unge P, Bayerdorffer E, Spiller RC, O'Morain C, Sipponen P, Wrangstadh M, Zeijlon L, Sinclair P: The DU-MACH study: eradication of *Helicobacter pylori* and ulcer healing in patients with acute duodenal ulcer using omeprazole-based triple therapy. Aliment Pharmacol Ther 1999;13:289–295.
12 Vallve M, Vergara M, Gisbert JP, Calvet X: Single vs. double dose of a proton-pump inhibitor in triple therapy for *Helicobacter pylori* eradication: a meta-analysis. Aliment Pharmacol Ther 2002;16:1149–1156.
13 Gisbert JP, Gonzalez L, Calvet X, Garcia N, Lopez T, Roque M, Gabriel R, Pajares JM: Proton-pump inhibitor, clarithromycin and either amoxicillin or nitroimidazole: a meta-analysis of eradi-cation of *Helicobacter pylori*. Aliment Pharmacol Ther 2000;14:1319–1328.
14 Vergara M, Vallvé M, Gisbert JP, Calvet X: Meta-analysis: comparative efficacy of different proton-pump inhibitors in triple therapy for *Helicobacter pylori* eradication. Aliment Pharmacol Ther 2003;18:647–654.
15 Calvet X, Garcia N, Lopez T, Gisbert JP, Gene E, Roque M: A meta-analysis of short versus long therapy with a proton-pump inhibitor, clarithromycin and either metronidazole or amoxicillin for treating *Helicobacter pylori* infection. Aliment Pharmacol Ther 2000;14:603–609.
16 de Boer WA, Tytgat GN: Regular review: treatment of *Helicobacter pylori* infection. BMJ 2000; 320:31–34.
17 Malfertheiner P, Megraud F, O'Morain C, Hungin AP, Jones R, Axon A, Graham DY, Tytgat G: Current concepts in the management of *Helicobacter pylori* infection – the Maastricht 2-2000 Consensus Report. Aliment Pharmacol Ther 2002;16:167–180.

18 Gisbert JP, Calvet X, Gomollon F, Sainz R: Treatment for the eradication of *Helicobacter pylori*. Recommendations of the Spanish consensus conference. Med Clin (Barc) 2000;114:185–195.

19 Ducons JA, Santolaria S, Guirao R, Ferrero M, Montoro M, Gomollon F: Impact of clarithromycin resistance on the effectiveness of a regimen for *Helicobacter pylori*: a prospective study of 1-week lansoprazole, amoxicillin and clarithromycin in active peptic ulcer. Aliment Pharmacol Ther 1999;13:775–780.

20 Gomollon F, Santolaria S, Sicilia B, Ferrero M, Revillo MJ, Ducons J, Villar M, Celaya MC, Montoro M: *Helicobacter pylori* resistance to metronidazole and clarithromycin: descriptive analysis 1997–2000. Med Clin (Barc) 2004;123:481–485.

21 Gisbert JP, Maria PJ: *Helicobacter pylori* resistance to metronidazole and to clarithromycin in Spain: a systematic review. Med Clin (Barc) 2001;116:111–116.

22 Cuchí E, Forné M, Quintana RS, Lite LJ, Garau AJ: Evolution of the sensitivity of 235 strains of *Helicobacter pylori* from 1995 to 1998 and impact of antibiotic treatment. Enferm Infecc Microbiol Clin 2002;20:157–160.

23 Chiba N, van Zanten SJOV, Sinclair P, Ferguson RA, Escobedo S, Grace E: Treating *Helicobacter pylori* infection in primary care patients with uninvestigated dyspepsia: the Canadian adult dyspepsia empiric treatment – *Helicobacter pylori* positive (CADET-Hp) randomised controlled trial. BMJ 2002;324:1012.

24 Manes G, Menchise A, de Nucci C, Balzano A: Empirical prescribing for dyspepsia: randomised controlled trial of test and treat versus omeprazole treatment. BMJ 2003;326:1118.

25 Heaney A, Collins JSA, Watson RGP, McFarland RJ, Bamford KB, Tham TCK: A prospective randomised trial of a 'test and treat' policy versus endoscopy based management in young *Helicobacter pylori*-positive patients with ulcer-like dyspepsia, referred to a hospital clinic. Gut 1999;45:186–190.

26 Moayyedi P, Deeks J, Talley NJ, Delaney B, Forman D: An update of the Cochrane systematic review of *Helicobacter pylori* eradication therapy in non-ulcer dyspepsia: resolving the discrepancy between systematic reviews. Am J Gastroenterol 2003;98:2621–2626.

27 Wong BC, Lam SK, Wong WM, Chen JS, Zheng TT, Feng RE, Lai KC, Hu WH, Yuen ST, Leung SY, Fong DY, Ho J, Ching CK, Chen JS: *Helicobacter pylori* eradication to prevent gastric cancer in a high-risk region of China: a randomized controlled trial. JAMA 2004;291:187–194.

28 Genta RM: Screening for gastric cancer: does it make sense? Aliment Pharmacol Ther 2004;20 (suppl 2):42–47.

29 Moayyedi P, Hunt RH: *Helicobacter pylori* public health implications. Helicobacter 2004;9(suppl 1): 67–72.

30 Schmid CH, Whiting G, Cory D, Ross SD, Chalmers TC: Omeprazole plus antibiotics in the eradication of *Helicobacter pylori* infection: a meta-regression analysis of randomized, controlled trials. Am J Ther 1999;6:25–36.

31 Gisbert JP, Marcos S, Gisbert JL, Pajares JM: *Helicobacter pylori* eradication therapy is more effective in peptic ulcer than in non-ulcer dyspepsia. Eur J Gastroenterol Hepatol 2001;13: 1303–1307.

32 Calvet X, Ducons J, Bujanda L, Bory F, Montserrat A, Gisbert JP, and the Helicobacter Study Group of the Asociación Española de Gastroenterología: seven *versus* ten days of rabeprazole triple therapy for *Helicobacter pylori* eradication: a multicenter randomized trial. Am J Gastroenterol 2005;100:1696–1701.

33 Gisbert JP, Gisbert JL, Marcos S, Pajares JM: Empirical *Helicobacter pylori* 'rescue' therapy after failure of two eradication treatments. Dig Liver Dis 2004;36:7–12.

34 Gomollon F, Sicilia B, Ducons JA, Sierra E, Revillo MJ, Ferrero M: Third-line treatment for *Helicobacter pylori*: a prospective, culture-guided study in peptic ulcer patients. Aliment Pharmacol Ther 2000;14:1335–1338.

35 Vicente R, Sicilia B, Gallego S, Revillo MJ, Ducons J, Gomollon F: *Helicobacter pylori* eradication in patients with peptic ulcer after two treatment failures: a prospective culture-guided study. Gastroenterol Hepatol 2002;25:438–442.

36 Vakil N: Are there geographical and regional differences in *Helicobacter pylori* eradication? Can J Gastroenterol 2003;17(suppl B):30B–32B.

37   Vakil N, Lanza F, Schwartz H, Barth J: Seven-day therapy for *Helicobacter pylori* in the United States. Aliment Pharmacol Ther 2004;20:99–107.

38   Laine L, Fennerty MB, Osato M, Sugg J, Suchower L, Probst P, Levine JG: Esomeprazole-based *Helicobacter pylori* eradication therapy and the effect of antibiotic resistance: results of three US multicenter, double-blind trials. Am J Gastroenterol 2000;95:3393–3398.

39   Laine L, Suchower L, Frantz J, Connors A, Neil G: Twice-daily, 10-day triple therapy with omeprazole, amoxicillin, and clarithromycin for *Helicobacter pylori* eradication in duodenal ulcer disease: results of three multicenter, double-blind, United States trials. Am J Gastroenterol 1998;93:2106–2112.

40   Marko D, Calvet X, Ducons J, Guardiola J, Tito H, Bory F: Comparison of two management strategies for *H. pylori* treatment: a clinical study and a cost effectiveness analysis. Helicobacter 2005;10:22–32.

41   Calvet X, Garcia N, Gené E, Campo R, Brullet E, Sanfeliu I: Modified seven-day, quadruple therapy as a first-line *Helicobacter pylori* treatment. Aliment Pharmacol Ther 2001;15:1061–1065.

42   Calvet X, Ducons J, Guardiola J, Tito L, Andreu V, Bory F, Guirao R: One-week triple vs. quadruple therapy for *Helicobacter pylori* infection – a randomized trial. Aliment Pharmacol Ther 2002; 16:1261–1267.

43   Katelaris PH, Forbes GM, Talley NJ, Crotty B: A randomized comparison of quadruple and triple therapies for *Helicobacter pylori* eradication: the quadrate study. Gastroenterology 2002;123: 1763–1769.

44   Laine L, Hunt R, El Zimaity H, Nguyen B, Osato M, Spenard J: Bismuth-based quadruple therapy using a single capsule of bismuth biskalcitrate, metronidazole, and tetracycline given with omeprazole versus omeprazole, amoxicillin, and clarithromycin for eradication of *Helicobacter pylori* in duodenal ulcer patients: a prospective, randomized, multicenter, North American trial. Am J Gastroenterol 2003;98:562–567.

45   Mantzaris GJ, Petraki K, Archavlis E, Amberiadis P, Christoforidis P, Kourtessas D, Chiotakakou E, Triantafyllou G: Omeprazole triple therapy versus omeprazole quadruple therapy for healing duodenal ulcer and eradication of *Helicobacter pylori* infection: a 24-month follow-up study. Eur J Gastroenterol Hepatol 2002;14:1237–1243.

46   Gomollon F, Valdeperez J, Garuz R, Fuentes J, Barrera F, Malo J, Tirado M, Simon MA: Cost-effectiveness analysis of two strategies of *Helicobacter pylori* eradication: results of a prospective and randomized study in primary care. Med Clin (Bar) 2000;115:1–6.

47   Gene E, Calvet X, Azagra R, Gisbert JP: Triple vs. quadruple therapy for treating *Helicobacter pylori* infection: an updated meta-analysis. Aliment Pharmacol Ther 2003;18:543–544.

48   Gene E, Calvet X, Azagra R, Gisbert JP: Triple vs. quadruple therapy for treating *Helicobacter pylori* infection: a meta-analysis. Aliment Pharmacol Ther 2003;17:1137–1143.

49   Hunt R, Fallone C, Veldhuyzan VZ, Sherman P, Smaill F, Flook N, Thomson A: Canadian *Helicobacter* study group consensus conference: update on the management of *Helicobacter pylori* – an evidence-based evaluation of six topics relevant to clinical outcomes in patients evaluated for *H pylori* infection. Can J Gastroenterol 2004;18:547–554.

50   Dial EJ, Romero JJ, Headon DR, Lichtenberger LM: Recombinant human lactoferrin is effective in the treatment of *Helicobacter felis*-infected mice. J Pharm Pharmacol 2000;52:1541–1546.

51   Dial EJ, Hall LR, Serna H, Romero JJ, Fox JG, Lichtenberger LM: Antibiotic properties of bovine lactoferrin on *Helicobacter pylori*. Dig Dis Sci 1998;43:2750–2756.

52   Miehlke S, Reddy R, Osato MS, Ward PP, Conneely OM, Graham DY: Direct activity of recombinant human lactoferrin against *Helicobacter pylori*. J Clin Microbiol 1996;34:2593–2594.

53   Guttner Y, Windsor HM, Viiala CH, Marshall BJ: Human recombinant lactoferrin is ineffective in the treatment of human *Helicobacter pylori* infection. Aliment Pharmacol Ther 2003;17:125–129.

54   Di Mario F, Aragona G, Dal Bò N, Cavestro GM, Cavallaro L, Iori V, Comparato G, Leandro G, Pilotto A, Franze A: Use of bovine lactoferrin for *Helicobacter pylori* eradication. Dig Liver Dis 2003;35:706–710.

55   Zullo A, De Francesco V, Scaccianoce G, Hassan C, Panarese A, Piglionica D, Panella C, Morini S, Ierardi E: Quadruple therapy with lactoferrin for *Helicobacter pylori* eradication: a randomised multicentre study. Dig Liver Dis 2005;37:496–500.

56 Di Mario F, Dal Bò N, Aragona G, Marconi V, Olivieri P, De Bastiani R, Marconi V, Olivieri PG, Marin R, De Bastiani R, Piazzi L, Chilovi F, Fedrizzi F, Tafner G, Vecchiati U, Monica F, Heras H, Franceschi M, Orzes N, Benedetti E, Fanigliulo L, Mazzocchi G, Cavallaro LG, Maino M, Iori V, Cavestro GM, Franzè A: Efficacy of bovine lactoferrin for *Helicobacter pylori* eradication: results of a multicentre study. Gut 2004;53(suppl VI):A123.

57 Borody TJ, Ashman O: Lactoferrin: milking ulcers? Dig Liver Dis 2003;35:691–693.

58 De Francesco V, Faleo D, Panella C, Ierardi E, Margiotta M: Sequential eradicating therapy: a treatment that does not discriminate *Helicobacter pylori* strains in patients with non-ulcer dyspepsia? Am J Gastroenterol 2002;97:2686–2687.

59 De Francesco V, Zullo A, Hassan C, Della VN, Pietrini L, Minenna MF, Winn S, Monno R, Stoppino V, Morini S, Panella C, Ierardi E: The prolongation of triple therapy for *Helicobacter pylori* does not allow reaching therapeutic outcome of sequential scheme: a prospective, randomised study. Dig Liver Dis 2004;36:322–326.

60 De Francesco V, Zullo A, Margiotta M, Marangi S, Burattini O, Berloco P, Russo F, Barone M, Di Leo A, Minenna MF, Stoppino V, Morini S, Panella C, Francavilla A, Ierardi E: Sequential treatment for *Helicobacter pylori* does not share the risk factors of triple therapy failure. Aliment Pharmacol Ther 2004;19:407–414.

61 De Francesco V, Della VN, Stoppino V, Amoruso A, Muscatiello N, Panella C, Ierardi E: Effectiveness and pharmaceutical cost of sequential treatment for *Helicobacter pylori* in patients with non-ulcer dyspepsia. Aliment Pharmacol Ther 2004;19:993–998.

62 Zullo A, Vaira D, Vakil N, Hassan C, Gatta L, Ricci C, De FV, Menegatti M, Tampieri A, Perna F, Rinaldi V, Perri F, Papadia C, Fornari F, Pilati S, Mete LS, Merla A, Poti R, Marinone G, Savioli A, Campo SM, Faleo D, Ierardi E, Miglioli M, Morini S: High eradication rates of *Helicobacter pylori* with a new sequential treatment. Aliment Pharmacol Ther 2003;17:719–726.

63 Cammarota G, Cianci R, Cannizzaro O, Cuoco L, Pirozzi G, Gasbarrini A, Armuzzi A, Zocco MA, Santarelli L, Arancio F, Gasbarrini G: Efficacy of two one-week rabeprazole/levofloxacin-based triple therapies for *Helicobacter pylori* infection. Aliment Pharmacol Ther 2000;14: 1339–1343.

64 Di Caro S, Ojetti V, Zocco MA, Cremonini F, Bartolozzi F, Candelli M, Lupascu A, Nista EC, Cammarota G, Gasbarrini A: Mono, dual and triple moxifloxacin-based therapies for *Helicobacter pylori* eradication. Aliment Pharmacol Ther 2002;16:527–532.

65 Di Caro S, Assunta ZM, Cremonini F, Candelli M, Nista EC, Bartolozzi F, Armuzzi A, Cammarota G, Santarelli L, Gasbarrini A: Levofloxacin based regimens for the eradication of *Helicobacter pylori*. Eur J Gastroenterol Hepatol 2002;14:1309–1312.

66 Wong WM, Gu Q, Lam SK, Fung FM, Lai KC, Hu WH, Yee YK, Chan CK, Xia HH, Yuen MF, Wong BC: Randomized controlled study of rabeprazole, levofloxacin and rifabutin triple therapy vs. quadruple therapy as second-line treatment for *Helicobacter pylori* infection. Aliment Pharmacol Ther 2003;17:553–560.

67 Zullo A, Hassan C, De Francesco, V, Lorenzetti R, Marignani M, Angeletti S, Ierardi E, Morini S: A third-line levofloxacin-based rescue therapy for *Helicobacter pylori* eradication. Dig Liver Dis 2003;35:232–236.

68 Nista EC, Candelli M, Cremonini F, Cazzato IA, di Caro S, Gabrielli M, Santarelli L, Zocco MA, Ojetti V, Carloni E, Cammarota G, Gasbarrini G, Gasbarrini A: Levofloxacin-based triple therapy vs. quadruple therapy in second-line *Helicobacter pylori* treatment: a randomized trial. Aliment Pharmacol Ther 2003;18:627–633.

69 Perri F, Festa V, Merla A, Barberani F, Pilotto A, Andriulli A: Randomized study of different 'second-line' therapies for *Helicobacter pylori* infection after failure of the standard 'Maastricht triple therapy'. Aliment Pharmacol Ther 2003;18:815–820.

70 Watanabe Y, Aoyama N, Shirasaka D, Maekawa S, Kuroda K, Miki I, Kachi M, Fukuda M, Wambura C, Tamura T, Kasuga M: Levofloxacin based triple therapy as a second-line treatment after failure of *Helicobacter pylori* eradication with standard triple therapy. Dig Liver Dis 2003; 35:711–715.

71 Cammarota G, Cianci R, Cannizzaro O, Martino A, Fedeli P, Lecca PG, di Caro S, Cesaro P, Branca G, Gasbarrini G: High-dose versus low-dose clarithromycin in 1-week triple therapy,

including rabeprazole and levofloxacin, for *Helicobacter pylori* eradication. J Clin Gastroenterol 2004;38:110–114.

72   Bilardi C, Dulbecco P, Zentilin P, Reglioni S, Iiritano E, Parodi A, Accornero L, Savarino E, Mansi C, Mamone M, Vigneri S, Savarino V: A 10-day levofloxacin-based therapy in patients with resistant *Helicobacter pylori* infection: a controlled trial. Clin Gastroenterol Hepatol 2004;2: 997–1002.

73   Sharara AI, Chaar HF, Racoubian E, Moukhachen O, Barada KA, Mourad FH, Araj GF: Efficacy of two rabeprazole/gatifloxacin-based triple therapies for Helicobacter pylori infection. Helicobacter 2004;9:255–261.

74   Iacopini F, Crispino P, Paoluzi OA, Consolazio A, Pica R, Rivera M, Palladini D, Nardi F, Paoluzi P: One-week once-daily triple therapy with esomeprazole, levofloxacin and azithromycin compared to a standard therapy for *Helicobacter pylori* eradication. Dig Liver Dis 2005;37:571–576.

75   Gatta L, Zullo A, Perna F, Ricci C, De Francesco V, Tampieri A, Bernabucci V, Cavina M, Hassan C, Ierardi E, Morini S, Vaira D: A 10-day levofloxacin-based triple therapy in patients who have failed two eradication courses. Aliment Pharmacol Ther 2005;22:45–49.

76   Nista EC, Candelli M, Zocco MA, Cazzato IA, Cremonini F, Ojetti V, Santero M, Finizio R, Pignataro G, Cammarota G, Gasbarrini G, Gasbarrini A: Moxifloxacin-based strategies for first-line treatment of *Helicobacter pylori* infection. Aliment Pharmacol Ther 2005;21:1241–1247.

77   Scarpignato C, Pelosini I: Rifaximin, a poorly absorbed antibiotic: pharmacology and clinical potential. Chemotherapy 2005;51(suppl 1):36–66.

78   Bock H, Koop H, Lehn N, Heep M: Rifabutin-based triple therapy after failure of *Helicobacter pylori* eradication treatment: preliminary experience. J Clin Gastroenterol 2000;31:222–225.

79   Gisbert JP, Calvet X, Bujanda L, Marcos S, Gisbert JL, Pajares JM: 'Rescue' therapy with rifabutin after multiple *Helicobacter pylori* treatment failures. Helicobacter 2003;8:90–94.

80   Perri F, Festa V, Clemente R, Villani MR, Quitadamo M, Caruso N, Bergoli ML, Andriulli A: Randomized study of two 'rescue' therapies for *Helicobacter pylori*-infected patients after failure of standard triple therapies. Am J Gastroenterol 2001;96:58–62.

81   Perri F, Festa V, Clemente R, Quitadamo M, Andriulli A: Rifabutin-based 'rescue therapy' for *Helicobacter pylori*-infected patients after failure of standard regimens. Aliment Pharmacol Ther 2000;14:311–316.

Xavier Calvet, MD, PhD
Unitat de Malalties Digestives, Hospital de Sabadell
Institut Universitari Parc Taulí, UAB, Parc Taulí, s/n
ES–08208 Sabadell/Barcelona (Spain)
Tel. +34 93 723 1010 (20101), Fax +34 93 716 0646
E-Mail xcalvet@cspt.es

This chapter should be cited as follows:

Calvet X: *Helicobacter pylori* Infection: Treatment Options. Digestion 2006;73(suppl 1):119–128.

Scarpignato C, Lanas Á (eds): Bacterial Flora in Digestive Disease.
Focus on Rifaximin.

....

Eradication of *Helicobacter pylori*: Are Rifaximin-Based Regimens Effective?

Antonio Gasbarrini[a], *Giovanni Gasbarrini*[a], *Iva Pelosini*[b],
Carmelo Scarpignato[b]

[a]Department of Internal Medicine, Gemelli University Hospital, Catholic University
of Sacred Heart, Rome, [b]Laboratory of Clinical Pharmacology, Department of Human
Anatomy, Pharmacology and Forensic Sciences, School of Medicine and Dentistry,
University of Parma, Parma, Italy

Abstract

Rifaximin is a non-absorbed semisynthetic rifamycin derivative with a broad spectrum
of antibacterial activity including Gram-positive and Gram-negative bacteria, both aerobes
and anaerobes. Although originally developed for the treatment of infectious diarrhea, the
appreciation of the pathogenic role of gut bacteria in several organic and functional gastrointestinal diseases has increasingly broadened its clinical use. Being the antibiotic active
against *Helicobacter pylori*, even towards clarithromycin-resistant strain, and being the primary resistance very rare, several investigations explored its potential use for eradication of
the microorganism. Rifaximin alone proved to be effective, but even the highest dose
(1,200 mg daily) gave a cure rate of only 30%. Dual and triple therapies were also studied,
with the better results obtained with rifaximin-clarithromycin and rifaximin-clarithromycin-
esomeprazole combinations. However, the eradication rates (60–70%) obtained with these
regimens were still below the standard set by the Maastricht Consensus guidelines. Although
rifaximin-based eradication therapies are promising, new antimicrobial combinations (with
and without proton pump inhibitors) need to be explored in well-designed clinical trials
including a large cohort of *H. pylori*-infected patients. The remarkable safety of rifaximin
will allow high-dose regimens of longer duration (e.g. 10 or 14 days) to be tested with confidence in the hope of achieving better eradication rates. A drawback of rifaximin could be its
inability to reach sufficiently high concentrations in the gastric mucus layer under and within
which *H. pylori* is commonly located and this would likely affect eradication rate. Taking
these considerations into account, bioadhesive rifaximin formulations able to better and persistently cover gastric mucosa, or combination with mucolytic agents, such as pronase or
acetylcysteine, need to be evaluated in order to better define the place of this antibiotic in our
therapeutic armamentarium.

Introduction

Helicobacter pylori infection is a long-lasting, transmissible, worldwide spread disease causing a significant morbidity and mortality with a relevant economic impact. Infection usually occurs during childhood and, when left untreated, results in lifelong colonization of the stomach.

Since Marshall and Warren [1] first described the infectious etiology of peptic ulcer disease in 1984, a great deal of evidence has accumulated to suggest that *H. pylori* eradication therapy cures peptic ulcer disease [2] and can be beneficial also to other *H. pylori*-related diseases [3]. Having been classified as a definite 'type I carcinogen' [4], this Gram-negative, microaerophile bacterium needs to be eradicated from the host at any time [5, 6] since this can prevent the development of dyspeptic symptoms and peptic ulcer disease in healthy asymptomatic subjects [7] and that of gastric cancer in dyspeptic patients [8].

The mechanisms whereby *H. pylori* may cause gastroduodenal disease and contribute to gastric carcinogenesis are still hypothetical [9–12]. However, the production of specific virulence factors by the bacterium, the inflammatory response of the host, and the association with environmental factors may all play a contributory role [9, 12, 19]. Gastric cancer develops through a stepwise progression from active gastritis, to atrophy and intestinal metaplasia, dysplasia and adenocarcinoma. This 'neoplastic cascade' was actually described before the discovery of *H. pylori* and, following its discovery, the microorganism was recognized as one of the key factors in driving the cascade [13].

H. pylori is a spiral-shaped bacterium that quickly adapts to a changing environment. The survival capabilities of this organism within the stomach make it therefore difficult to eradicate. The organism is able to survive over a wide pH range. It is found within the gastric mucus layer, deep within the mucus-secreting glands of the antrum, attached to cells, and even within cells [14]. The organism must be eradicated from each of these potential niches and this is a daunting task for any single antibiotic. Initial attempts to cure the infection showed that the presence of antibiotic susceptibility in vitro did not necessarily correlate with successful treatment. It was rapidly recognized that therapy with a single antibiotic led to a poor cure rate and various antimicrobial mixtures were tried resulting in several effective combinations of antibiotics, bismuth, and antisecretory drugs [15].

Therapy of *Helicobacter pylori* Infection

The management of *H. pylori* infection involves a three-step approach: diagnosis, treatment, and confirmation of successful eradication. The availability of accurate and non-invasive tests, such as the urea breath test (UBT) [16–18] or stool antigen test [16, 19, 20], has rendered confirmation of cure practical and reliable. Eradication is defined as the presence of negative tests for *H. pylori* 4 weeks or longer after the end of antimicrobial therapy. Clearance or suppression of *H. pylori* may occur during therapy, and failure to detect *H. pylori* on tests done within 4 weeks of the end of therapy may give false-negative results. The latter is because clearance or suppression is swiftly followed by recurrence of the original infection.

The location of *H. pylori* within the stomach (e.g., the mucus lining the surface epithelium or the surface of mucous cells) represents a challenge for antimicrobial therapy. Furthermore, the gastric lumen is a hostile environment for antimicrobials because the drugs must penetrate thick mucus and may need to be active at low pH values [14]. Successful therapy requires a combination of drugs that prevent the emergence of resistance and reach the bacteria within its various niches. An effective treatment must ensure that even a small population of bacteria does not remain viable.

Treatment regimens for *H. pylori* infection have been evolving since the early 1990s, when monotherapy was first recommended. Antimicrobial therapy for this infection is a complex issue, and the results from new combination treatments are often unpredictable. Errors that should be avoided include quick adoption of regimens tested only in small populations and substitution of a given well-studied, effective medication with another of the same class. Also, it is important to validate the success rate of a treatment regimen in each Country, and perhaps even in the specific region of each country, where its use is intended [21].

Several European guidelines [for reviews, see 15, 21–24] suggest the use of a 7-day triple therapy, comprising a proton pump inhibitor (or ranitidine bismuth citrate), clarithromycin and amoxicillin or metronidazole, as first-line therapy, whilst a 7-day quadruple therapy (proton pump inhibitor, bismuth salts, tetracycline, and metronidazole) is indicated for eradication failure patients. However, increasing evidence suggests that the success rate following such regimens is decreasing in several countries. Indeed, some systematic reviews showed that standard triple therapies fail to eradicate *H. pylori* in up to 20% of patients [15]. Moreover, even lower cure rates have been observed in primary medical care settings, bacterial eradication being achieved in only 61–76% of patients [25]. As a consequence, new therapeutic combinations to cure *H. pylori* infection have been pioneered in the last few years. Ten-day sequential treatment, for instance, is emerging as an alternative first-line therapy [26, 27]. In addition, some effective rescue therapies have been developed in order to overcome treatment failures [28–31].

Although there are several reasons accounting for the lack of efficacy of eradication regimens, the major cause was found to be *H. pylori* resistance to

Table 1. Genes affected by point mutations or other genetic events leading to antibiotic resistance in *H. pylori* and the frequency of resistance (from Mégraud and Lamouliatte [29])

Antibiotic group	Genes affected	Frequency of resistance
Macrolides	23S rRNA	0–20%
Metronidazole	*rdxA, frxA*	10–90%
Quinolones	*gyrA*	0–10%
Rifamycins	*rpoB*	0–5%
Amoxicillin	PBP-1A	few cases described
Tetracycline	16S rRNA	few cases described

antimicrobials (especially clarithromycin and metronidazole) [32–34]. The microorganism can become resistant to most antibiotics by chromosome mutation. This is the essential resistance mechanism found in this bacterial species, although genetic exchanges, especially transformation, have also been documented [29, 34]. The genes affected by point mutations together with the frequency of resistance for the commonly used classes of antimicrobials are shown in table 1.

Rifamycin derivatives (like rifampicin, rifabutin and rifaximin) display antibacterial activity against *H. pylori* [35–37]. Rifabutin [38], whose oral bioavailability is rather low (i.e. 20%), is being increasingly used in some 'rescue' therapies after failed eradication attempts [31, 39–41]. However, its use is in many countries restricted to mycobacterial infections and the drug is not devoid of systemic adverse effects, some of which could actually be serious [42, 43]. In addition, being a potent inducer of cytochrome P_{450} oxidative enzymes [44], rifabutin is endowed with several clinically relevant drug interactions. However, although a case of reversible myelotoxicity with leukopenia and thrombocytopenia has been reported [43], serious adverse effects associated with the short-term treatment used for *Helicobacter* eradication are generally rare [45].

The prevalence of *H. pylori* resistance to this group of antibiotics is not exactly known but is probably extremely low as these drugs have – until recently – only been used in a limited number of patients to treat mycobacterial infections. On these grounds, some new rifamycin derivatives that display a potent bactericidal activity against *H. pylori* have been patented by different pharmaceutical companies. More interesting, these compounds seem to be active also against those bacterial strains resistant to both metronidazole and clarithromycin [45].

Conversely from rifabutin, rifaximin is a poorly absorbed rifamycin derivative with a broad spectrum of antibacterial activity covering Gram-positive and

Table 2. Activity of rifaximin and other antimicrobial agents against *H. pylori* in vitro (from Mégraud et al. [52])

Antimicrobial	MIC$_{50}$ µg/ml	MIC$_{90}$ µg/ml	Range µg/ml
Rifaximin (pH 7.2)	1	2	0.25–4.00
Rifaximin (pH 6.0)	4	4	0.50–8.00
Rifampicin	2	4	0.25–4.00
Amoxicillin	<0.008	0.015	<0.008–0.06
CBS	16	32	8.00–32.00

Gram-negative organisms, both aerobes and anaerobes [46–50], including *H. pylori* [51–54]. Being virtually unabsorbed, its bioavailability within the gastrointestinal tract is rather high and the drug is almost completely devoid of adverse effects [46, 49]. Because of its antibacterial activity against the microorganism and the lack of strains with primary resistance [52, 54], the activity of rifaximin was explored in vivo in an attempt to find out a suitable antimicrobial combination for *H. pylori* eradication. The available in vitro and in vivo studies are summarized below.

In vitro Activity of Rifaximin against *Helicobacter pylori*

The antibacterial effect of rifaximin against *H. pylori* (still called *Campylobacter pyloridis* at that time) was first reported 16 years ago [51]. However, the first systematic investigation was performed in 1994 by Mégraud et al. [52], who found that this antibiotic was able to inhibit the growth of *H. pylori* with MIC values (table 2) intermediate between those of amoxicillin and colloidal bismuth subcitrate (CBS) [55]. In contrast to metronidazole, no strain tested exhibited primary resistance. Furthermore, the activity of rifaximin was only slightly affected by lowering the pH of the medium, conversely from what is currently observed with other antibiotics [14]. The lack of antagonism towards amoxicillin and CBS suggested that a combination of this rifamycin together with these antimicrobials could be used in vivo.

A subsequent study [53] confirmed the activity against the microorganism (table 3) and also showed the lack of antagonism towards metronidazole and omeprazole. Finally, Quesada et al. [54] – while supporting the antibacterial activity of rifaximin against 31 different strains of *H. pylori* – showed that this rifamycin derivative is active against clarithromycin-resistant strains.

The selection of rifaximin-resistant strains was also investigated on five different isolates of *H. pylori*. None of the strains exhibited primary resistance

Table 3. Activity of rifaximin, other antimicrobial agents and omeprazole against 40 strains (39 clinical isolates and the NCTC 11638 strain) of *H. pylori* at pH 7.0 (from Holton et al. [53])

Antimicrobial	MIC$_{50}$ μg/ml	MIC$_{90}$ μ/ml	Range μg/ml
Rifaximin	4	8	4.00–6.00
Ampicillin	0.03	0.25	0.03–0.50
Metronidazole	0.5	4	0.12–4.0
Omeprazole	32	>128	32 to >128

Table 4. Eradication rate and incidence of adverse events following administration of rifaximin and different rifaximin-based eradication regimens in *H. pylori*-positive patients (from Pretolani et al. [55])

Regimen	Eradication rate	Adverse events
Rifaximin 400 mg b.i.d.	40% (4/10)	0% (0/10)
Rifaximin + CBS 120 mg b.i.d.	50% (5/10)	20% (2/10)
Rifaximin + clarithromycin 500 mg b.i.d.	73% (8/11)	18% (2/11)
Rifaximin + metronidazole 250 mg b.i.d.	60% (6/10)	30% (3/10)

Drugs were given for 2 weeks and eradication checked 1 month after stopping treatment with either rapid urease test or histology on biopsy samples taken from the antrum and the corpus.

to rifaximin, but, after exposure to subinhibitory concentrations of the antibiotic, all five strains became resistant. The mutation frequency was similar to that observed with macrolides and quinolones, but was less frequent than that observed with metronidazole [52, 53].

In vivo *Helicobacter pylori* Eradication Trials

A first single-blind randomized study [55] evaluated the efficacy of rifaximin alone or in combination in *H. pylori*-positive patients with antral gastritis and found the dual therapy with clarithromycin particularly effective (table 4).

On the basis of these results, a triple therapy including rifaximin, amoxicillin and omeprazole was attempted [56]. However, results were disappointing since the eradication rate (i.e. 60%) did not differ from that observed with dual

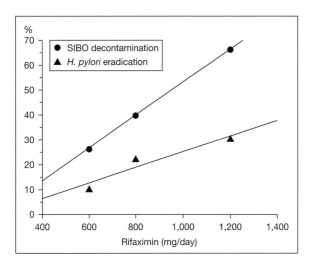

Fig. 1. Rifaximin dose-response curves for decontamination of SIBO (y = −13.571 + 6.6429e − 2x, r² = 1.000) and eradication of *H. pylori* (y = −6.5714 + 3.1429e − 2x, r² = 0.910) in the same (n = 63 out of 90) patients (from data in Lauritano et al. [61] and unpublished data by the same authors).

therapy. However, in this study, high doses (600 mg t.i.d.) of rifaximin suspension (2%) were used, which proved in a subsequent study [57] to be less effective than the tablet formulation. In addition, large volumes of the suspension had to be taken, which might have lowered patients' compliance and, consequently, the eradication rate [56]. Moreover, in the above study, drugs were given on an empty stomach. Since a meal markedly prolongs drug gastric residence time and improves its intragastric distribution to the body and fundus [58], postprandial dosing seems a more suitable strategy for improving topical delivery and mixing (thanks to increased antral motility) of antimicrobials [58,59], provided binding to or inactivation by food does not occur. An additional finding that would suggest postprandial dosing is that eating is associated with desquamation of gastric surface cells and discharge of mucus [60], possibly exposing the organisms to higher concentrations of the antimicrobial agent, or may expose a higher percentage of the organisms to it.

In a recent dose-finding study [61], performed to assess the efficacy of rifaximin in the treatment of small intestine bacterial overgrowth (SIBO), it was found that 70% of these patients were *H. pylori*-positive. This observation gave the opportunity to evaluate simultaneously the disappearance of SIBO and the eradication of the microorganism. As the dose of 1,200 mg daily was the most effective in achieving both end-points (fig. 1), it was combined with either

Table 5. SIBO decontamination and *H. pylori* eradication rates in patients given rifaximin plus either clarithromycin or levofloxacin for 1 week [from Gasbarrini et al., unpubl. results]

Antimicrobial combination (daily doses, mg)	SIBO decontamination rate, %	*H. pylori* eradication rate, %
Rifaximin (1,200) + clarithromycin (1,000)	75	60
Rifaximin (1,200) + levofloxacin (500)	78	50

clarithromycin or levofloxacin in an attempt to improve the results obtained with the rifamycin derivative alone. As shown in table 5, the rifaximin-clarithromycin combination reached the highest eradication rate.

Rifaximin was very well tolerated, with no difference in the safety profile amongst the three regimens studied. No abnormality of laboratory parameters was observed 3 days after the end of the treatment [61].

In a subsequent study [62] the effectiveness of two different triple therapies, both including rifaximin and a proton pump inhibitor (i.e. esomeprazole), combined with either clarithromycin or levofloxacin, were studied. Two groups of 24 naive *Helicobacter*-positive patients were randomized to receive one of the following treatments, all given for 7 days: (1) 24 patients were assigned to receive a triple therapy based on clarithromycin 500 mg b.i.d., rifaximin tablets 400 mg t.i.d., esomeprazole 40 mg o.d. (group CRE), and (2) 24 patients were assigned to receive a triple therapy based on levofloxacin 500 mg o.d., rifaximin tablets 400 mg t.i.d., esomeprazole 40 mg o.d. (group LRE).

H. pylori eradication was assessed using the UBT performed with citric acid and 75 mg of ^{13}C urea, 4 weeks after the end of therapy. A $\Delta^{13}C$-UBT over baseline value >3.5 was considered positive for active *H. pylori* infection.

Drug compliance was excellent and all the patients completed the study. The tolerability profile of both treatments was similar without significant difference between the two groups [62]. All the adverse events were reported as mild by the patients, the main complaint being taste disturbance.

As shown in figure 2, the clarithromycin-rifaximin-esomeprazole (CRE) regimen gave a reasonable eradication rate (although lower than that achieved when amoxicillin was used instead of rifaximin in a similar triple therapy), but the levofloxacin-rifaximin-esomeprazole (LRE) combination resulted in an unacceptably low cure rate. The incidence of gastrointestinal adverse events with CRE therapy was however considerably lower than that reported with the

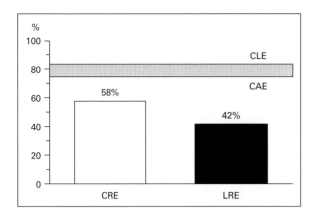

Fig. 2. *Helicobacter* eradication rate (on ITT analysis) obtained with the CRE (clarithromycin-rifaximin-esomeprazole) or LRE (levofloxacin-rifaximin-esomeprazole) regimens. The gray interval refers to the range of eradication rate obtained with CAE (clarithromycin-amoxicillin-esomeprazole) or CLE (levofloxacin-amoxicillin-esomeprazole) in the same Institution (from Gasbarrini et al. [62]).

standard triple therapy, being 53.3% with clarithromycin-amoxicillin-esomeprazole (CAE) and only 6.6% with CRE.

As expected from the in vitro data [52], the results obtained with the CRE triple regimen were similar to those obtained with dual (i.e. rifaximin-amoxicillin or rifaxi-min-metronidazole) therapies without a proton pump inhibitor [56, 63], thus confirming in vivo that the antibacterial activity of this rifamycin derivative is unaffected by intragastric pH.

Conclusions

Although several eradication regimens have been developed, the optimal treatment for *H. pylori* infection is not yet established. The very fact that new antimicrobial combinations are being explored, the results of which appear regularly in the medical literature, is evidence that no single regimen serves to provide the ideal treatment the clinicians require. Antimicrobial-related adverse effects represent the main cause of poor compliance, which often lead to eradication failure [21, 23, 64]. This is, for instance, the case of rifabutin-based regimens, which – despite the high cure rates [65–67] – are not devoid of serious adverse events [42, 43].

The excellent safety profile of rifaximin [46, 49], together with its activity against *H. pylori* strains [51–54], even resistant to clarithromycin [54], prompted several clinicians to investigate the rifaximin potential as a component of dual or triple eradication regimens. Taken together, all the above results suggest that rifaximin-based eradication therapies are promising but new antimicrobial combinations (with and without proton pump inhibitors) need to be explored in well-designed clinical trials including a large cohort of *H. pylori*-infected patients. The remarkable safety of rifaximin, confirmed in our own experience, will allow high-dose regimens of longer duration (e.g. 10 or 14 days) to be tested with confidence in the hope of achieving better eradication rates.

A drawback of rifaximin could be its inability to reach sufficiently high concentrations in the gastric mucus layer under and within which *H. pylori* is commonly located and this would likely affect eradication rate [68, 69]. Taking these considerations into account, bioadhesive rifaximin formulations able to better and persistently cover gastric mucosa [70, 71], or combination with mucolytic agents, such as pronase or acetylcysteine [72, 73], need to be evaluated in order to better define the place of this antibiotic in our therapeutic armamentarium.

References

1   Marshall BJ, Warren JR: Unidentified curved bacilli in the stomach of patients with gastritis and peptic ulceration. Lancet 1984;i:1311–1315.
2   Leodolter A, Kulig M, Brasch H, Meyer-Sabellek W, Willich SN, Malfertheiner P: A meta-analysis comparing eradication, healing and relapse rates in patients with *Helicobacter pylori*-associated gastric or duodenal ulcer. Aliment Pharmacol Ther 2001;15:1949–1958.
3   Cremonini F, Gasbarrini A, Armuzzi A, Gasbarrini G: *Helicobacter pylori*-related diseases. Eur J Clin Invest 2001;31:431–437.
4   International Agency for Research on Cancer: Infection with *Helicobacter pylori*; in IARC Monographs Vol. 61: Schistosomes, Liver Flukes and *Helicobacter pylori*. Lyon, IARC, 1994, pp 177–202.
5   Misiewicz JJ: Is the only good *Helicobacter* a dead *Helicobacter?* Helicobacter 1997;2(suppl 1):S89–S91.
6   Graham DY: The only good *Helicobacter pylori* is a dead *Helicobacter pylori*. Lancet 1997;350:70–71.
7   Vaira D, Vakil N, Rugge M, Gatta L, Ricci C, Menegatti M, Leandro G, Holton J, Russo VM, Miglioli M: Effect of *Helicobacter pylori* eradication on development of dyspeptic and reflux disease in healthy asymptomatic subjects. Gut 2003;52:1543–1547.
8   Uemura N, Okamoto S, Yamamoto S, Matsumura N, Yamaguchi S, Yamakido M, Taniyama K, Sasaki N, Schlemper RJ: *Helicobacter pylori* infection and the development of gastric cancer. N Engl J Med 2001;345:784–789.
9   Zarrilli R, Ricci V, Romano M: Molecular response of gastric epithelial cells to *Helicobacter pylori*-induced cell damage. Cell Microbiol 1999;1:93–99.
10   Ricci V, Zarrilli R, Romano M: Voyage *of Helicobacter pylori* in human stomach: odyssey of a bacterium. Dig Liver Dis 2002;34:2–8.
11   Uemura N, Okamoto S, Yamamoto S, et al: *Helicobacter pylori* infection and the development of gastric cancer. N Engl J Med 2001;345:784–789.

12 Peek RM Jr, Blaser MJ: *Helicobacter pylori* and gastrointestinal tract adenocarcinomas. Nat Rev Cancer 2002;2:28–37.

13 Helicobacter Cancer Collaborative Group: Gastric cancer and *Helicobacter pylori*: a combined analysis of 12 case-control studies nested within prospective cohorts. Gut 2001;49: 347–353.

14 Scarpignato C, Pelosini I: Antisecretory drugs for eradication of *Helicobacter pylori*: antibacterial activity and synergism with antimicrobial agents. Prog Basic Clin Pharmacol 1999;11:136–180.

15 Scarpignato C: Towards the ideal regimen for *Helicobacter pylori* eradication: the search continues. Dig Liver Dis 2004;36:243–247.

16 Makristathis A, Hirschl AM, Lehours P, Mégraud F: Diagnosis of *Helicobacter pylori* infection. Helicobacter 2004;9(suppl 1):7–14.

17 Gisbert JP, Pajares JM: Review article: ^{13}C-urea breath test in the diagnosis *of Helicobacter pylori* infection – a critical review. Aliment Pharmacol Ther 2004;20:1001–1017.

18 Parente F, Bianchi Porro G: The ^{13}C-urea breath test for non-invasive diagnosis of *Helicobacter pylori* infection: which procedure and which measuring equipment? Eur J Gastroenterol Hepatol 2001;13:803–806.

19 Gisbert JP, Pajares JM: Diagnosis of *Helicobacter pylori* infection by stool antigen determination: a systematic review. Am J Gastroenterol 2001;96:2829–2838.

20 Parente F, Maconi G, Porro GB, Caselli M: Stool test with polyclonal antibodies for monitoring *Helicobacter pylori* eradication in adults: a critical reappraisal. Scand J Gastroenterol 2002;37: 747–749.

21 Romano M, Cuomo A: Eradication of *Helicobacter pylori*: a clinical update. Med Gen Med 2004; 6:19 [available at http://www.pubmedcentral.gov/articlerender.fcgi?artid = 1140724].

22 McLoughlin RM, O'Morain CA, O'Connor HJ: Eradication of *Helicobacter pylori*: recent advances in treatment. Fundam Clin Pharmacol 2005;19:421–427.

23 Candelli M, Nista EC, Carloni E, Pignataro G, Zocco MA, Cazzato A, Di Campli C, Fini L, Gasbarrini G, Gasbarrini A: Treatment of *H. pylori* infection: a review. Curr Med Chem 2005;12: 375–384.

24 Ford AC, Delaney BC, Forman D, Moayyedi P: Eradication therapy in *Helicobacter pylori*-positive peptic ulcer disease: systematic review and economic analysis. Am J Gastroenterol 2004;99: 1833–1855.

25 Della Monica P, Lavagna A, Masoero G, Lombardo L, Crocella L, Pera A: Effectiveness of *Helicobacter pylori* eradication treatments in a primary care setting in Italy. Aliment Pharmacol Ther 2002;16:1269–1275.

26 Zullo A, Vaira D, Vakil N, Hassan C, Gatta L, Ricci C, De Francesco V, Menegatti M, Tampieri A, Perna F, Rinaldi V, Perri F, Papadia C, Fornari F, Pilati S, Mete LS, Merla A, Poti R, Marinone G, Savioli A, Campo SM, Faleo D, Ierardi E, Miglioli M, Morini S: High eradication rates of *Helicobacter pylori* with a new sequential treatment. Aliment Pharmacol Ther 2003;17:719–726.

27 De Boer WA, Kuipers EJ, Kusters JG: Sequential therapy: a new treatment for *Helicobacter pylori* infection. But is it ready for general use? Dig Liver Dis 2004;36:311–314.

28 Gisbert JP, Pajares JM: Review article: *Helicobacter pylori* 'rescue' regimen when proton pump inhibitor-based triple therapies fail. Aliment Pharmacol Ther 2002;16:1047–1057.

29 Mégraud F, Lamouliatte H: Review article: the treatment of refractory *Helicobacter pylori* infection. Aliment Pharmacol Ther 2003;17:1333–1343.

30 Parente F, Cucino C, Bianchi Porro G: Treatment options for patients with *Helicobacter pylori* infection resistant to one or more eradication attempts. Dig Liver Dis 2003;35:523–528.

31 Di Mario F, Cavallaro LG, Scarpignato C: Rescue therapies for management of *Helicobacter pylori* infection. Dig Dis 2006;24:in press.

32 Graham DY, de Boer WA, Tytgat GNJ: Choosing the best anti-*Helicobacter pylori* therapy: effect of antimicrobial resistance. Am J Gastroenterol 1996;91:1072–1076.

33 Houben MH, van de Beek D, Hensen EF, Craen AJ, Rauws EA, Tytgat GN: A systematic review of *Helicobacter pylori* eradication therapy – the impact of antimicrobial resistance on eradication rates. Aliment Pharmacol Ther 1999;13:1047–1055.

34 Mégraud F: Resistance of *Helicobacter pylori* to antibiotics and its impact on treatment options. Drug Resist Updat 2001;4:178–186.

35 Pilotto A, Franceschi M, Rassu M, Furlan F, Scagnelli M: In vitro activity of rifabutin against strains of *Helicobacter pylori* resistant to metronidazole and clarithromycin. Am J Gastroenterol 2000;95:833–834.

36 Heep M, Beck D, Bayerdorffer E, Lehn N: Rifampin and rifabutin resistance mechanism in *Helicobacter pylori*. Antimicrob Agents Chemother 1999;43:1497–1499.

37 Jiang ZD, DuPont HL: Rifaximin: in vitro and in vivo antibacterial activity. A review. Chemotherapy 2005;51(suppl 1):67–72.

38 Brogden RN, Fitton A: Rifabutin. A review of its antimicrobial activity, pharmacokinetic properties and therapeutic efficacy. Drugs 1994;47:983–1009.

39 Gisbert JP, Calvet X, Bujanda L, Marcos S, Gisbert JL, Pajares JM: 'Rescue' therapy with rifabutin after multiple *Helicobacter pylori* treatment failures. Helicobacter 2003;8:90–94.

40 Wong WM, Gu Q, Lam SK, Fung FM, Lai KC, Hu WH, Yee YK, Chan CK, Xia HH, Yuen MF, Wong BC: Randomized controlled study of rabeprazole, levofloxacin and rifabutin triple therapy vs. quadruple therapy as second-line treatment for *Helicobacter pylori* infection. Aliment Pharmacol Ther 2003;17:553–560.

41 Perri F, Festa V, Clemente R, Quitadamo M, Andriulli A: Rifabutin-based 'rescue therapy' for *Helicobacter pylori* infected patients after failure of standard regimens. Aliment Pharmacol Ther 2000;14:311–316.

42 Griffith DE, Brown BA, Girard WM, Wallace RJ Jr: Adverse events associated with high-dose ritabutin in macrolide-containing regimens for the treatment of *Mycobacterium avium* complex lung disease. Clin Infect Dis 1995;21:594–598.

43 Canducci F, Ojetti V, Pola P, Gasbarrini G, Gasbarrini A: Rifabutin-based *Helicobacter pylori* eradication rescue therapy. Aliment Pharmacol Ther 2001;15:143.

44 Finch CK, Chrisman CR, Baciewicz AM, Self TH: Rifampin and rifabutin drug interactions: an update. Arch Intern Med 2002;162:985–992.

45 Zullo A, Hassan C, Campo SMA, Morini S: Evolving therapy for *Helicobacter pylori* infection. Exp Opin Ther Patents 2004;14:1453–1464.

46 Scarpignato C, Pelosini I: Rifaximin, a poorly absorbed antibiotic: pharmacology and clinical potential. Chemotherapy 2005;51(suppl 21):36–66.

47 Ericsson CD, DuPont HL: Rifaximin in the treatment of infectious diarrhea. Chemotherapy 2005;51 (suppl 1):73–80.

48 Gerard L, Garey KW, DuPont HL: Rifaximin: a nonabsorbable rifamycin antibiotic for use in non-systemic gastrointestinal infections. Expert Rev Anti Infect Ther 2005;3:201–211.

49 Baker DE: Rifaximin: a nonabsorbed oral antibiotic. Rev Gastroenterol Disord 2005;5:19–30.

50 Huang DB, DuPont HL: Rifaximin – a novel antimicrobial for enteric infections. J Infect 2005;50:97–106.

51 Mignini F, Falcioni E, Prenna M, Santacroce F, Ripa S: In vitro antibacterial activity of rifaximin against *Campylobacter pylori* (*Campylobacter pyloridis*). Chemiotherapia (Florence) 1989;1(suppl 4):222–223.

52 Mégraud F, Bouffant F, Camou Juncas C: In vitro activity of rifaximin against *Helicobacter pylori*. Eur J Clin Microbiol Infect Dis 1994;13:184–186.

53 Holton J, Vaira D, Menegatti M, Barbara L: The susceptibility of *Helicobacter pylori* to the rifamycin, rifaximin. J Antimicrob Chemother 1995;35:545–549.

54 Quesada M, Sanfeliu I, Junquera F, Segura F, Calvet X: Evaluation of *Helicobacter pylori* susceptibility to rifaximin (in Spanish). Gastroenterol Hepatol 2004;27:393–396.

55 Pretolani S, Bonvicini F, Brocci E, Cilla D, Pasini P, Baldini L, Epifanio G, Miglio F, Gasbarrini G: Effect of rifaximin, a new non-absorbed antibiotic, in the treatment of *Helicobacter pylori* infection. Acta Gastroenterol Belg 1993;56:144A.

56 De Giorgio R, Stanghellini V, Barbara G, Guerrini S, Ferrieri A, Corinaldesi R: Rifaximin and *Helicobacter pylori* eradication. Eur Rev Med Pharmacol Sci 1997;1:105–110.

57 Dell'Anna A, Azzarone P, Ferrieri A: A randomized openly comparative study between rifaximin suspension versus rifaximin pills for the eradication of *Helicobacter pylori*. Eur Rev Med Pharmacol Sci 1999;3:105–110.

58 Atherton JC, Washington N, Bracewell MA, Sutton LJ, Greaves JL, Perkins AC, Hawkey CJ, Spiller RC: Scintigraphic assessment of the intragastric distribution and gastric emptying of an

encapsulated drug: the effect of feeding and of a proton pump inhibitor. Aliment Pharmacol Ther 1994;8:489–494.

59   Gottfries J, Svenheden A, Alpstein M, Bake B, Larsson A, Idstrom JP: Gastrointestinal transit of amoxicillin modified-release tablets and a placebo tablet including pharmacokinetic assessments of amoxicillin. Scand J Gastroenterol 1996;31:49–53.
60   Grant R, Grossman MI, Ivy AC: Histological changes in the gastric mucosa during digestion and their relationship to mucosal growth. Gastroenterology 1953;25:218–231.
61   Lauritano EC, Gabrielli M, Lupascu A, Santoliquido A, Nucera G, Scarpellini E, Vincenti F, Cammarota G, Flore R, Pola P, Gasbarrini G, Gasbarrini A: Rifaximin dose-finding study for the treatment of small intestinal bacterial overgrowth. Aliment Pharmacol Ther 2005;22:31–35.
62   Gasbarrini A, Lauritano EC, Nista EC, Candelli M, Gabrielli M, Santoro M, Zocco MA, Cazzato A, Finizio R, Ojetti V, Cammarota G, Gasbarrini G: Rifaximin-based regimens for eradication of *Helicobacter pylori*: a pilot study. Dig Dis 2006;24:in press.
63   Vaira D, Menegatti M, Miglioli M, Ferrieri A, et al: Rifaximin suspension for the eradication of *Helicobacter pylori*. Curr Ther Res 1997;58:300–308.
64   McLoughlin R, O'Morain C: Effectiveness of anti-infectives. Chemotherapy 2005;51:243–246.
65   Perri F, Festa V, Clemente R, Quitadamo M, Andriulli A: Rifabutin-based 'rescue therapy' for *Helicobacter pylori* infected patients after failure of standard regimens. Aliment Pharmacol Ther 2000;14:311–316.
66   Wong WM, Gu Q, Lam SK, Fung FM, Lai KC, Hu WH, Yee YK, Chan CK, Xia HH, Yuen MF, Wong BC: Randomized controlled study of rabeprazole, levofloxacin and rifabutin triple therapy vs. quadruple therapy as second-line treatment for *Helicobacter pylori* infection. Aliment Pharmacol Ther 2003;17:553–560.
67   Toracchio S, Capodicasa S, Soraja DB, Cellini L, Marzio L: Rifabutin-based triple therapy for eradication of *H. pylori* primary and secondary resistant to tinidazole and clarithromycin. Dig Liver Dis 2005;37:33–38.
68   Munoz DJB, Tasman Jones C, Pybus J: Effect of *Helicobacter pylori* infection on colloidal bismuth subcitrate concentration in gastric mucus. Gut 1992;33:592–596.
69   McNulty AM, Dent JC, Ford GA, Wilkinson SP: Inhibitory antimicrobial concentrations against *Campylobacter pylori* in gastric mucosa. J Antimicrob Chemother 1988;22:729–738.
70   Conway BR: Drug delivery strategies for the treatment of *Helicobacter pylori* infections. Curr Pharm Des 2005;11:775–790.
71   Wanlian Pharmaceutical Co Ltd: Rifaximin soft capsule composition [CN1451386] 2002.
72   Huynh HQ, Couper RT, Tran CD, Moore L, Kelso R, Butler RN: N-acetylcysteine, a novel treatment for *Helicobacter pylori* infection. Dig Dis Sci 2004;49:1853–1861.
73   Gotoh A, Akamatsu T, Shimizu T, Shimodaira K, Kaneko T, Kiyosawa K, Ishida K, Ikeno T, Sugiyama A, Kawakami Y, Ota H, Katsuyama T: Additive effect of pronase on the efficacy of eradication therapy against *Helicobacter pylori*. Helicobacter 2002;7:183–191.

Note Added in Proof

At the recent meeting of the *American College of Gastroenterology* in Honolulu (Hawaii, USA), Hilal and Hilal [1] presented the preliminary results of an open label study exploring the efficacy of a new rifaximin-based regimen in the eradication *of Helicobacter pylori*. Patients were given lansoprazole (30 mg b.i.d.), doxycycline (100 mg b.i.d.) and rifaximin (400 mg t.i.d.) for 14 days. Although this triple therapy was well tolerated, the eradication rate appeared to be rather low (i.e. 40%), especially when compared with the standard triple regimens.

Rifaximin for Eradication of *H. pylori*

Reference

1 Hilal RE, Hilal T: The efficacy and tolerability of riofaximin, doxycycline and lansoprazole in the treatment of *H. pylori* gastritis: an open label pilot study. Am J Gastroenterol 2005;100(suppl): S57.

Prof. Antonio Gasbarrini, MD, PhD
Department of Internal Medicine, Catholic University of Sacred Heart
Gemelli University Hospital, Largo A. Gemelli, 8
IT–00168 Rome (Italy)
Tel. +39 06 3015 4294
Fax +39 06 3550 2775
E-Mail agasbarrini@rm.unicatt.it

This chapter should be cited as follows:

Gasbarrini A, Gasbarrini G, Pelosini I, Scarpignato C: Eradication of *Helicobacter pylori*: Are Rifaximin-Based Regimens Effective? Digestion 2006;73(suppl 1):129–135.

Scarpignato C, Lanas Á (eds): Bacterial Flora in Digestive Disease.
Focus on Rifaximin.

·······················

Microbial Flora in NSAID-Induced Intestinal Damage: A Role for Antibiotics?

Ángel Lanas[a], *Carmelo Scarpignato*[b]

[a]Servicio de Aparato Digestivo, Hospital Clínico Universitario, Zaragoza, Spain;
[b]Laboratory of Clinical Pharmacology, Department of Human Anatomy,
Pharmacology and Forensic Sciences, School of Medicine and Dentistry,
University of Parma, Parma, Italy

Abstract

Upper gastrointestinal (GI) complications are well-recognized adverse events associated with non-steroidal anti-inflammatory drug (NSAID) use. However, NSAID-induced damage to the distal GI tract is also common and more frequent than previously recognized. These untoward effects include increased mucosal permeability, mucosal inflammation, anemia and occult blood loss, malabsorption, protein loss, ileal dysfunction, diarrhea, mucosal ulceration, strictures due to diaphragm disease as well as active bleeding and perforation. Studies with selective COX-2 inhibitors have shown that, in the short term, these agents do not increase mucosal permeability and display a reduced by 50% incidence of serious lower GI side effects compared to traditional NSAIDs. However, the long-term use of this therapeutic strategy is limited by the increased risk of serious cardiovascular events, especially in patients with multiple risk factors. Several studies have suggested that intraluminal bacteria play a significant role in the pathogenesis of small-bowel damage induced by NSAIDs and that enterobacterial translocation into the mucosa represents the first step that sets in motion a series of events leading to gross lesion formation. Experimental and clinical investigations indicate that in the short term, antibacterial agents either reduce or abolish NSAID enteropathy. However, potential adverse effects of systemic antimicrobials and the possible occurrence of drug resistance have so far precluded this interesting approach. The availability of poorly absorbed and effective antibiotics, like rifaximin, may represent an attractive alternative to prevent or limit NSAID-associated intestinal damage.

Non-steroidal anti-inflammatory drugs (NSAIDs) are widely used in patients suffering from different rheumatic and musculoskeletal conditions.

Across Europe, the proportion of drug prescribing accounted for by NSAIDs is variable but represents – on average – 7.7% of all prescriptions. In the USA, 20 million people regularly use NSAIDs, with a point prevalence of prescription of 10–15% in persons older than 65 years. A recent survey of people 65 years or older in Minnesota found that 70% of them had used NSAIDs and/or aspirin at least once weekly and 34% used them at least daily [1]. In Spain, 20% of the population uses this class of drugs at least 1 month per year. However, these figures might underestimate the actual dimension of NSAID use because they often exclude over-the-counter use of aspirin and other recently released non-aspirin NSAIDs [1].

Although NSAIDs represent a very effective class of drugs, their use is associated with a broad spectrum of untoward reactions in the liver, kidney, skin and gut. Upper gastrointestinal (GI) side effects are the most common adverse events associated with NSAID use [1, 2]. Indeed, although gastroduodenal mucosa possesses an array of defensive mechanisms, NSAIDs have a deleterious effect on most of them [3]. Although the upper GI toxicity of NSAIDs is well documented, the appreciation that NSAID damage extends beyond the duodenum is less well recognized. Upper GI effects are indeed the most known and most feared adverse events, but it is evident that NSAID therapy is also associated with lower GI complications, which contribute significantly to the morbidity and mortality associated with this class of drugs. NSAID-associated toxicity of the small and large bowel has several different manifestations and includes ulcerations, strictures, colitis, bleeding and perforation among others [4, 5]. In addition, NSAIDs may induce exacerbation of underlying diseases, like for instance inflammatory bowel disease (IBD), which is a difficult clinical problem since many patients suffer from both IBD and arthritic diseases [5].

Many of the above-mentioned clinical manifestations are believed to be the consequence of the inhibition of COX-1- and COX-2-driven prostaglandin (PG) synthesis by NSAID agents. However, other mechanisms may also be involved and the pathophysiology of NSAID-induced damage in the lower GI tract seems somehow different from that of the upper GI damage, where acid plays a pivotal role [1–3, 6].

Spectrum of Lesions and Symptoms Associated with GI Damage Induced by Non-Selective and COX-2 Selective NSAIDs

GI problems constitute a wide range of different clinical pictures, ranging from symptoms such as dyspepsia, heartburn and abdominal discomfort to more serious events, like mucosal erosions and peptic ulcer with its life-threatening complications, bleeding and perforation [1, 2]. It is now widely

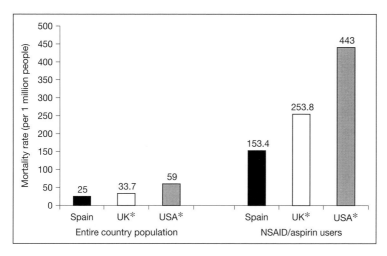

Fig. 1. Mortality rate attributed to NSAID/aspirin-associated GI complications in Spain and frequently reported estimates published in the USA and the UK [3, 4, 13, 15]. *Data estimated from the population registered in 1998. Estimations for mortality in NSAID/aspirin users have been calculated from the adult population with a NSAID of 20.6% use in Spain and 16.8% in the USA and the UK (from Lanas et al. [9]).

accepted that NSAID use increases the risk of upper GI bleeding and that the cumulative incidence of upper GI complications ranges between 0.92 and 1.4% after 12 months of NSAID use [7, 8]. The worst and undesirable outcome of GI complications is death. A recent study [9] has pointed out that 15.3 deaths per 100,000 NSAID/aspirin user-years occur in Spain as a consequence of GI complications, a figure which agrees with more recent estimates from the USA (fig. 1).

The use of COX-2-selective inhibitors has been associated with a significant reduction in the incidence of gastroduodenal ulcers when compared to traditional NSAIDs. Furthermore, high-dose rofecoxib and lumiracoxib use was associated with a 50–70% reduction of upper GI complications when compared to non-selective NSAIDs (namely naproxen and ibuprofen) [7, 8]. In the CLASS[1] study [10], high-dose celecoxib was better tolerated than non-selective NSAIDs in patients not taking low-dose aspirin. Although it is now becoming clear that coxibs lose their GI benefit over traditional NSAIDs when combined with low-dose aspirin [8, 10, 11] or in presence of multiple GI risk factors [12], recent epide-miological studies [13, 14] confirm that, in common clinical

---

[1] Celecoxib Long-term Arthritis Safety Study.

Table 1. Spectrum of lesions of the distal GI tract associated with NSAIDs

Subclinical damage	Clinical damage
Increase in mucosal permeability	Anemia
Mucosal inflammation	Mucosal diaphragms
Fecal occult blood loss	Strictures
Ileal dysfunction	Small bowel, colonic and rectal ulceration
Malabsorption	Colitis
	Bleeding
	Perforation
	Exacerbation of underlying diseases
	Chronic inflammatory bowel diseases
	Diverticulosis
	Angiodysplastic lesions

practice, these compounds are associated with the lowest risk of GI complications among all the available NSAIDs.

Although NSAID lesions located in the upper GI tract are common, it is now widely accepted that NSAID use is associated *both* with upper GI and lower GI complications [1, 2, 5, 15, 16]. The relatively small number of reports of toxic effects of NSAIDs to the small bowel may reflect primarily the lack of diagnostic tools. Indeed, push enteroscopy [17] and endoscopic capsule [18] have only recently been available to clinicians. Nevertheless, a host of small bowel manifestations have now been documented, ranging from strictures causing dramatic small-bowel obstruction and severe bleeding to low-grade 'NSAID enteropathy', a syndrome comprising increased intestinal permeability and low-grade inflammation with blood and protein loss [4–6]. The enteropathy, although not dramatic, may add to existing GI problems, especially in rheumatic patients, and contribute to iron-deficiency anemia or hypoalbuminemia. Autopsy studies [19] have also shown an increased incidence of small-bowel ulcers in long-term NSAID users.

Lesions Induced by NSAIDs in the Distal GI Tract

The prevalence of NSAID-associated lower GI side effects may exceed that detected in the upper GI tract and include a wide spectrum of lesions (table 1). In addition, the frequency of life-threatening complications due to the lower GI

Table 2. Intestinal inflammation in patients on long-term NSAIDs (from Sigthorsson et al. [20])

	Patients		4-day fecal excretion of ^{111}In white cells (% dose)
	studied	abnormal	
Controls	22	0	0.5 (0.2)*
Indomethacin	52	30	4.1 (2.9)*
Piroxicam	28	15	3.9 (1.1)*
Naproxen	58	42	3.9 (0.8)*
Ibuprofen	29	16	3.0 (1.2)*
Ketoprofen	14	9	3.5 (1.8)*
Diclofenac	38	24	4.4 (4.8)*
Aspirin	7	1	0.7 (0.3)
Sulindac	9	5	2.5 (2.9)*
Etodolac	11	7	3.7 (2.1)*
Nabumetone	13	2	1.1 (0.4)

*$p < 0.05$ vs. controls.

tract represents nowadays no less than a third of all GI complications associated with the use of these agents.

NSAID-Induced Increase in Gut Permeability and Inflammation

NSAIDs induce damage to both the small and the large bowel and at least 60–70% of patients taking NSAIDs develop enteropathy [5, 16]. In the small bowel, NSAIDs enhance gut permeability and induce mucosal inflammation (table 2) [20]. Increased gut permeability can be seen as soon as 12 h after the ingestion of single doses of ibuprofen, naproxen or indomethacin [21]. The process is rapidly (i.e. within 12 h) reverted, but it takes 4 days when the NSAID has been used repeatedly (1 week or more) [22]. The increase in gut permeability is observed with almost all NSAIDs, with the exception of those not undergoing enterohepatic recirculation [20, 23]. Being devoid of such a kinetic pattern and being non-acidic compounds, among other characteristics, COX-2-selective inhibitors rofecoxib and celecoxib do not increase intestinal permeability [2, 23, 24].

An initial increase in small intestine permeability is a prerequisite of the subsequent development of small intestine inflammation, which is associated with blood and protein loss [25]. Calprotectin is a neutrophil cytosolic protein that, being resistant to colonic bacterial degradation, can be measured in feces [26]. A landmark study [27], performed with 18 different NSAIDs, has shown

Table 3. Inflammation and blood loss in IBD and NSAID enteropathy (from Teahon et al. [30])

	Fecal excretion of ^{111}In-labeled neutrophils	Fecal excretion of ^{51}Cr-labeled red cells
Upper normal limit	<1%	<1 ml/day
Patients with UC	20.3% (8.3–53.1)	6.5 (1.8–29.2)
Patients with CD	17.0% (12.1–22.0)	2.1 (0.7–5.3)
Patients on NSAIDs	1.6% (0.7–3.0)	1.9 ml/day[1] (0.5–3.8)

CD = Crohn's disease; UC = ulcerative colitis.
[1]Value not significantly different from that found in patients with Crohn's disease.

that almost all these compounds significantly increase fecal calprotectin in patients with rheumatoid arthritis or osteoarthritis and that single stool fecal calprotectin concentrations are correlated with the 4-day fecal excretion of ^{111}In-labeled leukocytes.

All the above investigations [16, 20–25] have revealed that intestinal inflammation could be present in up to 60–70% of patients taking NSAIDs and that, once established, it may be detected up to 1–3 years after the NSAID has been stopped.

NSAID-Induced Anemia and Blood Loss

Anemia is frequent in patients taking NSAIDs and may be the consequence *of distal* GI tract blood loss. Different studies have shown that after NSAID ingestion the simultaneous intravenous injection of ^{111}In-labeled leukocytes and ^{99m}Tc-labeled erythrocytes revealed the identical location of both radioactive blood cell types in the intestine, thus suggesting a correlation between the inflammatory and hemorrhagic damage induced in the intestine by these agents [25, 27, 28]. Furthermore, approximately half of the patients with occult GI bleeding while on regular NSAIDs have jejunal or ileal ulcerations [29]. Although intestinal inflammation is lower in NSAID enteropathy compared with IBD, fecal blood loss appears to overlap that observed in Crohn's disease (table 3) [30].

NSAID-Associated Malabsorption, Protein Loss and Ileal Dysfunction

Patients taking long-term NSAIDs may also show intestinal malabsorption and protein-loss enteropathy [1, 5, 6]. The use of sulindac and fenamates has been associated with severe malabsorption and atrophic mucosa similar to that seen in celiac sprue. Loss of proteins has been shown at the ileal level and more

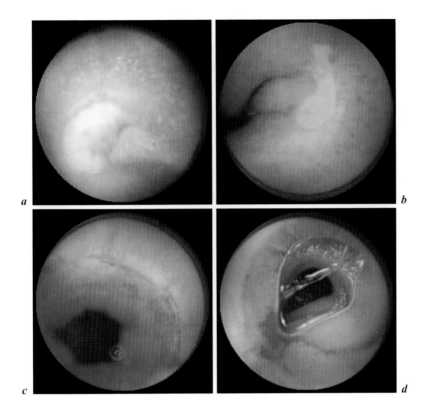

Fig. 2. Small intestine lesions seen with video-capsule in long-term users of NSAIDs. *a, b* Typical ulcer-like mucosal losses. *c* Image depicts a linear ulcer, almost healed. *d* A small bleeding lesion is evident. Courtesy of Given Imaging Ltd, Yoqneam, Israel.

recently it has been suggested that NSAIDs use increases the risk of acute diarrhea [5, 6] and that their use can be the responsible factor of many episodes seen in general practice [31].

NSAID-Associated Mucosal Ulceration and Intestinal Diaphragms

As already outlined, there is an increased incidence of small intestinal ulceration in long-term (>6 months) users of NSAIDs. Non-specific small-intestinal ulceration was found in 8.4% of the users of NSAIDs and 0.6% of the non-users (p < 0.001). Three patients taking NSAIDs were found to have died of perforated non-specific small-intestinal ulcers [19]. Imaging via the wire-less capsule endoscopy has revealed that NSAIDs induce several types of lesions, including intestinal ulceration, in the small bowel (fig. 2) [32, 33]. Colonoscopy studies have also shown that NSAID use is associated with isolated colonic ulcers, diffuse

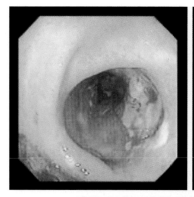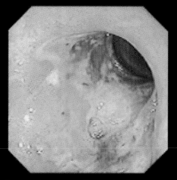

Fig. 3. Endoscopic appearance of colonic mucosal inflammation with ulceration in a 72-year-old woman who presented with abdominal pain, bloody diarrhea and weight loss. She had been taking significant amounts of NSAIDs for arthritis. Although grossly similar in appearance to ischemic colitis, the typical histological features of ischemic colitis (mucosal necrosis, fibrosis of the lamina propria and crypt atrophy, and overlying fibrinopurulent membrane) were not present on biopsy. Courtesy of Dr. David Martin, East Point, Ga., USA.

colonic ulceration that may or may not be associated with occult bleeding or complications, such as major intestinal bleeding and/or perforation (fig. 3). Diffuse colitis has been observed after the use of mefenamic acid, ibuprofen, piroxicam, naproxen or aspirin. NSAIDs may also exacerbate preexisting lesions including diverticulitis, reactivate IBD and trigger intestinal bleeding from angiodysplastic lesions [3–6, 16].

Strictures of the large or small intestine are a well-recognized side effect of NSAID-associated lower GI toxicity. The strictures are diaphragm-like rings of scar tissue (fig. 4) and represent a distinctive pathological entity that may have a silent clinical evolution or more often induce intermittent obstruction, anemia and or diarrhea and may require surgery for treatment and/or diagnosis [6, 16, 34].

NSAID-Associated Lower GI Complications

NSAID use increases the risk of lower GI bleeding and perforation to a similar extent to that seen in the upper GI tract. Two studies [35, 36] found that most patients with lower GI bleeding or perforation had evidence of recent aspirin or NSAID use. More recently, a large trial [15] has actually shown that the proportion of patients developing lower GI bleeding may be similar to that presenting with upper GI complications. In an attempt to spare gastroduodenal mucosa, an enteric-coated formulation of some NSAIDs has been developed in order to allow the release of the active drug into the small bowel. However,

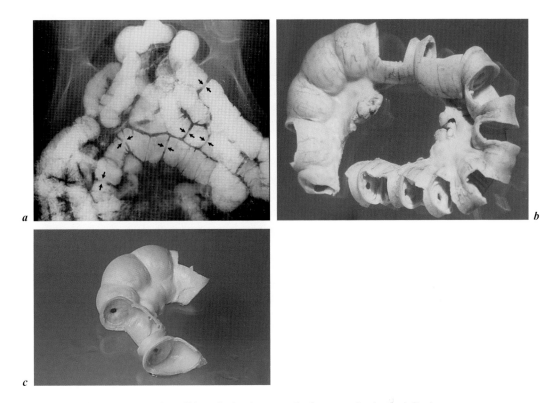

Fig. 4. Appearance of small intestinal strictures at barium examination and diaphragm-like rings in post-mortem specimens from long-term users of NSAIDs. Courtesy of Prof. Ingvar Bjarnason, Department of Medicine, Guy's, King's, St Thomas' Medical School, London, UK. *a* Small barium enema showing multiple NSAID-induced strictures marked by arrows on both sides. *b* Small-bowel loop where multiple NSAID-induced diaphragm-like rings can be clearly seen. *c* Detail of a small-bowel specimen showing the marked reduction of intestinal lumen.

endoscopic studies [1, 5, 37] have shown that, although these compounds are associated with reduced damage to the stomach and the duodenum, they do increase small intestinal damage [38], by enhancing the exposure of the distal GI tract to these noxious agents.

Effects of Selective COX-2 Inhibitors on the Small Bowel

COX-2 inhibitors may induce less or no damage to the intact distal GI tract compared to non-selective NSAIDs. The lack of intestinal damage with this class of drugs in animal experiments [24, 39, 40] has been confirmed in clinical studies [23, 41–43]. Most patients taking either meloxicam [27] or nimesulide [44], two preferential COX-2 inhibitors, had normal intestinal permeability and no increase in intestinal inflammation in comparison to control patients not taking the drug. In studies performed in healthy volunteers, rofecoxib [41] and etoricoxib [45] – conversely from traditional NSAIDs (namely indomethacin or ibuprofen) – proved to be unable of increasing fecal blood loss. Along the same lines, the incidence of anemia with celecoxib was significantly lower than that seen with traditional NSAIDs [10, 46]. Although some case reports of acute colitis or lower intestinal complication have been associated with administration of COX-2 inhibitors, data derived from the VIGOR[2] study have shown that the benefits of rofecoxib 50 mg/day over naproxen (500 mg b.i.d.) were present in *both* the upper and the lower GI tract with a risk reduction of 50 and 60%, respectively [7, 15]. Moreover, a retrospective study [47] reported the long-term (median 9 months) safety of these agents in patients with IBD.

Selective COX-2 Inhibitors: Gastrointestinal Benefits versus
Cardiovascular Risks

The main limitation to the use of this therapeutic strategy is the concern regarding the cardiovascular (CV) risk associated with the use of this new class of drugs. As a matter of fact, some publications [48–50] have raised concerns that coxibs may be prothrombotic and increase the risk of acute myocardial infarction (AMI). This has arisen because of the theoretical possibility that selective COX-2 inhibitors may affect the balance between prothrombotic and antithrombotic prostanoids [51]. And indeed, the CV safety of these agents has repeatedly been questioned. A subanalysis of the VIGOR trial [7] demonstrated a significant increase in the risk of AMI for rofecoxib users relative to naproxen users. The absence of a placebo group in this trial and the low event rate in this subgroup analysis make interpretation of these findings difficult. Possible explanations for these observations include an increased risk of AMI for rofecoxib, a cardioprotective effect of naproxen, or both. Alternatively, the findings of the VIGOR trial with respect to AMI may have simply occurred by chance and neither rofecoxib nor naproxen truly affects the risk of AMI. A thoughtful review discussing these issues, which the reader is referred to, has been published by Baigent and Patrono [52].

Subsequent to the publication of the VIGOR trial, a paper by Mukherjee et al. [53] extended the CV safety concern to celecoxib and potentially to all selective COX-2 inhibitors. After the appearance of this intriguing report, several analyses or meta-analyses providing evidence against [54–57] or for [58–62] an increase of CV risk during selective COX-2 therapy have been published. Since

---

[2]Vioxx Gastrointestinal Outcomes Research.

September 30, 2004, the day that rofecoxib was withdrawn from the market by Merck & Co. on the basis of the results of the APPROVe[3] trial, there has hardly been a day without significant news either in the scientific and the lay press on the general topic of COX-2 inhibitors. The release in the *New England Journal of Medicine* (March 17, 2005) of the results of three different studies [63–65] documenting the increase in AMI risk after administration of rofecoxib, celecoxib and parecoxib/valdecoxib confirmed that CV adverse events with these drugs is a class-dependent rather than a molecule-dependent effect. Meanwhile the *National Institutes of Health* decided to stop the ADAPT[4] trial because of an apparent increased incidence of IMA in patients treated with naproxen [66]. These results, unexpected especially in the light of the antiaggregant effect of naproxen [67–70], did suggest however that the CV risk of coxibs could also be shared by traditional NSAIDs. And indeed, recent observational studies [71–73] have concluded that both unselective and COX-2-selective NSAIDs share the same CV risks, i.e. increase in AMI, congestive hearth failure and sudden death risk. The lack of cardioprotective effect of naproxen and the inability of low-dose aspirin of counterbalancing the CV effects of coxibs, pointed out in the first study [71], challenge the hypothesis according to which the increase in CV risk by selective COX-2 inhibitors could be due to their 'prothrombotic' activity.

If a greater risk of AMI exists in patients receiving non-selective or COX-2-selective NSAIDs, it is possible that this is due to their ability to increase blood pressure (BP) [74, 75] rather than to a prothrombotic effect. Changes in coronary heart disease and stroke morbidity and mortality rates are directly related to changes in systolic BP, independent from changes in diastolic BP [76]. Even small differences from baseline measures have been shown to be of clinical relevance. For example, the ALLHAT[5] study [77] showed that additional reduction in systolic BP of only 3 mm Hg with chlorthalidone compared with doxazosin was associated with a 50% reduction in the development of new-onset congestive heart failure and a 19% reduction in strokes.

[3]Adenomatous Polyp Prevention on Vioxx, a 3-year trial with the primary aim of evaluating the efficacy of rofecoxib (25 mg daily) for the prophylaxis of colorectal polyps. The study was terminated early when the preliminary data from the study showed an increased relative risk of adverse thrombotic CV events beginning after 18 months of rofecoxib therapy.

[4]Alzheimer's Disease Anti-inflammatory Prevention Trial, a study designed to assess whether naproxen (220 mg b.i.d.) and celecoxib (200 mg b.i.d.) had potential benefit in preventing the onset of Alzheimer's disease. The study enrolled subjects 70 years of age or older who were considered to be at increased risk because of family history, but did not yet have symptoms of the disease. The planned duration of the study was 7 years, but the investigation was suspended after 3 years.

[5]Antihypertensive and Lipid-Lowering Treatment to Prevent Heart Attack Trial.

Data from clinical trials of coxibs indicate that these agents have effects on BP similar to those of traditional NSAIDs and the VIGOR trial [7] clearly showed that effect of rofecoxib on hypertension is dose-dependent as it is the increase in IMA risk in patients taking this drug [58]. It is unclear why rofecoxib is more likely to increase BP than celecoxib at the commonly used clinical doses [78, 79]. Possible explanations include inherent pharmacological differences between the two drugs or differences in the extent of COX-2 inhibition at doses considered to be clinically equivalent [80].

Hypertension seems therefore to be a dose-related, mechanism-based class effect of all NSAIDs, including coxibs. However, there is limited information from *prospective* clinical trials addressing the BP effects of coxibs, and more comparative data are needed. At this point, it is not clear which clinical characteristics represent risk factors for development of hypertension in patients receiving therapy with coxibs. Patients with renal impairment, heart failure, liver disease, and those of advanced age should be appropriately monitored for renal and BP abnormalities. As with traditional NSAIDs, hypertensive patients should be monitored for loss of BP control and the doses of antihypertensive medications should be adjusted if needed [74]. Extensive post-marketing surveillance is however needed especially because, according to one study [81], the presence of any cardiorenal risk factor is associated with an increase in coxib use.

Both the USA Food and Drug Administration (FDA) [82] and the European Medicine Agency (EMEA) [83], after a careful evaluation of the available data, concluded that CV adverse events associated with selective COX-2 inhibitors are both dose- and time-dependent and pointed out that the use of these drugs is contraindicated in patients with ischemic heart disease or stroke. A warning was also introduced for physicians to exercise caution when prescribing COX-2 inhibitors (EMEA and FDA) and non-selective NSAIDs (FDA) for patients with risk factors for heart disease, such as hypertension, hyperlipidemia (high cholesterol levels), diabetes and smoking, as well as for patients with peripheral arterial disease. Given the association between CV risk and exposure to COX-2 inhibitors, doctors were advised to use the lowest effective dose for the shortest possible duration of treatment.

Mechanisms of NSAID-Intestinal Damage

Although the inhibition of mucosal PG synthesis during NSAID use occurs along the entire digestive system, there are significant differences between the distal and the proximal GI tract in the concurrence of other pathogenic factors that may add to damage. Among them, the absence of acid and the

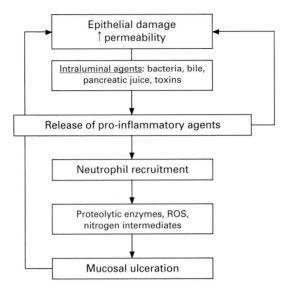

```
┌─────────────────────────────┐
│     Epithelial damage       │◄──────┐
│     ↑ permeability          │       │
└─────────────────────────────┘       │
       │                              │
       ▼                              │
  ┌──────────────────────────────┐   │
  │ Intraluminal agents: bacteria,│  │
  │ bile, pancreatic juice, toxins│  │
  └──────────────────────────────┘   │
       │                              │
       ▼                              │
┌─────────────────────────────────┐  │
│ Release of pro-inflammatory      │──┘
│ agents                           │
└─────────────────────────────────┘
       │
       ▼
  ┌──────────────────────────┐
  │  Neutrophil recruitment   │
  └──────────────────────────┘
       │
       ▼
  ┌──────────────────────────┐
  │ Proteolytic enzymes, ROS, │
  │ nitrogen intermediates    │
  └──────────────────────────┘
       │
       ▼
┌─────────────────────────────┐
│     Mucosal ulceration       │
└─────────────────────────────┘
```

Fig. 5. Mechanisms of intestinal mucosal damage induced by NSAIDs. Intraluminal factors, including bacteria, are key elements in the initiation event of damage, once the mucosal barrier has been disrupted by the local and systemic effects of NSAIDs as well as PG inhibition. Recruitment of neutrophils and consequent release of damaging agents induce ultimately inflammation and ulceration.

presence of bacteria and bile in the intestine are the most prominent ones, which may trigger specific NSAID-related pathogenic mechanisms at the distal GI tract level.

NSAID-induced damage to the intestinal epithelium is set in motion by a direct effect of the drug after oral administration, a persistent local action due to the enterohepatic recirculation of the compound, and the systemic effects carried out after its absorption (fig. 5) [5]. The initial biochemical local subcellular damage is due to the entrance of the usually acidic NSAID into the cell via damage of the brush border cell membrane, disruption of the mitochondrial metabolism, and enhancement of the oxidative phosphorylation process, with consequent ATP production. This leads to an increase in mucosal permeability [84], which facilitates the entrance and action of luminal factors such as dietary macromolecules, bile acids, components of pancreatic juice, and bacteria allowing them to promote the release of pro-inflammatory agents from the intestinal epithelium. These inflammatory agents attract neutrophils, which release proteolytic enzymes, reactive oxygen species, and nitrogen intermediates, that not only kill bacteria, but also contribute to inflammation and to the amplification of mucosal damage [85, 86]. The importance of neutrophils has been emphasized by the finding that NSAID-intestinal damage is almost completely abolished in neutropenic rats and animals treated with antimicrobials [85–87]. As in other body tissues, the neutrophil recruitment in the intestine is a process mainly mediated by (β_2 integrins CD 11/CD 18 upon stimulation of several cytokines [88]. TNF-α acts as a relevant cytokine promoting NSAID-induced neutrophil recruitment in the mucosa [87–90]. While in the stomach, where the bacterial load is minimal, the luminal hydrogen ions are crucial in the pathogenesis of gastric damage, at intestinal level the presence of bacteria and their toxic products play a prominent role. In this connection, it has been demonstrated that the damage induced by different NSAIDs to the intestine is attenuated in antimicrobial treated rats [85].

In addition to bacteria, other factors may also play a role. Enterohepatic recirculation seems to be important in the mechanisms of NSAID damage in the small intestine [91, 92]. Ligation of the common bile duct reduces the incidence of NSAID-induced lesions. Indeed, up to 60% of these compounds are excreted with the bile and released in the distal ileum by the action of bacteria, which may explain the higher drug concentration and the greater mucosal damage at that level. The inability of some drugs devoid of enterohepatic circulation to cause intestinal damage further underlines the importance of this pharmacokinetic feature [93]. Although the existence of two COX isoenzymes has long been known, it is still unclear whether the inhibition of one or both enzymatic activities is needed for the intestinal damage to develop. In COX-1-deficient mice there is no evidence of gastric and/or intestinal damage and these rodents are less prone to develop NSAID-induced mucosal ulceration [94]. Although these findings may suggest that NSAID-induced GI mucosal ulceration is derived from mechanisms other than COX-1 inhibition, it is conceivable that mice may have developed alternative mucosal defense mechanisms to counteract the genetically-induced mucosal PG deficiency. An increasing body of experimental evidence [95, 96] suggests that inhibition of both COX-1 and COX-2 is necessary to promote significant GI damage. The importance of PG deficiency in the pathogenesis of NSAID-induced intestinal damage is confirmed by the finding that administration of exogenous PGs before indomethacin either reduces or eliminates intestinal damage in rats [97, 98].

Prevention and Treatment of NSAID Enteropathy: Is There Room for Antibiotics?

As NSAID-associated intestinal damage is a pH-independent phenomenon, co-administration of antisecretory drugs is useless either in preventing or treating mucosal lesions. Not only were H_2-receptor antagonists (cimetidine and famotidine) unable to counterbalance the NSAID-induced increase of intestinal permeability but also mucosal protective compounds, like sucralfate and misoprostol, were similarly ineffective [99, 100]. Indeed, the potential beneficial effects of PGs on NSAID-induced intestinal permeability seem to be dose-dependent and of little benefit since the enterohepatic re-circulation of the NSAIDs overcomes the beneficial effect of (even high-dose) misoprostol [100].

Other potential approaches, including the administration of ω−3 fatty acids or glucose, are being tested, but none have proven to be effective during continuous NSAID therapy [5]. Much attention has focused on nitric oxide (NO) donating NSAIDs, the development of which was stimulated by the realization that there was mechanistic redundancy in gastroduodenal protection and that NO could stimulate the same gastroduodenal protective mechanisms as PGs. These drugs have recently been named COX-inhibiting NO donors (CINODs). The different NO-releasing moieties (nitroxybutyl or furoxan groups) added through a chemical spacer to standard NSAIDs result in different physicochemical properties and different NO-releasing capacities of the hybrid molecules [101]. As organic nitrates, NO-NSAIDs require metabolic degradation by tissue enzymes (mainly esterases of the intestinal wall and liver) to release NO, but the rate of NO release is much slower in comparison to other NO donors. Recent human studies with the nitroxybutyl derivative of naproxen (AZD-3582) [102] or aspirin (NCX-4016) [103] have pointed out not only the gastroduodenal but also the intestinal safety (i.e. lack of increase in intestinal permeability) of this new class of drugs, thus confirming a large number of animal data. Conversely from NSAIDs these compounds not only maintain gastric mucosal blood flow and reduce leukocyte-endothelial cell adherence but also reduce systemic BP [101]. While preclinical studies with these compounds have demonstrated reduced intestinal adverse effects (i.e. ulceration and bleeding) compared with parent compounds [104], no such data regarding the lower GI tract in humans are available. NSAID transition metalloelement complexes [5] do not display GI or renal toxicity while maintaining anti-inflammatory activity. These new complexes have been investigated in animals, but clinical studies are lacking. Phosphodiesterase inhibitors (like theophylline or pentoxifylline) improve indomethacin-induced enteropathy in rats, via reduction of tissue TNF-α, IL-1β and iNOS expression [105]. As these drugs are available for human use, a clinical trial exploring their usefulness in preventing NSAID enteropathy appears worthwhile.

Antimicrobial Therapy

There is sufficient animal evidence to support a key role of bacteria in the induction of damage in the intestine by NSAIDs. Several investigations [50, 106, 107] have suggested that bacterial flora may play a role on the pathogenesis

Table 4. Reduction of intestinal inflammation and blood loss by metronidazole in patients on NSAIDs (from Bjarnason et al. [113])

Parameter	Metronidazole 800 mg/day		Significance
	before	after	
Fecal excretion of ^{111}In-labeled neutrophils, %	4.7 ± 1.30	1.5 ± 0.36	p < 0.001
Fecal excretion of ^{51}Cr-labeled red cells, ml	2.6 ± 0.44	0.9 ± 0.13	p < 0.001
5-hour urinary excretion ratio ^{51}Cr-EDTA/*L*-rhamnose	0.133 ± 0.012	0.1154 ± 0.017	NS

Intestinal inflammation was assessed by fecal excretion of ^{111}In-labeled neutrophils while blood loss was quantitated via fecal excretion of ^{51}Cr-labeled red cells. The urinary excretion ratio or ^{51}Cr-EDTA/L-rhamnose was used as an index of intestinal permeability.

of NSAID bowel injury and Robert and Asano [91] did show more than 25 years ago that germ-free rats are resistant to indomethacin-induced intestinal lesions. A recent paper [108] found an unbalanced growth of Gram-negative bacteria in the ileum of NSAID-treated animals and showed that heat-killed *Escherichia coli* cells and their purified lipopolysaccharide (LPS) caused deterioration of NSAID-induced ulcers. Additional studies demonstrated that antimicrobials, like tetracycline [107], kanamycin [109, 110], metronidazole [50, 110] and neomycin + bacitracin [109] attenuate NSAID enteropathy, thus giving further support to the pathogenic role of enteric bacteria. The evidence from animal experiments has been confirmed in human studies, showing that metronidazole, an antimicrobial mainly targeted against anaerobic organisms [111], significantly prevented indomethacin-induced increase of intestinal permeability in healthy volunteers [112] and reduced inflammation and blood loss in rheumatic patients taking NSAIDs (table 4) [113]. Although metronidazole is able to protect against mitochondrial uncoupling induced by indomethacin [114], it does not possess any 'intrinsic' anti-inflammatory activity [115]. Its beneficial effect on NSAID enteropathy is therefore likely to be due to the antibacterial action. In this connection, an elegant study [116] with microbiological cultures of luminal aspirates was able to show that small intestinal permeability is increased in subjects with small intestine bacterial overgrowth (SIBO). This finding can easily explain how antibacterial agents, by correcting SIBO, could counterbalance intestinal permeability changes which set in motion a series of pathophysiological events leading to gross lesion formation.

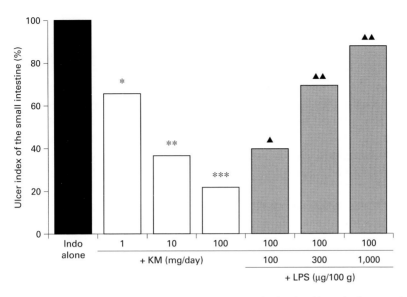

Fig. 6. Dose-dependent inhibition by kanamycin (KM) of intestinal mucosal damage induced by indomethacin in rats. The beneficial effect of the antibiotic was reversed by the concomitant administration of lipopolysaccharide (LPS) (from Koga et al. [109]). *$p < 0.05$. **$p < 0.01$. ***$p < 0.001$. ▲$p < 0.05$ and ▲▲p 0.001 vs. 100 mg KM-pretreated rats vs. indomethacin alone.

A recent and interesting study [109] has shown that both euthymic and athymic nude rats developed intestinal ulcers following administration of indomethacin to the same degree under conventional conditions, but no or minimal ulcer under specific pathogen-free conditions. Pretreatment of conventional rats with intragastric kanamycin sulfate, an aminoglycoside, attenuated indomethacin enteropathy in a dose-dependent fashion. Interestingly, when LPS was injected intraperitoneally in kanamycin-pretreated rats, it fully restored enteropathy in a dose-dependent manner, indicating that indomethacin enteropathy is dependent on bacterial load (fig. 6) and does not require a T-cell function. It has also been shown that some of the pathogenic mechanisms involved in NSAID-induced intestinal damage may be consequence of bacterial invasion [117] and that enterobacterial trans-location to the mucosa represents the first step required for activation of various factors such as iNOS/NO system and neutrophils, all of which play a role in the pathogenesis of NSAID enteropathy. In this connection, it has been shown that following indomethacin, the number of enterobacteria, inducible NO synthase activity and NO production in the intestinal mucosa increase with time, and these changes *precede* the occurrence of intestinal damage. Treatment of the animals with both N^G-nitro-L-arginine methyl ester (L-NAME) and aminoguanidine prevented indomethacin-induced intestinal lesions, with suppression of NO production. Both dexamethasone and an inhibitor of interleukin-1 β/TNF-α production also reduce the severity of intestinal lesions as well as the increase in iNOS activity following administration of indomethacin [117]. Likewise, the occurrence of intestinal damage is attenuated by pretreatment of the animals with anti-neutrophil serum, but none of these treatments, however, affected the translocation of enterobacteria to the mucosa. By contrast, ampicillin suppressed the increase in mucosal iNOS activity as well as the enterobacterial numbers invaded in the mucosa and inhibited the occurrence of intestinal lesions after administration of indomethacin [117].

Besides metronidazole, which also acts by reducing leukocyte adherence and migration and scavenging free radicals [118–120], sulfasalazine (a drug widely used in the treatment of IBD), was shown to prevent acute increments in intestinal permeability, and to reduce intestinal inflammation and blood loss induced by different NSAIDs [121]. Conversely from sulfasalazine, other DMARDs[6] (like penicillamine, chlorochine and aurum salts) proved to be completely ineffective [5, 121].

Despite all the above evidence, no clinical trials have been formally carried out in humans in order to evaluate the effect of antibiotics in the prevention of intestinal damage induced by NSAIDs. Several barriers, including the absence of clear relevant endpoints, the potential of adverse effects and drug resistance associated with long-term antimicrobial treatment, have precluded this interesting approach. The current advancements in GI diagnostics and therapeutics have now changed the old scenario. On the one hand, actual mucosal damage can now be evaluated non-invasively by capsule enteroscopy that can demonstrate the effect of the therapy on subclinical markers (erosions, ulcers, mucosal bleeding) of potential development of serious clinical events. On the other hand, the availability of poorly absorbed and effective antibiotics, like rifaximin [122], allows nowadays to take this therapeutic approach into consideration amongst the strategies to limit the extent of intestinal damage in some patients.

Conclusions

It is today clear that NSAIDs also damage the lower GI tract and that this damage is of clinical relevance. Unfortunately, current prevention strategies that reduce the extent of damage in the upper GI tract are not effective in the

---

[6] Disease-Modifying Anti-Rheumatic Drugs.

lower GI one. Only therapy with selective COX-2 inhibitors may represent an alternative when the intestine is the target for prevention. However, the increase of severe CV events associated with long-term therapy with this class of drugs may be of concern in patients with CV risk factors. New alternatives, including antibiotic prophylaxis with poorly absorbed compounds, need therefore to be evaluated. One could actually speculate that cyclic antibiotic administration, getting rid of enteric pathogenic bacteria, would protect in this way the intestine from the damaging effect of anti-inflammatory compounds. This could be particularly useful in elderly patients, in whom a co-existence of osteoarthritis and colonic diverticular disease [123] would make rifaximin administration very cost-effective.

Acknowledgement

Dr. Ángel Lanas' work is supported in part by a grant from the Instituto de Salud Carlos III (C03/02).

References

1   Lanas A: NSAIDs and ulcer disease: scope of the problem, NSAIDS vs. COX-2 selective inhibitors, role of PPIs, risk factors and strategies for management. Post J Med 2005;117:23–28.
2   Scarpignato C, Bjarnason I, Bretagne JF, De Pouvourville G, García Rodríguez LA, Goldstein JL, Müller PA, Simon B: Working Team Report: towards a GI safer antiinflammatory therapy. Gastroenterol Int 1999;12:186–215.
3   Scarpignato C: Nonsteroidal anti-inflammatory drugs: how do they damage gastroduodenal mucosa? Dig Dis 1995;13(suppl 1):9–39.
4   Houchen CW: Clinical implications of prostaglandin inhibition in the small bowel. Gastroenterol Clin North Am 2001;4:953–969.
5   Lanas A, Panés J, Pique JM: Clinical implications of COX-1 and/or COX-2 inhibition for the distal gastrointestinal tract. Curr Pharm Des 2003;9:2253–2266.
6   Fortun PJ, Hawkey CJ: Nonsteroidal anti-inflammatory drugs and the small intestine. Curr Opin Gastroenterol 2005;21:169–175.
7   Bombardier C, Laine L, Reicin A, Shapiro D, Burgos-Vargas R, Davis B, Day R, Ferraz MB, Hawkey CJ, Hochberg MC, Kvien TK, Schnitzer TJ, VIGOR Study Group: comparison of upper gastrointestinal toxicity of rofecoxib and naproxen in patients with rheumatoid arthritis. N Engl J Med 2000;343:1520–1528.
8   Schnitzer TJ, Burmester GR, Mysler E, Hochberg MC, Doherty M, Ehrsam E, Gitton X, Krammer G, Mellein B, Matchaba P, Gimona A, Hawkey CJ, TARGET Study Group: Comparison of lumiracoxib with naproxen and ibuprofen in the Therapeutic Arthritis Research and Gastrointestinal Event Trial (TARGET), reduction in ulcer complications: randomised controlled trial. Lancet 2004;364:665–674.
9   Lanas A, Perez-Aisa MA, Feu F, Ponce J, Saperas E, Santolaria S, Rodrigo L, Balanzo J, Bajador E, Almela P, Navarro JM, Carballo F, Castro M, Quintero E, Investigators of the Asociacion Espanola de Gastroenterologia (AEG): A nationwide study of mortality associated with hospital admission due to severe gastrointestinal events and those associated with non-steroidal anti-inflammatory drug use. Am J Gastroenterol 2005;100:1685–1693.

10   Silverstein FE, Faich G, Goldstein JL, Simon LS, Pincus T, Whelton A, Makuch R, Eisen G, Agrawal NM, Stenson WF, Burr AM, Zhao WW, Kent JD, Lefkowith JB, Verburg KM, Geis GS: Gastrointestinal toxicity with celecoxib vs. nonsteroidal anti-inflammatory drugs for osteoarthritis and rheumatoid arthritis. The CLASS study: a randomized controlled trial. Celecoxib Long-Term Arthritis Safety Study. JAMA 2000;284:1247–1255.

11   Laine L, Maller ES, Yu C, Quan H, Simon T: Ulcer formation with low-dose enteric-coated aspirin and the effect of COX-2-selective inhibition: a double-blind trial. Gastroenterology 2004;127: 395–402.

12   Skelly MM, Hawkey CJ: Dual COX inhibition and upper gastrointestinal damage. Curr Pharm Des 2003;9:2191–2195.

13   Mamdani M, Rochon PA, Juurlink DN, Kopp A, Anderson GM, Naglie G, Austin PC, Laupacis A: Observational study of upper gastrointestinal haemorrhage in elderly patients given selective cyclo-oxygenase-2 inhibitors or conventional non-steroidal anti-inflammatory drugs. BMJ 2002;325:624.

14   Norgard B, Pedersen L, Johnsen SP, Tarone RE, McLaughlin JK, Friis S, Sorensen HT: COX-2-selective inhibitors and the risk of upper gastrointestinal bleeding in high-risk patients with previous gastrointestinal diseases: a population-based case-control study. Aliment Pharmacol Ther 2004;19:817–825.

15   Laine L, Connors LG, Reicin A, Hawkey CJ, Burgos-Vargas R, Schnitzer TJ, Yu K, Bombardier C: Serious lower gastrointestinal clinical events with nonselective NSAID or coxib use. Gastroenterology 2003;124:288–292.

16   Bjorkman D: Nonsteroidal anti-inflammatory drug-associated toxicity of the liver, lower gastrointestinal tract, and esophagus. Am J Med 1989;2:17S–21S.

17   Rossini FP, Pennazio M: Small-bowel endoscopy. Endoscopy 2002;34:13–20.

18   Maiden L, Thjodleifsson B, Theodors A, Gonzalez J, Bjarnason I: A quantitative analysis of NSAID-induced small bowel pathology by capsule enteroscopy. Gastroenterology 2005;128: 1172–1178.

19   Allison MC, Howatson AG, Torrance CJ, Lee FD, Russell RI: Gastrointestinal damage associated with the use of nonsteroidal anti-inflammatory drugs. N Engl J Med 1992;327:749–754.

20   Sigthorsson G, Tibble J, Hayllar J, Menzies I, Macpherson A, Moots R, Scott D, Gumpel MJ, Bjarnason I: Intestinal permeability and inflammation in patients on NSAIDs. Gut 1998;43: 506–511.

21   Bjarnason I, Smethurst P, Macpherson A, Walker F, McElnay JC, Passmore AP, Menzies IS: Glucose and citrate reduce the permeability changes caused by indomethacin in humans. Gastroenterology 1992;102:1546–1550.

22   Bjarnason I, Williams P, Smethurst P, Peters TJ, Levi AJ: Effect of non-steroidal anti-inflammatory drugs and prostaglandins on the permeability of the human small intestine. Gut 1986;27: 1292–1297.

23   Smecuol E, Bai JC, Sugai E, Vázquez H, Niveloni S, Pedreira S, Maurino E, Meddings J: Acute gastrointestinal permeability responses to different nonsteroidal anti-inflammatory drugs. Gut 2001;49:650–655.

24   Tibble JA, Sigthorsson G, Foster R, Bjarnason I: Comparison of the intestinal toxicity of celecoxib, a selective COX-2 inhibitor, and indomethacin in the experimental rat. Scand J Gastroenterol 2000;35:802–807.

25   Bjarnason I, Zanelli G, Prouse P, Smethurst P, Smith T, Levi S, Gumpel MJ, Levi AJ: Blood and protein loss via small-intestinal inflammation induced by non-steroidal anti-inflammatory drugs. Lancet 1987;ii:711–714.

26   Poullis A, Foster R, Mendall MA, Fagerhol MK: Emerging role of calprotectin in gastroenterology. J Gastroenterol Hepatol 2003;18:756–762.

27   Tibble JA, Sigthorsson G, Foster R, Scott D, Fagerhol MK, Roseth A, Bjarnason I: High prevalence of NSAID enteropathy as shown by a simple faecal test. Gut 1999;45:362–366.

28   Bjarnason I, Zanelli G, Smith T, Smethurst P, Price AB, Gumpel MJ, Levi AJ: The pathogenesis and consequence of non-steroidal anti-inflammatory drug induced small intestinal inflammation. Scand J Rheumatol 1987;22(suppl 64):55–62.

29   Morris AJ, Madhok R, Sturrock RD, Capell HA, Mackenzie JF: Enteroscopic diagnosis of small bowel ulceration in patients receiving non-steroidal anti-inflammatory drugs. Lancet 1991; 337:520.

30   Teahon K, Bjarnason I: Comparison of leukocyte excretion and blood loss in inflammatory disease of the bowel. Gut 1993;34:1535–1538.

31   Etienney I, Beaugerie L, Viboud C, Flahault A: Non-steroidal anti-inflammatory drugs as a risk factor for acute diarrhoea: a case crossover study. Gut 2003;52:260–263.

32   Chutkan R, Toubia N: Effect of nonsteroidal anti-inflammatory drugs on the gastrointestinal tract: diagnosis by wireless capsule endoscopy. Gastrointest Endosc Clin N Am 2004;14:67–85.

33   Goldstein JL, Eisen GM, Lewis B, Gralnek IM, Zlotnick S, Fort JG: Video capsule endoscopy to prospectively assess small bowel injury with celecoxib, naproxen plus omeprazole, and placebo. Clin Gastroenterol Hepatol 2005;3:133–141.

34   Halter F, Weber B, Huber T, Eigenmann F, Frey MP, Ruchti C: Diaphragm disease of the ascending colon. J Clin Gastroenterol 1993;16:74–80.

35   Lanas A, Sekar MC, Hirschowitz BI: Objective evidence of aspirin use in both ulcer and non-ulcer upper and lower gastrointestinal bleeding. Gastroenterology 1992;103:862–869.

36   Lanas A, Serrano P, Bajador E, Esteva F, Benito R, Sainz R: Evidence of aspirin use in both upper and lower gastrointestinal perforation. Gastroenterology 1997;112:683–689.

37   Day TK: Intestinal perforation associated with osmotic slow release indomethacin capsules. Br Med J 1983;287:1671–1672.

38   Davies NM: Sustained release and enteric coated NSAIDs: are they really GI safe? J Pharm Pharm Sci 1999;2:5–14.

39   Masferrer JL, Zweifel BS, Manning PT, Hauser SD, Leahy KM, Smith WG, Isakson PC, Seibert K: Selective inhibition of inducible cyclooxygenase in vivo is anti-inflammatory and nonulcerogenic. Proc Natl Acad Sci USA 1994;91:3228–3232.

40   Yokota A, Taniguchi M, Takahira Y, Tanaka A, Takeuchi K: Rofecoxib produces intestinal but not gastric damage in the presence of a low dose of indomethacin in rats. J Pharmacol Exp Ther 2005;314:302–309.

41   Hunt RH, Bowen B, Mortensen ER, Simon TJ, James C, Cagliola A, Quan H, Bolognese JA: A randomized trial measuring fecal blood loss after treatment with rofecoxib, ibuprofen, or placebo in healthy subjects. Am J Med 2000;109:201–206.

42   Sigthorsson G, Crane R, Simon T, Hoover M, Quan H, Bolognese J, Bjarnason I: COX-2 inhibition with rofecoxib does not increase intestinal permeability in healthy subjects: a double-blind crossover study comparing rofecoxib with placebo and indomethacin. Gut 2000;47:527–532.

43   Atherton C, Jones J, McKaig B, Bebb J, Cunliffe R, Burdsall J, Brough J, Stevenson D, Bonner J, Rordorf C, Scott G, Branson J, Hawkey CJ: Pharmacology and gastrointestinal safety of lumiracoxib, a novel cyclooxygenase-2 selective inhibitor: an integrated study. Clin Gastroenterol Hepatol 2004;2:113–120.

44   Shah AA, Thjodleifsson B, Murray FE, Kay E, Barry M, Sigthorsson G, Gudjonsson H, Oddsson E, Price AB, Fitzgerald DJ, Bjarnason I: Selective inhibition of COX-2 in humans is associated with less gastrointestinal injury: a comparison of nimesulide and naproxen. Gut 2001;48:339–346.

45   Hunt RH, Harper S, Callegari P, Yu C, Quan H, Evans J, James C, Bowen B, Rashid F: Complementary studies of the gastrointestinal safety of the cyclooxygenase-2-selective inhibitor etoricoxib. Aliment Pharmacol Ther 2003;17:201–210.

46   Burke TA, Zabinski RA, Pettitt D, Maniadakis N, Maurath CJ, Goldstein JL: A framework for evaluating the clinical consequences of initial therapy with NSAIDs, NSAIDs plus gastroprotective agents, or celecoxib in the treatment of arthritis. Pharmacoeconomics 2001;19(suppl 1): 33–47.

47   Mahadevan U, Loftus EV Jr, Tremaine WJ, Sandborn WJ: Safety of selective cyclooxygenase-2 inhibitors in inflammatory bowel disease. Am J Gastroenterol 2002;97:910–914.

48   Cleland LG, James MJ, Stamp LK, Penglis PS: COX-2 inhibition and thrombotic tendency: a need for surveillance. Med J Aust 2001;175:214–217.

49   Boers M: NSAIDS and selective COX-2 inhibitors: competition between gastroprotection and cardioprotection. Lancet 2001;357:1222–1223.

50 Justice E, Carruthers DM: Cardiovascular risk and COX-2 inhibition in rheumatological practice. J Hum Hypertens 2005;19:1–5.

51 Catella-Lawson F, Crofford LJ: Cyclooxygenase inhibition and thrombogenicity. Am J Med 2001;110(suppl 3A):28S–32S.

52 Baigent C, Patrono C: Selective cyclooxygenase-2 inhibitors, aspirin, and cardiovascular disease: a reappraisal. Arthritis Rheum 2003;48:12–20.

53 Mukherjee D, Nissen SE, Topol RJ: Risk of cardiovascular events associated with selective COX-2 inhibitors. JAMA 2001;286:954–959.

54 Konstam MA, Weir MR, Reicin A, Shapiro D, Sperling RS, Barr E, Gertz BJ: Cardiovascular thrombotic events in controlled, clinical trials of rofecoxib. Circulation 2001;104:2280–2288.

55 White WB, Faich G, Whelton A, Maurath C, Ridge NJ, Verburg KM, Geis GS, Lefkowith JB: Comparison of thromboembolic events in patients treated with celecoxib, a cyclooxygenase-2 specific inhibitor, versus ibuprofen or diclofenac. Am J Cardiol 2002;89:425–430.

56 Mamdani M, Rochon P, Juurlink DN, Anderson GM, Kopp A, Naglie G, Austin PC, Laupacis A: Effect of selective cyclooxygenase-2 inhibitors and naproxen on short-term risk of acute myocardial infarction in the elderly. Arch Intern Med 2003;163:481–486.

57 Shaya FT, Blume SW, Blanchette CM, Weir MR, Mullins CD: Selective cyclooxygenase-2 inhibition and cardiovascular effects: an observational study of a Medicaid population. Arch Intern Med 2005;165:181–186.

58 Ray WA, Stein CM, Daugherty JR, Hall K, Arbogast PG, Griffin MR: COX-2 selective non-steroidal anti-inflammatory drugs and risk of serious coronary heart disease. Lancet 2002;360:1071–1073.

59 Solomon DH, Schneeweiss S, Glynn RJ, Kiyota Y, Levin R, Mogun H, Avorn J: Relationship between selective cyclooxygenase-2 inhibitors and acute myocardial infarction in older adults. Circulation 2004;109:2068–2073.

60 Kimmel SE, Berlin JA, Reilly M, Jaskowiak J, Kishel L, Chittams J, Strom BL: Patients exposed to rofecoxib and celecoxib have different odds of nonfatal myocardial infarction. Ann Intern Med 2005;142:157–164.

61 Graham DJ, Campen D, Hui R, Spence M, Cheetham C, Levy G, Shoor S, Ray WA: Risk of acute myocardial infarction and sudden cardiac death in patients treated with cyclooxygenase-2-selective and non-selective non-steroidal anti-inflammatory drugs: nested case-control study. Lancet 2005;365:475–481.

62 Lévesque LE, Brophy JM, Zhang B: The risk for myocardial infarction with cyclooxygenase-2 inhibitors: a population study of elderly adults. Ann Intern Med 2005;142:481–489.

63 Solomon SD, McMurray JJ, Pfeffer MA, Wittes J, Fowler R, Finn P, Anderson WF, Zauber A, Hawk E, Bertagnolli M, Adenoma Prevention with Celecoxib (APC) Study Investigators: Cardiovascular risk associated with celecoxib in a clinical trial for colorectal adenoma prevention. N Engl J Med 2005;352:1071–1080.

64 Nussmeier NA, Whelton AA, Brown MT, Langford RM, Hoeft A, Parlow JL, Boyce SW, Verburg KM: Complications of the COX-2 inhibitors parecoxib and valdecoxib after cardiac surgery. N Engl J Med 2005;352:1081–1091.

65 Bresalier RS, Sandler RS, Quan H, Bolognese JA, Oxenius B, Horgan K, Lines C, Riddell R, Morton D, Lanas A, Konstam MA, Baron JA, Adenomatous Polyp Prevention on Vioxx (APPROVe) Trial Investigators: Cardiovascular events associated with rofecoxib in a colorectal adenoma chemoprevention trial. N Engl J Med 2005;352:1092–1102.

66 FDA Alert for Health Care Provider: Naproxen [http://www.fda.gov/cder/drug/InfoSheets/HCP/Naproxen-hcp.pdf].

67 Shah AA, Thjodleifsson B, Murray FE, Kay E, Barry M, Sigthorsson G, Gudjonsson H, Oddsson E, Price AB, Fitzgerald DJ, Bjarnason I: Selective inhibition of COX-2 in humans is associated with less gastrointestinal injury: a comparison of nimesulide and naproxen. Gut 2001;48:339–346.

68 Knijff-Dutmer EA, Kalsbeek-Batenburg EM, Koerts J, van de Laar MA: Platelet function is inhibited by non-selective non-steroidal anti-inflammatory drugs but not by cyclooxygenase-2-selective inhibitors in patients with rheumatoid arthritis. Rheumatology (Oxford) 2002;41:458–461.

69 Rothschild BM: Comparative antiplatelet activity of COX1 NSAIDS versus aspirin, encompassing regimen simplification and gastroprotection: a call for a controlled study. Reumatismo 2004;56:89–93.

70   Capone ML, Tacconelli S, Sciulli MG, Grana M, Ricciotti E, Minuz P, Di Gregorio P, Merciaro G, Patrono C, Patrignani P: Clinical pharmacology of platelet, monocyte, and vascular cyclooxyge-nase inhibition by naproxen and low-dose aspirin in healthy subjects. Circulation 2004;109: 1468–1471.

71   Hippisley-Cox J, Coupland C: Risk of myocardial infarction in patients taking cyclooxygenase-2 inhibitors or conventional non-steroidal anti-inflammatory drugs: population-based nested case-control analysis. BMJ 2005;330:1366–1372.

72   Hudson M, Richard H, Pilote L: Differences in outcomes of patients with congestive heart failure prescribed celecoxib, rofecoxib, or non-steroidal anti-inflammatory drugs: population-based study. BMJ 2005;330:1370–1375.

73   Johnsen SP, Larsson H, Tarone RE, McLaughlin JK, Norgard B, Friis S, Sorensen HT: Risk of hospitalization for myocardial infarction among users of rofecoxib, celecoxib, and other NSAIDs: a population-based case-control study. Arch Intern Med 2005;165:978–984.

74   Brater DC: Anti-inflammatory agents and renal function. Semin Arthritis Rheum 2002;32(suppl 1): 33–42.

75   Armstrong EP, Malone DC: The impact of nonsteroidal anti-inflammatory drugs on blood pres-sure, with an emphasis on newer agents. ClinTher 2003;25:1–18.

76   Izzo JL, Levy D, Black HR: Importance of systolic blood pressure in older Americans. Clinical advisory statement. Hypertension 2000;35:1021–1024.

77   ALLHAT Collaborative Research Group: Major cardiovascular events in hypertensive patients randomized to doxazosin vs. chlorthalidone. The antihypertensive and lipid-lowering treatment to prevent heart attack trial (ALLHAT). JAMA 2000;283:1967–1975.

78   Whelton A, Fort JG, Puma JA, Normandin D, Bello AE, Verburg KM, SUCCESS VI Study Group: Cyclooxygenase-2-specific inhibitors and cardiorenal function: a randomized, controlled trial of celecoxib and rofecoxib in older hypertensive osteoarthritis patients. Am J Ther 2001;8:85–95.

79   Whelton A, White WB, Bello AE, Puma JA, Fort JG: Effects of celecoxib and rofecoxib on blood pressure and edema in patients> or = 65 years of age with systemic hypertension and osteoarthri-tis. Am J Cardiol 2002;90:959–963.

80   Hawkey CJ: Cyclooxygenase inhibition: between the devil and the deep blue sea. Gut 2002;50 (suppl 3):25–30.

81   Harley C, Wagner S: The prevalence of cardiorenal risk factors in patients prescribed non-steroidal anti-inflammatory drugs: data from managed care. Clin Ther 2003;25:139–149.

82   FDA Public Health Advisory: FDA announces important changes and additional warnings for COX-2-selective and non-selective non-steroidal anti-Inflammatory drugs (NSAIDs) [http://www. fda.gov/cder/drug/ advisory/COX2. htm].

83   EMEA/62838/2005 Public Statement – European Medicines Agency announces regulatory action on COX-2 inhibitors [http://www.emea.eu.int/htms/hotpress/d6275705.htm].

84   Somasundaram S, Sigthorsson G, Simpson RJ, Watts J, Jacob M, Tavares IA, Rafi S, Roseth A, Foster R, Price AB, Wrigglesworth JM, Bjarnason I: Uncoupling of intestinal mitochondrial oxidative phosphorylation and inhibition of cyclooxygenase are required for the development of NSAID enteropathy in the rat. Aliment Pharmacol Ther 2000;14:639–650.

85   Davies NM, Jamali F: Pharmacological protection of NSAID-induced intestinal permeability in the rat: effect of tempo and metronidazole as potential free radical scavengers: Hum Exp Toxicol 1997;16:345–349.

86   Bjarnason I, Hayllar J, Macpherson AJ, Russell AS: Side effects of non-steroidal anti-inflammatory drugs on the small and large intestine in humans. Gastroenterology 1993;104:1832–1847.

87   Bertrand V, Guimbaud R, Tulliez M, Mauprivez C, Sogni P, Couturier D, Giroud JP, Chaussade S, Chauvelot-Moachon L: Increase in tumour necrosis factor-α production linked to the toxicity of indomethacin for the rat small intestine. Br J Pharmacol 1998;124:1385–1394.

88   Stadnyk AW, Dollard C, Issekutz TB, Issekutz AC: Neutrophil migration into indomethacin induced rat small intestinal injury is CD11a/CD18 and CD11b/CD18 co-dependent. Gut 2002;50: 629–635.

89   Appleyard CB, McCafferty DM, Tigley AW, Swain MG, Wallace JL: Tumour necrosis factor mediation of NSAID-induced gastric damage: role of leukocyte adherence. Am J Physiol 1996; 270:G42–G48.

90   Reuter BK, Wallace JL: Phosphodiesterase inhibitors prevent NSAID enteropathy independently of effects on TNF-a release. Am J Physiol 1999;277:G847–G854.

91   Robert A, Asano T: Resistance of germ-free rats to indomethacin-induced intestinal lesions. Prostaglandins 1977;14:333–341.

92   Wax J, Clinger WA, Varner P, Bass P, Winder CV: Relationship of the enterohepatic cycle to ulcerogenesis in the rat small bowel with flufenamic acid. Gastroenterology 1970;58:772–780.

93   Reuter BK, Davies NM, Wallace JL: Nonsteroidal anti-inflammatory drug enteropathy in rats: role of permeability, bacteria, and enterohepatic recirculation. Gastroenterology 1997;112:109–117.

94   Langenbach R, Morham SG, Tiano HF, Loftin CD, Ghanayem BI, Chulada PC, Mahler JF, Lee CA, Goulding EH, Kluckman KD, Kim HS, Smithies O: Prostaglandin synthase-1 gene disruption in mice reduces arachidonic acid-induced inflammation and indomethacin induced gastric ulceration. Cell 1995;83:483–492.

95   Sigthorsson G, Simpson RJ, Walley M, Anthony A, Foster R, Hotz-Behoftsitz C, Palizban A, Pombo J, Watts J, Morham SG, Bjarnason I: COX-1 and 2, intestinal integrity, and pathogenesis of nonsteroidal anti-inflammatory drug enteropathy in mice. Gastroenterology 2002;122: 1913–1923.

96   Takeuchi K, Tanaka A, Ohno R, Yokota A: Role of COX inhibition in pathogenesis of NSAID-induced small intestinal damage. J Physiol Pharmacol 2003;54(suppl 4):165–182.

97   Houchen CW, Stenson WF, Cohn SM: Disruption of cyclooxygenase-1 gene results in an impaired response to radiation injury. Am J Physiol 2000;279:G858–G865.

98   Redfern JS, Feldman M: Role of endogenous prostaglandins in preventing gastrointestinal ulceration: induction of ulcers by antibodies to prostaglandins. Gastroenterology 1989;96:596–605.

99   Davies GR, Wilkie ME, Rampton DS: Effects of metronidazole and misoprostol on indomethacin-induced changes in intestinal permeability. Dig Dis Sci 1993;38:417–425.

100   Jenkins RT, Rooney PJ, Hunt RH: Increased bowel permeability to ^{51}Cr-EDTA in controls caused by naproxen is not prevented by cyto-protection. Arthritis Rheum 1998;31(suppl 1):R11.

101   Wallace JL, Del Soldato P: The therapeutic potential of NO-NSAIDs. Fundam Clin Pharmacol 2003;17:11–20.

102   Hawkey CJ, Jones JI, Atherton CT, Skelly MM, Bebb JR, Fagerholm U, Jonzon B, Karlsson P, Bjarnason IT: Gastrointestinal safety of AZD3582, a cyclooxygenase inhibiting nitric oxide donator: proof of concept study in humans. Gut 2003;52:1537–1542.

103   Fiorucci S, Santucci L, Gresele P, Faccino RM, Del Soldato P, Morelli A: Gastrointestinal safety of NO-aspirin (NCX-4016) in healthy human volunteers: a proof of concept endoscopic study. Gastroenterology 2003;124:600–607.

104   Conforti A, Donini M, Brocco G, De Soldato P, Benoni G, Cuzzolin L: Acute anti-inflammatory activity and gastrointestinal tolerability of diclofenac and nitrofenac. Agents Actions 1993;40: 176–180.

105   Saud B, Nandi J, Ong G, Finocchiaro S, Levine RA: Inhibition of TNF-α improves indomethacin-induced enteropathy in rats by modulating iNOS expression. Dig Dis Sci 2005;50:1677–1683.

106   Davies NM, Jamali F: Pharmacological protection of NSAID-induced intestinal permeability in the rat: effect of tempo and metronidazole as potential free radical scavengers. Hum ExpToxicol 1997;16:345–349.

107   Banerjee AK, Peters TJ: Experimental nonsteroidal anti-inflammatory drug-induced enteropathy in the rat: similarities to inflammatory bowel disease and effect of thromboxane synthetase inhibitors. Gut 1990;31:1358–1364.

108   Hagiwara M, Kataoka K, Arimochi H, Kuwahara T, Ohnishi Y: Role of unbalanced growth of Gram-negative bacteria in ileal ulcer formation in rats treated with a nonsteroidal anti-inflammatory drug. J Med Invest 2004;51:43–51.

109   Koga H, Aoyagi K, Matsumoto T, Iida M, Fujishima M: Experimental enteropathy in athymic and euthymic rats: synergistic role of lipopolysaccharide and indomethacin. Am J Physiol 1999; 276:G576–G582.

110   Kinouchi T, Kataoka K, Bing SR, Nakayama H, Uejima M, Shimono K, Kuwahara T, Akimoto S, Hiraoka I, Ohnishi Y: Culture supernatants of *Lactobacillus acidophilus* and *Bifidobacterium adolescentis* repress ileal ulcer formation in rats treated with a nonsteroidal anti-inflammatory

drug by suppressing unbalanced growth of aerobic bacteria and lipid peroxidation. Microbiol Immunol 1998;42:347–355.

111 Freeman CD, Klutman NE, Lamp KC: Metronidazole: a therapeutic review and update. Drugs 1997;54:679–708.

112 Bjarnason I, Smethurst P, Fenn CG, Lee CE, Menzies IS, Levi AJ: Misoprostol reduces indomethacin-induced changes in human small intestinal permeability. Dig Dis Sci 1989;34:407–411.

113 Bjarnason I, Hayllar J, Smethurst P, Price A, Gumpel MJ: Metronidazole reduces intestinal inflammation and blood loss in non-steroidal anti-inflammatory drug induced enteropathy. Gut 1992;33:1204–1208.

114 Leite AZ, Sipahi AM, Damiao AO, Coelho AM, Garcez AT, Machado MC, Buchpiguel CA, Lopasso FP, Lordello ML, Agostinho CL, Laudanna AA: Protective effect of metronidazole on uncoupling mitochondrial oxidative phosphorylation induced by NSAID: a new mechanism. Gut 2001;48:163–167.

115 Ganrot-Norlin K, Stalhandske T, Karlstrom R: Lack of anti-inflammatory activity of metronidazole. Acta Pharmacol Toxicol (Copenh) 1981;49:130–133.

116 Riordan SM, McIver CJ, Thomas DH, Duncombe VM, Bolin TD, Thomas MC: Luminal bacteria and small-intestinal permeability. Scand J Gastroenterol 1997;32:556–563.

117 Konaka A, Kato S, Tanaka A, Kunikata T, Korolkiewicz R, Takeuchi K: Roles of enterobacteria, nitric oxide and neutrophil in pathogenesis of indomethacin-induced small intestinal lesions in rats. Pharmacol Res 1999;40:517–524.

118 Müller M: Reductive activation of nitroimidazoles in anaerobic microorganisms. Biochem Pharmacol 1986;35:37–41.

119 Akamatsu H, Oguchi M, Nishijima S, Asada Y, Takahashi M, Ushijima T, Niwa Y: The inhibition of free radical generation by human neutrophils through the synergistic effects of metronidazole with palmitoleic acid: a possible mechanism of action of metronidazole in rosacea and acne. Arch Dermatol Res 1991;282:449–454.

120 Arndt H, Paltisch KD, Grisham MB, Granger DN: Metronidazole inhibits leukocyteendothelial cell adhesion in rat mesenteric venules. Gastroenterology 1994;106:1271–1276.

121 Hayllar J, Smith T, Macpherson A, Price AB, Gumpel M, Bjarnason I: Nonsteroidal anti-inflammatory drug-induced small intestinal inflammation and blood loss. Effects of sulfasalazine and other disease-modifying anti-rheumatic drugs. Arthritis Rheum 1994;37:1146–1150.

122 Scarpignato C, Pelosini I: Rifaximin, a poorly absorbed antibiotic: pharmacology and clinical potential. Chemotherapy 2005;51(suppl 1):36–66.

123 Kadam UT, Jordan K, Croft PR: Clinical co-morbidity in patients with osteoarthritis: a case-control study of general practice consult-ers in England and Wales. Ann Rheum Dis 2004;63: 408–414.

Note Added in Proof

While this review was being submitted, we came across an interesting case report [1] showing how difficult the diagnosis of NSAID-induced small bowel diaphragmatic strictures could be. In a patient on long-term low-dose (81 mg daily) aspirin for coronary heart disease (CHD) presenting with intermittent episodes of periumbilical pain lasting approximately 12 h, associated with bloating, nausea, vomiting, and diarrhea, an extensive GI evaluation (including EGD, colonoscopy with ileoscopy, barium contrast radiography of the small bowel, and push enteroscopy with an overtube to 130 cm distal to the ligament of Treitz) was negative. Only capsule endoscopy revealed multiple ileal membranous strictures with circumferential ulcerations that were oozing blood. The diaphragm-like strictures demonstrated by the video capsule in the ileum were not apparent to visual inspection or by palpation of the length of the small bowel and only intraoperative endoscopy demonstrated multiple ileal diaphragms with ulceration and active bleeding.

Prevention and treatment of NSAID-enteropathy continues to be a challenge and effective agents are needed. Oral recombinant human lactoferrin (RHLF) supplementation during a short-term indomethacin challenge reduced the NSAID-mediated increase in small intestinal permeability [2] and may therefore provide a nutritional tool in the treatment of hyperpermeability-associated disorders. In a recent rodent study [3] this milk protein was effective in preventing acute NSAID-induced increases in gut bleeding and myeloperoxidase activity and also capable of blocking some chronic manifestations associated with indomethacin administration. Protection by RHLF of the intestinal tract from NSAIDs was independent of prostaglandins and nitric oxide and appeared to be linked to attenuation of neutrophil migration to the intestine [3]. On the other hand, besides being an anti-inflammatory compound [4], lactoferrin displays prebiotic properties [5]. The well-known capacity of lactoferrin-derived peptides to stimulate the growth of bifidobacteria [6] may also be responsible for such protective effect and further supports the manipulation of bacterial flora as a means of preventing NSAID-induced damage to the small bowel.

In addition to non-selective CINODs, a series of proprietary nitric oxide-enhancing COX-2 inhibitors has been synthesized [7] in the hope of improving the efficacy and safety of this class of drugs. A phase II study on the lead compound (a rofecoxib derivative), started in mid 2004 [8], has been halted after Vioxx® withdrawal [9]. However, the search for new drug candidates continues.

References

1   Manetas M, O'Loughlin C, Kelemen K, Barkin JS: Multiple small-bowel diaphragms: a cause of obscure GI bleeding diagnosed by capsule endoscopy. Gastrointest Endosc 2004;60:848–851.
2   Troost FJ, Saris WH, Brummer RJ: Recombinant human lactoferrin ingestion attenuates indomethacin-induced enteropathy in vivo in healthy volunteers. Eur J Clin Nutr 2003;57: 1579–1585.
3   Dial EJ, Dohrman AJ, Romero JJ, Lichtenberger LM: Recombinant human lactoferrin prevents NSAID-induced intestinal bleeding in rodents. J Pharm Pharmacol 2005;57:93–99.
4   Conneely OM: Anti-inflammatory activities of lactoferrin. J Am Coll Nutr 2001;20(suppl 5): 389S–395S.
5   Lonnerdal B: Nutritional and physiologic significance of human milk proteins. Am J Clin Nutr 2003;77:1537S–1543S.
6   Liepke C, Adermann K, Raida M, Mägert HJ, Forssmann WG, Zucht HD: Human milk provides peptides highly stimulating the growth of bifidobacteria. Eur J Biochem 2002;269:712–718.

7   Nitromed: Nitric oxide-enhancing NSAIDs for inflammation [http://www.nitromed.com/ pain_ inflammation.asp].

8   Nitromed® Press Release: Merck and Nitro-Med advance first nitric oxide-enhancing COX-2 inhibitor into phase II clinical testing [http://www.nitromed.com/06_22_04.shtml].

9   NewsRx: Merck halts trial of lead candidate in nitric oxide-enhancing COX-2 inhibitors [http://www.newsrx.com/issue_article/Health-and-Medicine-Week/2004-10-25/102520043334 665W.html].

Ángel Lanas, MD, PhD
Servicio de Aparato Digestivo, Hospital Clínico 'Lozano Blesa'
ES–50009 Zaragoza (Spain)
Tel. +34 976 762 538, Fax +34 976 762 539
E-Mail alanas@unizar.es

This chapter should be cited as follows:

Lanas Á, Scarpignato C: Microbial Flora in NSAID-Induced Intestinal Damage: A Role for Antibiotics? Digestion 2006;73(suppl 1):136–150.

Author Index

Subject Index